BSAVA Manual of Canine and Feline Wound Management and Reconstruction

Second edition

Editors:

John Williams
MA VetMB LLB CertVR DipECVS FRCVS
European Specialist in Small Animal Surgery
Oakwood Veterinary Referrals, Cheshire CW8 1LP

and

Alison Moores
BVSc(Hons) CertSAS DipECVS MRCVS
RCVS and ECVS Specialist in Small Animal Surgery
Anderson Sturgess Veterinary Specialists,
Winchester SO21 2LL

Published by:

British Small Animal Veterinary Association
Woodrow House, 1 Telford Way, Waterwells
Business Park, Quedgeley, Gloucester GL2 2AB

A Company Limited by Guarantee in England.
Registered Company No. 2837793.
Registered as a Charity.

Other titles in the BSAVA Manuals series:

Manual of Avian Practice: A Foundation Manual
Manual of Backyard Poultry Medicine and Surgery
Manual of Canine & Feline Abdominal Imaging
Manual of Canine & Feline Abdominal Surgery
Manual of Canine & Feline Advanced Veterinary Nursing
Manual of Canine & Feline Anaesthesia and Analgesia
Manual of Canine & Feline Behavioural Medicine
Manual of Canine & Feline Cardiorespiratory Medicine
Manual of Canine & Feline Clinical Pathology
Manual of Canine & Feline Dentistry and Oral Surgery
Manual of Canine & Feline Dermatology
Manual of Canine & Feline Emergency and Critical Care
Manual of Canine & Feline Endocrinology
Manual of Canine & Feline Endoscopy and Endosurgery
Manual of Canine & Feline Fracture Repair and Management
Manual of Canine & Feline Gastroenterology
Manual of Canine & Feline Haematology and Transfusion Medicine
Manual of Canine & Feline Head, Neck and Thoracic Surgery
Manual of Canine & Feline Musculoskeletal Disorders
Manual of Canine & Feline Musculoskeletal Imaging
Manual of Canine & Feline Nephrology and Urology
Manual of Canine & Feline Neurology
Manual of Canine & Feline Oncology
Manual of Canine & Feline Ophthalmology
Manual of Canine & Feline Radiography and Radiology: A Foundation Manual
Manual of Canine & Feline Rehabilitation, Supportive and Palliative Care: Case Studies in Patient Management
Manual of Canine & Feline Reproduction and Neonatology
Manual of Canine & Feline Shelter Medicine: Principles of Health and Welfare in a Multi-animal Environment
Manual of Canine & Feline Surgical Principles: A Foundation Manual
Manual of Canine & Feline Thoracic Imaging
Manual of Canine & Feline Ultrasonography
Manual of Canine & Feline Wound Management and Reconstruction
Manual of Canine Practice: A Foundation Manual
Manual of Exotic Pet and Wildlife Nursing
Manual of Exotic Pets: A Foundation Manual
Manual of Feline Practice: A Foundation Manual
Manual of Practical Animal Care
Manual of Practical Veterinary Nursing
Manual of Practical Veterinary Welfare
Manual of Psittacine Birds
Manual of Rabbit Medicine
Manual of Rabbit Surgery, Dentistry and Imaging
Manual of Raptors, Pigeons and Passerine Birds
Manual of Reptiles
Manual of Rodents and Ferrets
Manual of Small Animal Practice Management and Development
Manual of Wildlife Casualties

For further information on these and all BSAVA publications, please visit our website:
www.bsava.com

Contents

Contributors

Davina Anderson MA VetMB PhD DipECVS DSAS(Soft Tissue) MRCVS
RCVS and European Specialist in Small Animal Surgery
Anderson Sturgess Veterinary Specialists, The Granary, Poles Lane, Hursley, Winchester SO21 2LL

Stephen J. Baines MA VetMB PhD CertVR CertSAS DipECVS MRCVS
RCVS and European Specialist in Small Animal Surgery
Department of Veterinary Clinical Sciences, Royal Veterinary College, Hawkshead Lane,
North Mymms, Herts AL9 7TA

David Fowler DVM MVetSc Diplomate ACVS
Western Veterinary Specialist Center, Calgary, Alberta, Canada

Ed Friend BVetMed CertSAS DipECVS MRCVS
European Specialist in Small Animal Surgery
Wey Referrals, 125/129 Chertsey Road, Woking, Surrey GU21 5BP

Giselle Hosgood BVSc MS PhD Diplomate ACVS FACVSc
Department of Veterinary Clinical Sciences, School of Veterinary Medicine,
Louisiana State University, Baton Rouge, LA 70803, USA

Jane Ladlow MA Vet MB Cert VR Cert SAS DipECVS MRCVS
European Specialist in Small Animal Surgery
Department of Veterinary Medicine, University of Cambridge, Madingley Road, Cambridge CB3 0ES

Philipp D. Mayhew BVM&S Diplomate ACVS MRCVS
Columbia River Veterinary Specialists, 6818 NE 4th Plain Blvd, Vancouver, WA 98661, USA

Alison Moores BVSc (Hons) CertSAS DipECVS MRCVS
RCVS and European Specialist in Small Animal Surgery
Anderson Sturgess Veterinary Specialists, The Granary, Poles Lane, Hursley, Winchester SO21 2LL

Jacqui D. Niles BVetMed CertSAS Diplomate ACVS MRCVS
Metropolitan Veterinary Associates, 2626 Van Buren Avenue, Box 881, Valley Forge,
PA 19482, USA

Juliet Pope BVSc CertSAS MRCVS
Highcroft Veterinary Group, 615 Wells Rd, Whitchurch, Bristol BS14 9BE

Richard A.S. White BVetMed PhD DSAS DVR Diplomate ACVS DipECVS FRCVS
RCVS and European Specialist in Small Animal Surgery; RCVS Specialist in Veterinary Oncology
Dick White Referrals, Station Farm, Six Mile Bottom, Newmarket CB8 0UH

John Williams MA VetMB LLB CertVR DipECVS FRCVS
European Specialist in Small Animal Surgery
Oakwood Veterinary Referrals, 267 Chester Road, Hartford, Northwich, Cheshire CW8 1LP

Forewords

I am delighted to have been asked by the Editors to write a Foreword for the new *BSAVA Manual of Canine and Feline Wound Management and Reconstruction*. As a soft tissue surgeon, I have found these cases to be amongst my most rewarding, and most frustrating. Key elements of successful wound management include providing an environment conducive to wound healing, defect closure using sound surgical principles, and support of the patient's systemic health. The contributing authors are internationally recognised as excellent surgeons and teachers, and their text is liberally punctuated by helpful diagrams and practical hints. These people know as well as anyone how difficult it can be to bring all the pieces of the puzzle together (literally!). The techniques they have chosen to describe are supported by up-to-date research and a lot of 'on the job' observation.

This Manual addresses all aspects of wound management from a sound basis of fundamental principles, using current scientific literature combined with years of practical experience to help the reader understand why issues with wound healing arise, and how to diagnose and address those issues.

The approach used in constructing this Manual can best be described as putting philosophy into practice, allowing anyone who owns it to understand these sometimes complex conditions and approach their management in a scholarly, yet pragmatic way. It can be used as a reference text for basic principles, a 'cook book' for surgical procedures, and a resource to help explain the intricacies of wound management to owners and students. It should be present on the shelf of every small animal surgeon.

Geraldine B. Hunt ACVSc Fellow and Specialist in Small Animal Surgery
Visiting Professor, UC Davis, California

Sir Archibald McIndoe was one of the pioneers of human reconstructive surgery, helping hundreds of fighter pilots severely burned and disfigured during action in World War II. His patients established the famous 'Guinea Pig Club'. Such successes, and the raised expectations of pet owners, have led to the establishment of similar techniques in veterinary surgery – not just for guinea pigs but for all animals injured in accidents and fires, or undergoing extensive surgery.

Ten years ago our knowledge of wound management and reconstructive surgery in animals was brought together in the first edition of this Manual, which has since been an invaluable resource for practitioners dealing with such distressing cases. A decade later, a second edition is timely as our understanding of the wound healing process, right down to the molecular level, has advanced immeasurably. Recommendations on how to treat wounds and perform reconstruction have been refined based on this new understanding.

The editors are highly qualified and well respected surgeons, and have assembled an array of equally talented surgeons to write this edition. Their writing is as meticulous as their surgical technique, and is beautifully illustrated by colour photographs and line drawings – even if the actual content is not aesthetic. Pages describing and illustrating operative techniques are in a format that provides immediate help to the practitioner. Thus, within this Manual, readers are going to find not only the theory of how to manage wounds but also the practical tips designed to improve success.

Ed Hall MA VetMB PhD DipECVIM MRCVS
BSAVA President 2008–2009

Preface

Since the publication, 10 years ago, of the first edition of the *BSAVA Manual of Canine and Feline Wound Management and Reconstruction*, there have been many advances in wound management, and particularly in oncological surgery, that have led to veterinary surgeons being presented with larger and more complex wounds. At the same time, the understanding of the physiology of wound healing has advanced, and the techniques available for wound closure have multiplied, with greater use of the already described axial pattern flaps and increasing use and description of muscle flaps. Other challenges facing the veterinary surgeon include the recognition of multi-drug-resistant bacteria and nosocomial infections.

We therefore set out to provide an up-to-date book containing detailed surgical descriptions, with surgical illustrations and photographs of case examples. In particular, the understanding of local subdermal plexus flaps, axial pattern flaps and muscle flaps has been enhanced with step-by-step descriptions of the surgical techniques, including planning, lifting and rotating flaps, as well as closing defects at the donor site. The illustrations in this Manual follow a similar format to those in other recent BSAVA Manuals of soft tissue surgery.

Complications are often overlooked in veterinary textbooks and it was a conscious decision of the Editors to include them in this Manual. It is particularly important for veterinary surgeons not only to consider potential complications before treatment but also, importantly, to recognize when they occur and to provide appropriate management. Similarly, there are some specific wounds, such as axillary wounds or burns, that may require a different approach to management, such as omentalization, and these are also covered in detail.

The Manual is useful for all veterinary surgeons presented with a challenging wound. It provides information in a readily accessible manner on wound management and dressings of open wounds. The chapter on tension-relieving techniques is applicable to the management of small wounds treated in everyday practice, as well as larger wounds treated less often or on a more specialist basis. There are more advanced chapters on skin grafts, axial pattern flaps and muscle flaps, for those with a caseload of larger and more complex wounds. Although microvascular techniques are still not routinely performed in veterinary practice, it is expected that during the lifetime of this Manual these techniques may become more commonplace.

The authors have been chosen from the UK and North America and represent a group of individuals with an interest and many years of experience and recognized expertise in wound management and reconstruction. Their remit was to produce a Manual that would discuss all the aspects of wound management that a veterinary practitioner might need, and provide a wealth of treatment options to provide expedient and cost-effective wound closure with minimal complications and morbidity – a task which we believe they have effectively achieved. We are grateful for their hard work and dedication, and their practical approach to the topic.

The Editors are particularly grateful to the publishing team at BSAVA. Finally, our thanks go to Samantha Elmhurst for the surgical illustrations, which are invaluable for this Manual.

John Williams and Alison Moores
February 2009

BSAVA Manuals

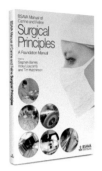
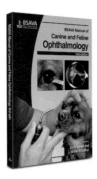
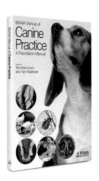
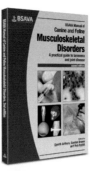
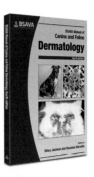
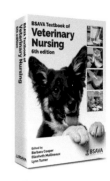

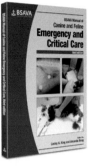
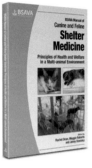
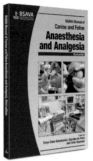
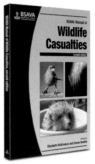
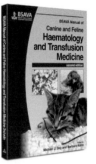
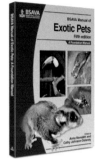

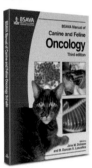
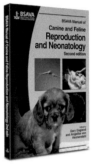
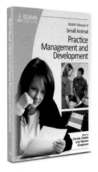
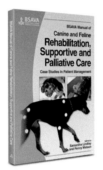
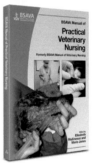
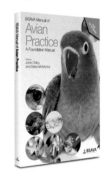

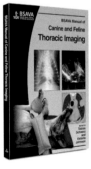
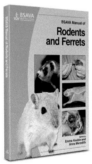
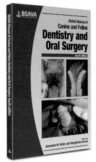
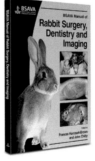
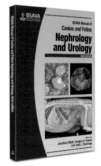
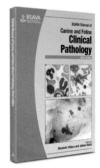

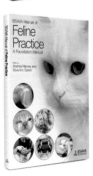
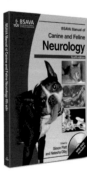
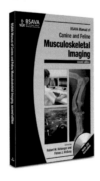
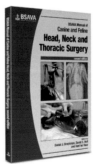
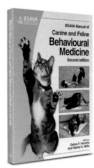
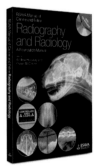

Tel: 01452 726700   Fax: 01452 726701

Email: administration@bsava.com   Web: www.bsava.com

The biology of wound healing

Giselle Hosgood

Introduction

Wound healing is a normal physiological function that restores the continuity of tissues after injury. It is a complex process characterized by macroscopic, microscopic and biochemical events. Considerable advances in molecular technology have enhanced our understanding. Through a knowledge of the processes involved, the clinician should be able to appreciate the role they can play in wound healing and understand current and future treatment options that may modulate the healing process. Particular emphasis is given here to cytokine messaging because this is the key that unlocks the mystery to understanding wound healing.

Phases of wound healing

Wound healing is described in phases (haemostasis, inflammation, repair and maturation) based on microscopic changes. These phases have corresponding macroscopic characteristics that are recognized by the clinician. Wound healing is dynamic, with the timing of the phases imprecise and overlapping to some degree; e.g. repair will start before the inflammation phase has ended (Figure 1.1).

Notably, the microscopic events are initiated, mediated and sustained by biochemical mediators known as cytokines and growth factors (Figure 1.2). The biochemical events of wound healing are complex.

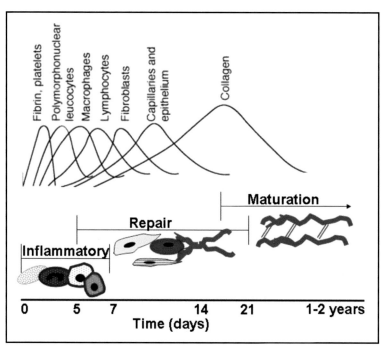

1.1 Cellular content and matrix accumulation within a wound during the phases of wound healing. Note the overlap of these events during the phases of wound healing (axis not to scale).

KEY			
Collagen	ᴡᴡᴡ	Endothelial cell	●
Fibroblast	⬭	Macrophage	◉
Monocyte	⊙	Myofibroblast	⬱
Neutrophil	◉	Platelet	⬭

Mediator	Abbreviation	Source(s)	Functions
Connective tissue growth factor	CTGF	Endothelial cells, fibroblasts	Chemotactic and mitogenic for various connective tissue cells
Epidermal growth factor	EGF	Platelets, macrophages, saliva, urine, milk, plasma	Mitogenic for epidermal cells and fibroblasts Stimulates epidermal cell migration and extracellular matrix (ECM) formation

1.2 Mediators and regulators of wound healing. (continues) ▶

Mediator	Abbreviation	Source(s)	Functions
Fibroblast growth factor	FGF	Macrophages, mast cells, T lymphocytes, endothelial cells, fibroblasts, and many tissues	Chemotactic for fibroblasts Mitogenic for fibroblasts and epidermal cells Stimulates epidermal cell migration, angiogenesis, wound contraction and ECM formation
Granulocyte/macrophage colony stimulating factor	GM-CSF	Multiple cells	Induces differentiation and proliferation of granulocytes Modulates monocyte and macrophage function Mitogenic for epidermal and endothelial cells
Heparin-binding epidermal growth factor	HB-EGF	Macrophages	Stimulates epidermal cell migration, proliferation, fibroblast proliferation, ECM formation
Insulin-like growth factor-1	IGF-1	Macrophages, fibroblasts, epidermal cells, liver, other tissue	Stimulates synthesis of sulphated proteoglycans, collagen, epidermal cell migration and fibroblast proliferation Has endocrine effects similar to growth hormone
Interferons	IFNs	Lymphocytes and fibroblasts	Activates macrophages Inhibits fibroblast proliferation and synthesis of MMPs Regulates other cytokines
Interleukins	ILs	Macrophages, mast cells, epidermal cells, lymphocytes, and many tissues	Chemotactic for leucocytes (IL-1) and fibroblasts (IL-4) Stimulates MMP-1 synthesis (IL-1), angiogenesis (IL-1, -8), TIMP synthesis (IL-6) Regulates other cytokines
Keratinocyte growth factor (also called FGF-7)	KGF	Fibroblasts	Stimulates epidermal cell migration, proliferation, and differentiation
Macrophage chemoattractant protein	MCP	Epidermal cell	Chemotactic for leucocytes, macrophages
Macrophage inflammatory protein	MIP	Macrophage	Chemotactic for leucocytes
Matrix metalloproteinases	MMPs	Multiple families including collagenases, gelatinases, and stromelysins; numerous cell sources within the ECM including macrophages, epidermal cells, endothelial cells and fibroblasts	Activate other MMPs, degrade cell basement membranes, collagen, and other proteins. Important in cell migration and collagen remodelling
Nerve growth factor	NGF	Neural and glial cells	A neurotrophic factor that modulates neuronal cell survival by both positive and negative regulation May alter VEGF expression
Nitric oxide	NO	Leucocytes Endothelial cells Many tissues	Vasodilation, antimicrobial activity, induces vascular permeability Regulation of cell proliferation Modulates ECM formation
Platelet-derived growth factor (including isoforms PDGF-AA, -AB and -BB)	PDGF	Platelets, macrophages, endothelial cells, epidermal cells, smooth muscle cells	Chemotactic for leucocytes, macrophages, fibroblasts, and smooth muscle cells Activates leucocytes, macrophages and fibroblasts Mitogenic for fibroblasts, endothelial cells, and smooth muscle cells Stimulates production of MMPs, fibronectin, and hyaluronic acid Stimulates angiogenesis and wound contraction, and remodelling Inhibits platelet aggregation Regulates integrin expression
Tissue inhibitors of matrix metalloproteinases (TIMP-1, -2, -3, -4)	TIMPs	Fibroblasts, macrophages, endothelial cells	TIMPs inhibit MMPs; important for balance between collagen deposition and removal in ECM remodelling; TIMPs involved in vascular smooth muscle migration and apoptosis
Transforming growth factor alpha	TGF-α	T lymphocytes, macrophages, epidermal cells, and many tissues	Similar to EGF
Transforming growth factor beta (including isoforms TGF-β1, -β2, and -β3)	TGF-β	Platelets, T lymphocytes, macrophages, endothelial cells, epidermal cells, smooth muscle cells, fibroblasts	Chemotactic for leucocytes, macrophages, lymphocytes, fibroblasts and smooth muscle cells Stimulates TIMP synthesis, epidermal cell migration, angiogenesis and fibroplasia Induces differentiation of fibrocyte to myofibroblast Inhibits production of MMPs and epidermal cell proliferation Regulates integrin expression and other cytokines Induces TGF-β production

1.2   (continued) Mediators and regulators of wound healing. (continues) ▶

Mediator	Abbreviation	Source(s)	Functions
Tumour necrosis factor	TNF	Macrophages, mast cells, T lymphocytes	Activates macrophages Mitogenic for fibroblasts Stimulates angiogenesis Regulates other cytokines
Vascular endothelial cell growth factor	VEGF	Epidermal cells	Increases vascular permeability Mitogenic for endothelial cells

1.2 (continued) Mediators and regulators of wound healing.

The platelet is the key cell in the initiation of wound healing and releases cytokines and essential growth factors that stimulate the process. The events of healing are then amplified, sustained and modified by wound macrophages, endothelial cells and fibroblasts. The wound matrix plays an important role in sustaining and modifying repair and maturation.

Haemostasis

The first response to injury is haemostasis (Figure 1.3), which is attempted in three steps: (1) vasoconstriction; (2) formation of the platelet plug; and (3) activation of the coagulation cascade with formation of the fibrin plug (blood clot).

Blood and lymph flows from damaged blood vessels and lymphatics to fill the wound and cleanse the wound surface. Almost immediately the blood vessels undergo a reflex constriction, and endothelial damage activates the platelet with subsequent formation of the platelet plug. Vasoconstriction is mediated by local release of bradykinin, serotonin, catecholamines and endothelin, and production of thromboxane A_2 through activation of the arachidonic pathway. Vasoconstriction lasts only 5–10 minutes, by which time the platelet plug has formed.

The blood vessels then dilate, and intravascular cells and fluid pass through the vessel walls into the extravascular space. Vasodilation is mediated by histamine released from local mast cells activated by tissue damage. Prostaglandins from the arachidonic pathway, kinins from the coagulation cascade, and complement factors also contribute to vasodilation. Endothelial damage results in exposure of tissue factor (tissue thromboplastin, factor III) and activation of the intrinsic coagulation cascade during which soluble fibrinogen is converted to a network of insoluble fibrin fibres. The resulting combination of activated platelets, red blood cells, fluid and fibrin forms the fibrin plug within the wound defect (Figure 1.4).

Insoluble fibrin monomers within the clot, in the presence of activated factor XIII, become covalently cross-linked and directly bind to platelets via their $\alpha_{11b}\beta_3$ integrin receptors to form the provisional extracellular matrix (ECM). Notably, factor XIII

Phase	Timing	Visual characteristics	Key cells	ECM components	Microscopic features	Key regulators/mediators
Haemostasis	Immediate	Bleeding				
	0–10 minutes	Blanching	Endothelial cells			Catecholamines, prostaglandins, thromboxanes
		Clot formation	Platelets, endothelial cells	Fibrin, fibronectin	Formation of fibrin plug	Intrinsic coagulation cascade – tissue factor, thrombin

1.3 Haemostasis: timing, visual changes, microscopic features and key biochemical events.

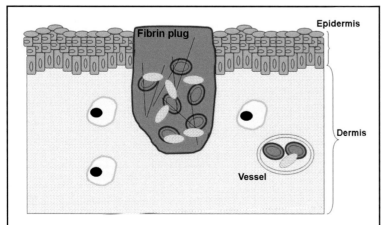

1.4 Haemostasis. Blood and lymph from damaged vessels and lymphatics fill the wound immediately after injury. The platelets, in combination with the red blood cells, fluid and fibrin, form a plug in the wound. (Modified with permission from Hosgood, 2006)

KEY			
Dermis		Epidermal cell	
Fibrin	—	Mast cell	•
Platelet		Red blood cell	

deficiency will result in impaired wound healing while the absence of fibrinogen does not prevent wound healing but will result in disorganized epidermal cell migration and decreased wound strength.

The provisional ECM facilitates entry of cells into the wound through its binding sites for adhesion molecules (integrins, selectins) on the surface of migrating neutrophils, macrophages, endothelial cells and fibroblasts. For example, fibrin will bind monocytes and neutrophils at their CD 11b/CD 18 integrin receptor, and bind endothelial cells and fibroblasts via $\alpha_5\beta_3$ integrin receptors.

- **Integrins are adhesion molecules (cell receptors) on the surface of cells that can bind to components of the ECM. This binding will trigger a reaction in the cell leading to changes in cell adhesion, growth or migration. Changes that occur within cells can also alter the affinity of integrins for components of the ECM.**
- **Selectins are a family of single chain, transmembrane glycoproteins that mediate adhesion of neutrophils to endothelial cells during inflammation; however, the binding is of low affinity.**

Thus, the fibrin plug not only acts as a haemostatic plug and an immediate barrier to infection and fluid loss, but also provides a substrate for early organization of wound healing. It stabilizes the wound edges and the provisional ECM provides some wound strength. The surface of the fibrin plug will dry and form a scab or *eschar* that protects the wound, prevents further haemorrhage, and allows wound healing to continue underneath. The scab does not provide any wound strength and will eventually slough, along with dead inflammatory cells and dead bacteria.

The role of the provisional ECM:
- **Facilitates entry of migrating neutrophils, macrophages, endothelial cells and fibroblasts into the wound**
- **Reservoir for growth factors and cytokines which bind to fibrin within the matrix**
- **Haemostatic plug**
- **Immediate barrier to infection and fluid loss**
- **Substrate for early organization of wound healing**
- **Provides some wound strength**

Inflammation

Inflammation (Figure 1.5) is characterized by migration of leucocytes into the wound (Figure 1.6), which occurs within 6 hours of injury. Inflammation begins with activation of the complement system at the time of injury. Complement degradation products attract neutrophils to the wound and are opsonins for phagocytosis. An opsonin is a molecule that binds to bacteria and foreign cells and enhances their uptake by phagocytes.

The neutrophil is the first cell to enter the wound and is the predominant cell type for the first 3 days, peaking at 24–48 hours. Fibrinopeptides released by the conversion of fibrinogen into fibrin (see Haemostasis, above) are potent chemoattractants for neutrophils. Other substances such as leucotrienes

Phase	Timing	Visual characteristics	Key cells	ECM components	Microscopic features	Cell adhesion molecules	Key regulators/mediators
Inflammation	Days 0–6	Erythema, heat, swelling, pain, exudation	Endothelial cells, mast cells, neutrophils, macrophages, T lymphocytes	Provisional ECM – fibrin	Vascular vasodilation, cellular infiltration	Integrin and selectin receptors on inflammatory cells, platelets	Histamine, kinins, leucotrienes, thrombin, complement, PDGF, TGF-β, VEGF, IGF-1, MCP-1, MIP-1α, IL-1α, IL-1β, IL-6, IL-8, TNF-α

1.5 Inflammation: timing, visual changes, microscopic features and key biochemical events.

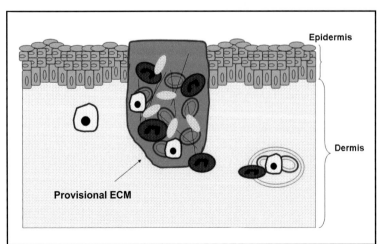

1.6 Inflammation. Leucocytes migrate into the wound soon after injury. Tissue damage releases mediators that are potent chemoattractants for neutrophils. (Modified with permission from Hosgood, 2006)

KEY			
Blood vessel	◯	Dermis	▨
Epidermal cell	▱	Fibrin	—
Monocyte	⊙	Neutrophil	⬤
Platelet	◌	Red blood cell	⬭

and bacterial peptides are also chemoattractants for leucocytes. Activated platelets degranulate and release substances such as platelet-derived growth factor (PDGF) and transforming growth factor beta (TGF-β), which are potent attractants for macrophages and fibroblasts. Interestingly, while the platelet appears vital to wound healing, absence of platelets did not affect the overall outcome of wound healing in a rat model though it did affect the inflammatory response; reduced numbers of macrophages and T lymphocytes were observed in wounds of thrombogenic rats (Szpaderska et al., 2003).

Neutrophils

Mediators in the provisional ECM promote the adhesion, margination and extravasation of neutrophils from blood vessels into the wound. Proteinases released by neutrophils to degrade necrotic tissue attract more neutrophils. The neutrophil phagocytoses bacteria and extracellular debris, removing them from the wound. The neutrophil releases toxic oxygen species including nitric oxide to kill bacteria, and degrade bacterial macromolecules, denatured ECM and damaged cells. Nitric oxide is an important mediator of vasodilation and increased vascular permeability in the early inflammatory phase. The neutrophil is also a source of pro-inflammatory mediators such as interleukins (IL-1α, IL-1β, IL-6, IL-8) and tumour necrosis factor alpha (TNF-α). The neutrophil, while integral to wound healing, is not essential and can be detrimental: open wounds in rats epithelialized faster in neutrophil-depleted mice, and had similar wound strength and similar collagen content to those in normal mice (Dovi et al., 2003).

The combination of wound fluid, degrading neutrophils and denatured tissue comprises the wound exudate, also referred to as pus. The presence of wound exudate gives the wound a mistakenly unhealthy appearance but is in fact vital to the healing process. Exudate does not imply infection. Note that neutrophils are present in sterile wounds.

The role of neutrophils in inflammation:
- **Kill bacteria and remove extracellular debris by**
  - **Phagocytosis**
  - **Release of toxic oxygen species**
- **Mediate vasodilation and increased vascular permeability**
- **Produce pro-inflammatory cytokines**

Monocytes and macrophages

Monocytes migrate into the wound with neutrophils in the same proportion as peripheral blood. While the neutrophil predominates in early inflammation, its presence is short-lived and monocytes predominate in older wounds. The concentration of monocytes in the wound peaks at 48–72 hours but the cells can remain in the wound for weeks. Cytokines released from activated neutrophils combined with degradation products and inflammatory proteins in the provisional ECM attract circulating monocytes into the wound. Many growth factors and cytokines are attractants for monocytes including PDGF, TGF-α, TGF-β, vascular endothelial growth factor (VEGF), insulin-like growth factor-1 (IGF-1), nerve growth factor (NGF), macrophage chemoattractant protein 1 (MCP-1) and macrophage inflammatory protein 1 alpha (MIP-1α) (Werner and Grose, 2003). Once acute inflammation subsides, local vascular permeability is restored and blood cells cease to pass into the extravascular space. If foreign material or bacteria remain in the wound, the monocytes undergo proliferation.

Monocytes are essential to wound healing and proliferation of monocytes is characteristic of chronic inflammation.

Monocytes transform into activated wound macrophages and reside within the provisional ECM, becoming an important source of growth factors and cytokines that sustain wound healing. The macrophage perpetuates the inflammatory process by the production and release of pro-inflammatory cytokines such as IL-1α, IL-1β, IL-6 and TNF-α. The macrophage also stimulates and modulates the repair process (fibroplasia, angiogenesis and epithelialization) through the release of fibroblast growth factor 2 (FGF-2), TGF-α, TGF-β, epidermal growth factor (EGF), IGF, PDGF, VEGF, and matrix metalloproteinases (MMPs) and their tissue inhibitors (TIMPs). Macrophages present early in wound healing are important in debridement of the wound through their phagocytic activity. Macrophages present later in the wound, along with neutrophils, are important in modification of the provisional ECM. The provisional ECM will become the wound ECM, which is described and recognized as granulation tissue.

Monocytes may also coalesce and form multinucleated giant cells, which also have phagocytic functions, or may evolve into epidermal cells and histiocytes.

The role of macrophages in inflammation:
- **Produce pro-inflammatory cytokines**
- **Stimulate and modulate repair**
- **Modify provisional ECM to form granulation tissue**
- **Phagocytosis (multinucleated giant cells)**
- **Evolve into epidermal cells and histiocytes**

Lymphocytes

The link between inflammation, phagocytosis and wound healing involves innate and adaptive immune responses. The innate immune system provides a non-specific immediate defence from infection by inflammatory reactions and the action of leucocytes, including neutrophils and macrophages. The adaptive immune system is activated when the innate immune response fails to eliminate a pathogen; it is specific to individual pathogens. The lymphocyte is the major cell of the adaptive immune system

At injury, invading pathogens are recognized by their highly conserved structure, known as pathogen-associated molecular patterns (PAMPs), e.g. the lipopolysaccharides of Gram-negative bacteria.

Among the receptors for PAMPs are the toll-like receptors (TLRs) expressed on neutrophils, macrophages, epidermal and endothelial cells. When the TLRs of a cell bind foreign products, the cell is activated to produce pro-inflammatory mediators including cytokines (TNF-α, IL-1), adhesion molecules (integrins, selectins) and growth factors.

> **The T lymphocyte is important in wound healing and the depletion of all subsets of T lymphocytes will impair wound healing.**

The role of each T lymphocyte subset may be opposing. Rats depleted of CD4+ T cells had a significant decrease in wound strength, while rats depleted of CD8+ T cells had a significant increase in wound strength (Davis *et al.,* 2001). The CD4$^+$ cells are characterized by two subpopulations: a CD4$^+$ immature effector T cell (T$_H$0) has the potential to differentiate into an inflammatory T cell (T$_H$1) or a helper T cell (T$_H$2), each secreting distinct cytokine profiles (Figure 1.7). The T$_H$1 cytokines activate macrophages (cellular immunity) and the T$_H$2 cytokines activate B cells (humoral immunity). The T$_H$1 cytokine interferon gamma (IFN-γ) will induce the expression of inducible nitric oxide (iNOS) in macrophages; thus the effect of T cells on wound healing may be mediated through nitric oxide (Munder *et al.,* 1998).

The role of lymphocytes in healing:
- **Inflammatory T lymphocytes (T$_H$1): macrophage activation (cellular immunity), probably mediated via nitric oxide**
- **Helper T lymphocytes (T$_H$2): B cell activation (humoral immunity)**

Nitric oxide (NO)

The role of nitric oxide in wound healing is complicated. It may be due to its chemical reaction with oxygen, leading to formation of reactive oxygen species, or to its interaction with heme or metal-containing enzymes (Luo and Chen, 2005). Nitric oxide is a small radical formed from L-arginine by three distinct isoforms of nitric oxide synthase (NOS); two of these (cNOS) are constitutively expressed (i.e. expressed regardless of surrounding conditions) and are found in many cell types including endothelial cells. Inducible nitric oxide synthase (iNOS) is not typically expressed in cells in their basal state but is expressed in activated cells under certain conditions. The cytokines IL-1, TNF-α and IFN-γ are inducers of iNOS. Expression of iNOS is high during early wound healing, peaking about 48–72 hours after injury and then decreasing.

The effects of NO during the inflammatory phase include vasodilation, antimicrobial activity, antiplatelet aggregation and induction of vascular permeability. Nitric oxide has the capacity to regulate cell proliferation during the repair phase and the net effect may depend on its concentration. Low doses of NO stimulate proliferation of fibroblasts, endothelial and epidermal cells but higher concentrations are inhibitory. NO may protect endothelial cells from apoptosis. Interaction between growth factors and NO occur during the repair phase. VEGF is dependent on NO, and VEGF can self-regulate itself by upregulating the expression of cNOS in endothelial cells. Collagen deposition in the ECM appears dependent on NO, with deposition enhanced by the presence of NO, arginine or iNOS overexpression. The cause of downregulation of iNOS is unclear but TGF-β is a strong inhibitor of iNOS. Inhibition of NOS will reduce collagen deposition.

The role of nitric oxide in inflammation:
- **Vasodilation**
- **Antimicrobial activity**
- **Antiplatelet aggregation**
- **Induction of vascular permeability**
- **Regulation of cell proliferation during the repair phase**
  - **Stimulation at low doses**
  - **Inhibition at high doses**
- **Protects endothelial cells from apoptosis**
- **Collagen deposition in the ECM**

Repair

Angiogenesis, fibroplasia, and epithelialization are all proliferative processes that occur during the repair phase (Figure 1.8). Wound contraction also occurs during this phase. The transition from the inflammatory to the repair phase is marked by the invasion of fibroblasts and an increased accumulation of collagen in the wound (Figure 1.9). In addition, there is migration and formation of new endothelial structures within the wound. The combination of new capillaries, fibroblasts and fibrous connective tissue forms the characteristic red fleshy granulation tissue that fills the wound.

The role of granulation tissue:
- **Fills the tissue defect**
- **Protects the wound**
- **Provides a barrier to infection**
- **Provides a surface for epithelialization**
- **Contains myofibroblasts that are important in wound contraction**

Cell type	Common secreted cytokine profile	Cell-specific secreted cytokine profile
T$_H$1	IL-3, GM-CSF	IL-2, IFN-γ, TNF-β
T$_H$2	IL-3, GM-CSF	IL-4, IL-5, IL-6, IL-10, IL-13

1.7 Cytokine profiles of T lymphocytes.

Phase	Timing	Visual characteristics	Key cells	ECM components	Microscopic features	Cell adhesion molecules	Key regulators/mediators
Repair	24–48 hours	Eschar (scab) sloughing	Epidermal cells	Provisional ECM, collagen, fibronectin, vitronectin, tenascin E	Re-epithelialization	Integrins – $\alpha_5\beta_1$, $\alpha_5\beta_5$, $\alpha_5\beta_6$, β_1	FGF-2, FGF-7, FGF-10, TGF-β, NGF, HGF, HB-EGF, KGF, nitric oxide, leptin, MMP/TIMP, IL-6, GM-CSF
	Days 4–7	Granulation tissue, visible epithelium at wound edge	Fibroblasts, endothelial cells	Provisional ECM → ECM, fibrin, collagen, glycosaminoglycan (GAG), proteoglycan	Fibroblast migration and replication within ECM, collagen deposition, endothelial migration and replication with new capillary formation	Integrins – $\alpha_5\beta_1$, $\alpha_5\beta_3$, $\alpha_5\beta_9$,	PDGF, TGF-β, FGF-2, ECF, IGF-1, connective tissue growth factor (CTGF), HB-EGF, VEGF, angiopoietin, MMP/TIMP
	Days 5–9	Visible wound contraction	Fibrocyte → myofibroblast		Appearance of phenotypically unique myofibroblasts in wound, wound contraction	Integrin-actin signalling → actin-associated cell-matrix adhesions (AACMAs)	TGF-β_1, TGF-β_2, PDGF
	Days 3–21		Fibroblasts, macrophages	Net collagen production	Collagen deposition		PDGF, TGF-β, FGF, VEGF, IGF-1, MCP-1, CTGF

1.8 Repair: timing, visual changes, microscopic features and key biochemical events.

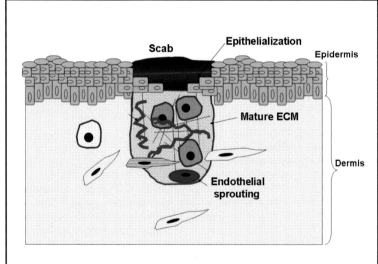

1.9 Repair. Angiogenesis and fibroplasia result in the formation of the mature extracellular matrix. Epithelialization also occurs. The macrophage, derived from the wound monocyte, is integral to stimulation of the process. The myofibroblast is essential to wound contraction and ECM modulation. (Modified with permission from Hosgood, 2006)

The transition from provisional ECM to mature ECM or granulation tissue is very active by 3–5 days after injury, and hence the first 3–5 days is sometimes referred to as the 'lag' phase of healing. This reflects a lag in gain in wound strength and not a lag in wound healing. It is clear that wound elements are considerably active during this time.

In order for new cells to enter the wound the following processes (Figure 1.10) must occur:

- A biochemical signal or cytokine is sent to local cells to stimulate cell proliferation and migration
- Cells express integrin and selectin receptors that will interact with the ECM to guide them into the wound
- Proteolytic enzymes known as matrix metalloproteinases (MMPs) degrade ECM in front of the migrating cells to allow them to enter the ECM.

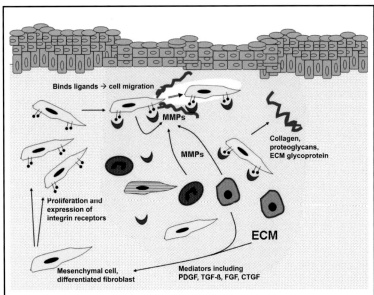

1.10 Repair. Complex interactions within the ECM allow movement of cells into the wound and the formation of new structures. Ligands within the ECM bind integrin receptors on the fibroblasts to facilitate cell migration through a path cleaved by proteases (MMPs).

KEY			
Collagen	⋎⋏⋎	Dermis	▨
Epidermal cell	⬭	Fibroblast	⬳
Integrin receptor	⥜	Ligands	⌣
Macrophage	⬤	Myofibroblast	⬱
Neutrophil	⬤		

Fibroplasia

The fibroblast population begins to increase about 3–4 days after wounding and is very active by 7 days. The fibroblasts synthesize the true ECM of the wound, which includes the building blocks of collagen, proteoglycans and ECM glycoproteins.

The connection between the inflammatory and repair phases is through cytokine and growth factor activity, which stimulates fibroblast migration into the provisional ECM. One or more populations of mesenchymal cells move into the wound with the endothelial cells. Sources of fibroblasts include differentiated fibroblasts and undifferentiated mesenchymal cells close to the wound. Mediators produced by macrophages, including PDGF, TGF-β, FGF and connective tissue growth factor (CTGF), in concert with ECM molecules such as fibronectin, stimulate fibroblasts in the surrounding tissue to proliferate, express appropriate integrin receptors and migrate into the wound. Integrins are adhesion molecules essential to cell migration, which promote cell–cell and cell–matrix interactions. They are a family of transmembrane proteins, composed of two polypeptide chains (α and β) that are expressed on the migrating cells. The protein binds to ligands or molecules expressed on various surfaces, such as activated endothelium, and components of the ECM (fibrin, fibrinogen, vitronectin). Fibrin, fibronectin and hyaluronan within the provisional ECM provide a conduit for cell migration. The appearance of fibronectin and the appropriate integrin receptors that bind the fibroblasts is the rate-limiting step in the formation of granulation tissue.

Fibroblast movement into the tightly woven provisional ECM requires active proteolytic enzymes, known as matrix metalloproteinase (MMPs) to cleave a path for cell migration. Sources of MMPs include neutrophils, macrophages, endothelial cells and fibroblasts. ECM fragments released after MMP proteolysis further regulate cell activities and are termed matrikines (Maquart *et al.,* 2005).

The MMPs include six families of zinc-dependent enzymes, including collagenases, stromolysins, metalloelastins, matrilysin, matrix-type metalloproteinases (MT-MMPs) (Figure 1.11) and gelatinases. Gene expression of MMP is regulated by cytokines and growth factors including interleukins, interferon, keratinocyte growth factor (KGF), EGF, bFGF, VEGF, PDGF, TGF-β, TNF-α and extracellular matrix metalloproteinase inducer (EMMPRIN). All MMPs are secreted, except for MT-MMPs, which exist as membrane-bound proteins attached to the surface of the cell membrane. Activation of MMPs is mostly extracellular, activated by other activated MMPs, or serine proteases that cleave the peptide bonds within the MMP prodomain.

Common name	MMP	Substrate specificity	Activated by	Activator of	Function
Collagenases					
Collagenase 1 (Fibroblast collagenase)	MMP-1	Fibrillar collagens – predominantly III, also I, II, VII, VIII, X	Kallikrein, chymase, plasmin, MMP-3, MMP-10	MMP-2	Re-epithelialization – epidermal migration, proliferation
Collagenase 2 (Neutrophil collagenase)	MMP-8	Fibrillar collagens – predominantly I, also III, II	Plasmin, MMP-3, MMP-10	Unknown	Prevents apoptosis, regulates inflammation

1.11 Characteristics of matrix metalloproteinases (MMPs). (continues) ▶

Common name	MMP	Substrate specificity	Activated by	Activator of	Function
Collagenases continued					
Collagenase 3	MMP-13	Fibrillar collagens – predominantly II, also I, III, IV, IX, X, XI, gelatin, laminin, tenascin	Plasmin, MMP-2, MMP-3, MMP-10	MMP-2, MMP-9	Endothelial cell migration
Collagenase 4	MMP-18	Fibrillar collagens – predominantly III	Unknown	Unknown	May act as MT-MMP
Gelatinases					
Gelatinase A	MMP-2	Gelatin, collagen type IV, I, fibronectin, tenascin	MMP-1, MMP-7, MT1-MMP, MMP-13	MMP-9, MMP-13	Epidermal migration, modulates inflammation
Gelatinase B	MMP-9	Gelatin, collagen type IV, I, XIV,	Plasmin, MMP-3, MMP-2	Unknown	Promotes inflammation, promotes migration of neutrophils
Stromelysins					
Stromelysin 1	MMP-3	Collagen type IV, fibronectin, aggrecan, nidogen	Plasmin, kallikrein, chymase, tryptase, elastase, cathepsin G	MMP-1, MMP-9	Promotes cell migration
Stromelysin 2	MMP-10	Collagen type IV, fibronectin, aggrecan, nidogen	Plasmin, kallikrein, chymase, tryptase, elastase, cathepsin G	MMP-8, MMP-13	Promotes cell migration Re-epithelialization
Stromelysin 3	MMP-11	Alpha1 proteinase inhibitor	Furin	Unknown	Unknown
Matrolysin 1	MMP-7	Collagen type IV, fibronectin, aggrecan, nidogen, elastin	Plasmin, MMP-3	MMP-2	Modulates inflammation, stimulates re-epithelialization, inhibits apoptosis
Matrolysin 2	MMP-26	Collagen type IV, gelatin, fibronectin			May affect cell migration
Membrane-type MMPs					
MT1-MMP	MMP-14	Collagen type I, II, III, gelatin, fibronectin, laminin, vitronectin, aggrecan	Plasmin, furin	MMP-2, MMP-13	Epidermal cell regulation
MT2-MMP	MMP-15	Large tenascin C, fibronectin, laminin, entactin, aggrecan and perlecan	Unknown	MMP-2, MMP-13	Inhibits apoptosis
MT3-MMP	MMP-16	Collagen type III, gelatin, casein, fibronectin	Unknown	MMP-2	Reduces cell adhesion and migration
MT4-MMP	MMP-24	Unknown	Unknown	MMP-2	
MT5-MMP	MMP-17	Unknown	Unknown	MMP-2	
MT6-MMP	MMP-25	Unknown	Unknown	MMP-2	Promotes neutrophil migration
Novel MMP					
Macrophage elastase (Metalloelastase)	MMP-12	Collagen type IV, fibronectin, vitronectin, laminin, aggrecan, nidogen, elastin	Unknown	Unknown	Stimulates corneal epithelial proliferation

1.11 (continued) Characteristics of matrix metalloproteinases (MMPs).

The increase in the fibroblast population within the provisional ECM due to both the migration and proliferation of cells sets the stage for collagen deposition in the wound during the repair phase. Many growth factors are involved in fibroblastic proliferation and stimulation including PDGF, TGF-β, EGF, FGF-2, IGF-1, CTGF, and heparin-binding epidermal growth factor (HB-EGF). Collagen peptides (procollagens) are synthesized within the fibroblast and exported to the ECM. A critical step in procollagen production is the hydroxylation of lysine and proline residues in the endoplasmic reticulum. This hydroxylation is necessary for the processing of the procollagen molecules into fibrils and is dependent on a number of cofactors including oxygen, vitamin C, ferrous iron and α-ketoglutarate. The procollagen chains are secreted into the ECM where they are aggregated into fibrils, facilitated in part by proteoglycans that are also secreted by the fibroblast.

In normal skin, type III collagen comprises only 10–20% of all collagen, while type I collagen comprises 80–90%. In the early wound, type III collagen predominates; it is replaced by type I collagen produced by fibroblasts, with a marked increase in the type I:type III ratio as the wound matures. The elaboration, orientation and contraction of the ECM components by the fibroblast organize the fibrin-filled wound into a durable connective tissue. The myofibroblast is also integral to this process. The greatest rate of accumulation of connective tissue occurs in the wound between 7 and 14 days after injury with the net production of collagen peaking at day 21, after which the collagen content stabilizes. Increasing quantities of collagen in the ECM signal fibroblasts to decrease collagen production. IFN-γ and TNF-α also modulate this process. Regression of the capillary content of the granulation tissue is also observed at this time, and the once fibroblast-rich granulation tissue becomes a relatively acellular scar as cells in the wound undergo apoptosis. Thus, there is a transition to maturation and remodelling, which will ultimately enhance wound strength.

Summary of the stages of fibroplasia:
- **Local fibroblasts are stimulated to proliferate, express integrin receptors and migrate into the wound**
- **Myofibroblasts develop, probably from fibrocytes which are stem cells from the bone marrow, and infiltrate the wound**
- **ECM products provide a conduit for fibroblast migration**
- **MMPs cleave a path in the ECM for fibroblast migration**
- **Fibroblasts synthesize and release collagen and other components of the true ECM**
- **The ECM is organized into durable connective tissue**
- **Eventually collagen production slows**
- **Capillaries regress to an acellular scar**

Angiogenesis

Angiogenesis is the development of new capillaries into areas previously unoccupied by vascular tissue. New capillaries develop from pre-existing vessels at the wound edges and endothelial cells that have migrated into the extracellular matrix.

Angiogenesis is a complex event, relying on interaction of the ECM with mediators that stimulate the migration and proliferation of endothelial cells (see Figure 1.9). The earliest phase of angiogenesis involves cell migration rather than cell division; intact or recently broken capillary blood vessels are stimulated by angiogenic factors to allow migration of columns of endothelial cells towards the wound. The endothelial cells migrate into the provisional ECM as early as 2 days after wounding. Strong stimuli for endothelial migration include VEGF, FGF, TGF-β and angiopoietin. Critical factors for angiogenesis include the presence of the provisional ECM and the expression of integrins and MMPs by the endothelial cells (Serini *et al.*, 2006). The integrins are the major cell surface receptors of the endothelial cells for the ECM and their expression is stimulated by VEGF, FGF and TGF-β. Many integrins appear important, especially integrin $\alpha_5\beta_1$, $\alpha_5\beta_3$ and $\alpha_5\beta_9$. The expression of MMPs is also stimulated by VEGF, FGF-2 and TGF-β. The role of the MMPs is to degrade the basement membrane and the ECM to allow the endothelial cells to migrate, form tubes and eventually form new

capillaries. Endothelial cells typically migrate in sheets whereas fibroblasts migrate individually. While endothelial cell invasion into the wound is occurring, endothelial proliferation also begins. Continued angiogenesis is stimulated by mitogenic factors for the endothelial cells produced by the macrophage, the endothelial cells themselves, and factors reposited in the ECM. Mitogenic factors include FGF, VEGF, TGF-β, angiogenin, angiotropin, angiopectin 1, thrombospondin and endothelin. Local wound changes such as low oxygen tension, increased lactate and low pH are also a stimulus for angiogenesis, through their effects on mediator production.

Early granulation tissue has a rich capillary bed with a characteristic deep red colour. The immature capillaries are quite porous but become 'non-leaky' as they mature, stimulated by angiopoietins. As the ECM matures, the new blood vessels disintegrate due to apoptosis and the redness of the wound is reduced. Many ECM molecules regulate this cell death, including thrombospondin 1 and 2, and anti-angiogenic factors such as angiostatin, endostatin, angiopoietin 2 and angiotensinogen.

Summary of the stages of angiogenesis:
- **Production of angiogenic factors**
- **Early endothelial cell migration into the provisional ECM leading to capillary formation**
- **Concurrent degradation of basement membrane and ECM by MMPs to allow endothelial cell migration**
- **Endothelial cell proliferation then commences**
- **Maturation of capillaries**
- **Late apoptosis of new blood vessels during ECM maturation**

Epithelialization

- **The predominant early activity in epithelialization is one of mobilization and migration of epidermal cells at the margin of the wound, followed by proliferation of epidermal cells behind these leading cells. Epidermal cells behind the migrating cells begin to proliferate 1–2 days after injury.**
- **In an incised wound that is sutured with the skin edges apposed, epithelialization may be complete as early as 24–48 hours after injury.**
- **In partial thickness skin wounds, epidermal migration over the wound surface begins almost immediately from both the wound margins and adnexal appendages such as hair follicles and sweat glands.**
- **In full-thickness skin wounds, the epidermis can only be resurfaced from the wound margins after adequate granulation tissue has formed. Generally, new epidermis is not visible at the wound edges until 4–5 days after injury.**

Soon after injury, the epidermal cells at the margin of the wound undergo phenotypic alteration that includes retraction of intracellular monofilaments, dissolution of most desmosomes that provide physical connections between the cells, and formation of peripheral cytoplasmic actin filaments, which allow cell movement. Lateral movement of the epidermal cells is facilitated by the lack of adherence between epidermal and dermal cells to one another, because of the dissolution of hemidesmosomal links between the epidermis and the basement membrane induced by collagenases and MMPs produced by the epidermal cells. Urokinase plasminogen activator produced by epidermal cells under the stimulus of hypoxia is also important in migration of epidermal cells across the ECM. Urokinase plasminogen activator converts plasminogen to plasmin which is capable of degrading the ECM (Daniel and Groves, 2002). Integrin receptors on the epidermal cells allow them to interact with a variety of ECM proteins including fibronectin and vitronectin, which are interspersed in the type I collagen at the margin of the wound, and in the provisional ECM in the wound. The path of migration of the epidermal cells is determined by integrins expressed on the membranes of migrating epidermal cells (Watt, 2002). Major integrins expressed in the intact epidermis include $\alpha_2\beta_1$, $\alpha_3\beta_1$ and $\alpha_9\beta_1$. After injury, expression of $\alpha_5\beta_1$ integrin (fibrin receptor), $\alpha_5\beta_5$ integrin (fibrin and vitronectin receptor) $\alpha_5\beta_6$ integrin (fibronectin, vitronectin, tenascin C and TGF-β receptor) and β_1 integrin are upregulated.

Stimuli for the migration and proliferation of epidermal cells include EGF, TGF-α and KGF produced by epidermal cells, wound fibroblasts and wound macrophages. As re-epithelialization occurs, there is progressive accumulation of new basement membrane material (laminin) under the migrating cells, starting at the margin of the wound and continuing inward. The epidermal cells revert to their normal phenotype and become firmly attached to the basement membrane and the underlying dermis. Over time, the epidermal layer will stratify. In general, melanocytes in the skin adjacent to the wound will undergo mitosis and migrate into the regenerating epidermis. Integrin receptors on the melanocytes appear important in modulating the migration of melanocytes along the basement membrane of the newly formed epithelium and in the intercellular recognition of epidermal cells. Repigmentation is progressive from the periphery of the wound to the centre and there is a lag of 1–2 weeks before pigmentation is noted. Maximal melanocyte proliferation may not be seen for several months.

Incomplete or complicated epithelialization occurs in:

- Large open wounds where:
    - Stratification of the epidermal layer may take weeks to months
    - Re-epithelialization may not be complete, leaving exposed granulation tissue in the centre of the wound
    - Epidermis towards the centre of the wound may be thin and easily traumatized

- Full-thickness wounds, since adnexal structures do not regenerate
- Pigmented skin, since repigmentation of the epidemis is variable and inconsistent across subjects.

Summary of the stages of epithelialization:
- **Movement of epidermal cells at the edge of the wound facilitated by:**
    - **Loss of contact with adjacent cells and basement membrane**
    - **Ability to move**
- **Proliferation of epidermal cells behind the migrating epidermal cells**
- **Accumulation of basement membrane under migrating cells**
- **Attachment of epidermal cells to basement membrane as the wound defect is covered with epidermal cells**
- **Epidermal cell stratification**
- **Melanocyte mitosis and migration into new epidermis**

Contraction

Contraction refers to the reduction in wound size that corresponds to changes in the tension of the wound and surrounding tissue. Visible wound contraction is evident by 5–9 days after injury.

There is a unique population of fibroblast-like cells within the wound that differ from the normal fibroblast of healthy mesenchymal tissue and may differ from tissue fibroblasts that migrate into the wound (Eyden, 2005). These cells are called myofibroblasts and they have a characteristic appearance, with phenotypic features of abundant contractile filaments, intercellular tight junctions and a distorted nuclear envelope. The myofibroblasts contain varying amounts of actin, a smooth muscle protein, and intermediate filament proteins, desmin and vimentin. The source of these cells is unclear, with local resident fibroblasts (Faggian et al., 1998), smooth-muscle cells (Gabbiani, 1996) and pericytes (Desmouliere et al., 1993) implicated. The most recent evidence suggests that the fibrocyte is the primary source (Hong et al., 2007).

Fibrocytes are a distinct population of circulating cells originating from the bone marrow that infiltrate the wound during the inflammatory phase. The fibrocyte was initially described as a subset of the leucocyte, since it expressed a common leucocyte antigen (CD45); it also exhibits fibroblast-like characteristics and is capable of collagen production, which is sufficient to distinguish it from a leucocyte. However, the fibrocyte also has a cell surface phenotype that differentiates it from the tissue fibroblast (Bellini and Mattoli, 2007). The fibrocyte is considered a progenitor cell and can differentiate into a number of cells including myofibroblasts, osteoblasts, chondroctyes, and adipocytes.

The differentiation of fibrocytes into myofibroblasts is induced by TGF-β1, which mediates α-smooth muscle actin (SMA) gene expression. The expression of SMA peaked between 4 and 67 days after wounding in mice, which coincided with an increase in activated TGF-β1 in the wounds (Mori *et al.*, 2005). During the second week of healing, appearance of myofibroblasts corresponds to contraction of the wound. Wound contraction and ECM remodelling is a function of the myofibroblast and its complex interaction with other cells and the ECM, involving mediators such as TGF-β_1, TGF-β_2, and PDGF. The expression of α-SMA in the stress fibres of the myofibroblast is essential for acquisition of its high contractile ability. Actin-associated cell-matrix adhesions (AACMAs) provide the interface between ECM components and intracellular stress fibres. These complex adhesions with the ECM, originally called fibronexus, are important for the efficient transmission of myofibroblast contractile forces to the ECM to promote wound contraction. The exact nature of the adhesions is unclear but complex integrin–actin signalling is involved. The term AACMAs is used to encompass all adhesions as they become identified. Adhesions identified include fibrillar adhesions, immature focal adhesions, mature focal adhesions and fibronexus, all of which have been described with varying molecular compositions.

During wound contraction the surrounding skin stretches (intussusceptive growth) and the wound takes on a stellate appearance. Contraction will continue until the wound edges meet and negative feedback from touching cells halts the process. Contraction will also cease if the tension of the surrounding skin equals or exceeds the force of contraction. If contraction ceases and the wound has remaining exposed granulation tissue, epithelialization may continue to occur and cover the wound.

A low myofibroblast content in the granulation tissue may result in failure of a wound to contract despite laxity in the surrounding skin. Once the epidermis has been re-formed, the number of myofibroblasts rapidly decreases due to apoptosis, the stimulus for which is unknown.

Maturation

Summary of the events of maturation (Figure 1.12):
- **The cellularity of the granulation tissue is reduced as fibroblasts and endothelial cells die**
- **The collagen fibre bundles become thicker, show increased cross-linking, and take on specific orientation along the lines of tension**
- **A reduction in the collagen content of the ECM by decreased production and increased degradation**

The transition from ECM to scar requires remodelling of the connective tissue content of the wound. The random haphazard appearance of the cellular and collagen fibre content of the granulation tissue is altered (Figure 1.13). The reorganization of the connective tissue and rearrangement of collagen bundles may take months, even years. The growth in mechanical strength is extremely slow.

Phase	Timing	Visual characteristics	Key cells	ECM components	Microscopic features	Key regulators/mediators
Maturation	Day 21+	Visible wound contraction, complete epithelialization	Fibroblasts	Stabilization of collagen production → reduction of collagen content	ECM remodelling, collagen cross-linking	PDGF, TGF-β, NGF, IL-1, IL-6, IL-10, TNF-α, IFN-γ, ECM components, MMP/TIMP
		Reduced redness	Endothelial cells	Endothelial cell apoptosis, reduction in capillary density		Thrombospondin, angiostatin, endostatin

1.12   Maturation: timing, visual changes, microscopic features and key biochemical events.

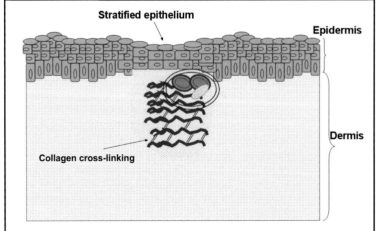

1.13   Maturation. Remodelling of the ECM reduces the cellular, collagen and vascular content of the matrix. Collagen reorientation and cross-linking increases wound strength. (Modified with permission from Hosgood, 2006)

KEY			
Blood vessel		Collagen	
Dermis		Epidermal cell	
Platelet		Red blood cell	

Remodelling is also characterized by a reduction in the collagen content of the ECM. Collagen already deposited within the ECM provides negative feedback, first reducing the rate of collagen deposition and then decreasing the overall collagen content. IFN-γ and TNF-α also cause fibroblasts to reduce collagen production. Collagen is degraded by proteolytic enzymes (MMPs) secreted by macrophages, epidermal cells, endothelial cells and fibroblasts within the ECM. Remodelling is a balance between MMP and TIMP expression, over which the ECM has a key role. Growth factors involved in this modulation include TGF-β, PDGF, and IL-1 (Chakraborti et al., 2003).

The TIMPs are important inhibitors of MMPs since they irreversibly bind to active MMPs. There are four structurally related members of the TIMP family (TIMP-1 to TIMP-4), which show a certain degree of specificity in their inhibitory action (Figure 1.14). The role of the TIMPs in normal wound healing is not only in the remodelling of the ECM, but also in inhibition of angiogenesis and induction of apoptosis. An imbalance between MMPs and TIMPs may play a role in delayed wound healing. The TIMPs are expressed by a variety of cell types including the fibroblast, epidermal, endothelial, osteoclast, chondrocyte, smooth muscle cell and many tumour cells. Expression can be affected by many growth factors (FGF, PDGF, EGF) and cytokines (IL-6, IL-1, IL-1β).

Wound strength

Although there is no dramatic gain in wound strength in the first 3–5 days after injury, some strength is provided by the fibrin in the fibrin plug (Figure 1.15). In addition, early ingrowth of capillaries and any epithelialization across an apposed wound provides some strength. There is no evidence that the other elements of the provisional ECM contribute to wound strength. The most rapid gain in wound strength occurs between 7 and 14 days after injury, corresponding to the rapid accumulation of collagen in the wound. By 21 days, the collagen content of the wound is at its maximum; however, the wound strength is only about 20% of its final strength. Thereafter the gain in wound strength is slow, reflecting the collagen breakdown and rearrangement during the process of remodelling.

Wounds never attain the tensile strength of normal tissue – at maximum strength a scar is only 70% to 80% as strong as normal tissue.

TIMP	Source	Characteristics
TIMP-1	Inducible, secreted in soluble form Expressed in fibroblasts, macrophages, endothelial cells	Potently inhibits most MMPs except MT1-MMP, MMP-2
TIMP-2	Constitutive, secreted in soluble form Expressed in fibroblasts, macrophages, endothelial cells	Potently inhibits most MMPs except MMP-9
TIMP-3	Inducible Exclusively associated with the ECM May play a role in cell detachment and migration	Inhibits MMP-1,-2,-3,-9 and -13
TIMP-4	Inducible Endothelial cell	Inhibits MMP-1,-2,-3,-7, and -9

1.14 Characteristics of tissue inhibitors of metalloproteinases (TIMPs).

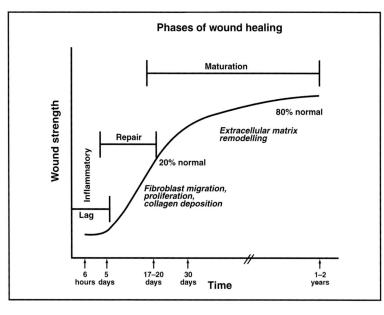

Phases of wound healing

1.15 Changes in wound strength during wound healing. Axes not to scale. (Modified with permission from Hosgood, 2006)

References and further reading

Bellini A and Mattoli S (2007) The role of the fibrocyte, a bone marrow-derived mesenchymal progenitor, in reactive and reparative fibroses. *Laboratory Investigations* **87,** 858–870

Chakraborti S, Mandal M, Das S *et al.* (2003) Regulation of matrix metalloproteinases: an overview. *Molecular Cell Biochemistry* **253,** 269–285

Daniel RJ and Groves RW (2002) Increased migration of murine keratinocytes under hypoxia is mediated by induction of urokinase plasminogen activator. *Journal of Investigative Dermatology* **119,** 1304–1309

Davis PA, Corless DJ, Aspinall R *et al.* (2001) Effect of CD4(+) and CD8(+) cell depletion on wound healing. *British Journal of Surgery* **88,** 298–304

Desmouliere A, Geinoz A, Gabbiani F *et al.* (1993) Transforming growth factor-β1 induced -α smooth muscle actin expression in granulation tissue myofibroblasts and in quiescent and growing cultured fibroblasts. *Journal of Cell Biology* **122,** 103–111

Dovi JV, He LK and DiPietro LA (2003) Accelerated wound closure in neutrophil-depleted mice. *Journal of Leukocyte Biology* **74,** 448–455

Eyden B (2005) The myofibroblast: a study of normal, reactive and neoplastic tissues with an emphasis on ultrastructure. Part 1. Normal and reactive cells. *Journal of Submicroscopic Cytology and Pathology* **37,** 109–204

Faggian L, Pampinella F, Roelofs M *et al.* (1998) Phenotypic changes in the regenerating rabbit bladder muscle. Role of interstitial cells and innervation on smooth muscle cell differentiation. *Histochemistry and Cell Biology* **109,** 25–39

Gabbiani G (1996) The cellular derivation and the life span of the myofibroblast. *Pathology, Research and Practice* **192,** 708–711

Hong KM, Belperio JB, Keane MP *et al.* (2007) Differentiation of human circulating fibrocytes as mediated by transforming growth factor-beta and peroxisome proliferator activated receptor-gamma. *Journal of Biological Chemistry* **282,** 22910–229120

Hosgood G (2006) Stages of wound healing and their clinical relevance. *Veterinary Clinics of North America: Small Animal Practice* **36,** 667–685

Luo JD and Chen AF (2005) Nitric oxide: a newly discovered function in wound healing. *Acta Pharmacologica Sinica* **26,** 259–264

Maquart FX, Bellon G, Pasco S *et al.* (2005) Matrikines in the regulation of extracellular matrix degradation. *Biochimie* **87,** 353–360

Mori L, Bellini A, Stacey MA *et al.* (2005) Fibrocytes contribute to the myofibroblast population in wounded skin and originate from the bone marrow. *Experimental Cell Research* **304,** 81–90

Munder M, Eichmann K and Modolell M (1998) Alternative metabolic states in murine macrophages reflected by the nitric oxide synthase/arginase balance: competitive regulation by CD4+ T cells correlates with Th1/Th2 phenotype. *Journal of Immunology* **160,** 5347–5354

Serini GD, Valdembri D and Bussolino F (2006) Integrins and angiogenesis: a sticky business. *Experimental Cell Research* **312,** 651–658

Szpaderska AM, Egozi EI, Gamelli RL *et al.* (2003) The effect of thrombocytopenia on dermal wound healing. *Journal of Investigative Dermatology* **120,** 1130–1137

Tsirogianni AK, Moutsopoulos NM and Moutsopoulos HM (2006) Wound healing: immunological aspects. *Injury, International Journal of the Care of the Injured* **37S,** S5–S12

Watt FM (2002) Role of integrins in regulating epidermal adhesion, growth and differentiation. *EMBO Journal* **21,** 3919–3926

Werner S and Grose R (2003) Regulation of wound healing by growth factors and cytokines. *Physiology Review* **83,** 835–870

2

Wound aetiology and classification

Juliet Pope

'For violence, like Achilles' lance, can heal the wounds that it has inflicted.'

Jean-Paul Sartre, from the preface to **The Wretched of the Earth** *by Frantz Fanon, 1961*

Introduction

This chapter examines those aspects of the aetiology and classification of wounds that relate specifically to the external surface and its associated structures. Since wounds have a wide variety of aetiologies and their patterns of tissue trauma vary considerably, it follows that the clinician's ability to appreciate the cause, likely progression, options for treatment and possible complications are of paramount importance.

Wound classification

Wounds can be classified in several ways, none of which is universally accepted. Some classifications begin with differentiating between open and closed wounds (Figure 2.1); others concentrate on aetiology or level of contamination. Whichever classification is preferred, a thorough and careful examination allows an assessment of possible aetiology and the extent of the damage to the skin and its surrounding and deeper

Open wounds
Surgical incision
Laceration
Abrasion
Avulsion
Degloving
Shearing
Puncture
• Bite/sting: cat/dog; snake; insect; spider; tick
• Firearm
Burn: thermal; chemical; electrical; radiation
Pressure sores
Cast- and bandage-related

Closed wounds
Contusion
Haematoma
Crush injury
Hygroma

2.1 One method of wound classification: open *versus* closed.

structures. Once the likely aetiology is known, either through clinical history or examination, possible complications can be taken into consideration when choosing treatment.

Wound complications and assessment

There are a multitude of possible complications for any wound. Most of these can be considered at presentation, and treatment altered to make allowance for them. There are three primary considerations: the wound itself; the patient; and the time lapsed since the injury occurred (Figure 2.2).

Wound factors
Degree of obvious contamination:
• Foreign material
• Bacteria
Aetiology:
• Devitalized tissue
• Necrotic tissue
• Risk of foreign material
• Risk of bacterial contamination

Patient factors
Concurrent injuries
Concurrent disease
Concurrent medication

Length of time since injury occurred
Peracute wound
Acute wound
Chronic wound

2.2 Factors determining possible complications.

If a wound is grossly contaminated, as is often seen with road traffic accidents, then attempting primary closure is clearly likely to fail. If the patient has suffered major blood loss due to concurrent injuries then any wound, whether clean or contaminated, will need delayed closure. A freshly incised wound can be simply closed with minimal risk of complication, but if the same wound is not presented for a week the risk of complications is likely to be greatly increased.

It would be easy to assume that a closed wound may not require any specific treatment but some of these wounds progress to open wounds due to devitalization of deep tissue, causing delayed necrosis. For example, a dog bite that causes a crush injury without breaking through the dermis can result in skin necrosis several days later and become secondarily infected if left untreated.

In human wound management the TIME acronym is used as a method for judging wounds, independent of aetiology:

- **T**issue
- **I**nfection and **I**nflammation
- **M**oisture
- **E**pithelialization.

Using this system, the presenting wound is assessed methodically and treated to maximize healing potential by:

1. Removing non-viable tissue
2. Removing factors predisposing to infection or treating established infection
3. Correcting any moisture imbalance preventing epithelial healing
4. Identifying wounds that are not continuing to full healing.

Incisional injuries and lacerations

These injuries can be surgical or traumatic. In surgery, the incising object is most commonly a scalpel blade, whereas traumatic wounds may be due to sharp objects as disparate as a kitchen knife, broken glass or a rusty piece of tin and are classed as lacerations.

The edges of an incisional wound are generally clean and free from tissue damage. The size of the wound is determined by the characteristics of the skin surrounding it: freely mobile skin with high elasticity tends to give a much larger open area than would be seen where the skin is more tightly attached to the underlying structures and where elasticity may be less (Figure 2.3). There are significant differences in elasticity between different breeds and some concurrent medical conditions can affect skin elasticity.

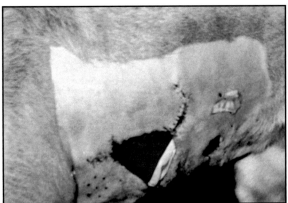

2.3 Laceration from an unknown object sustained by a dog during a walk. The mobility of the skin on the lateral thorax results in a large gaping wound. Wounds in this area are prone to breakdown due to tension and the pulling effect of the front leg to the relatively loosely adhered skin.

Complications

Incisional wounds tend not to become infected because:

- Most have minimal contamination with low bacterial numbers
- They often involve superficial veins and the subdermal plexus, resulting in sufficient bleeding to decrease tissue colonization by endogenous bacteria
- There is rarely significant damage to surrounding tissues, which might become devitalized and vulnerable to bacterial invasion.

Exceptions are where patients have impaired resistance to infection or where the incising object was heavily contaminated.

Depending upon the incising object there may be damage to deeper structures, so consideration should be given to physical exploration and/or imaging to identify damage to muscles, tendons or nerves. Lacerations extending into a body cavity and/or viscus can be classified as puncture wounds (see later).

Abrasions

Skin is damaged by frictional forces when it moves parallel to a rough surface, usually at speed. An abrasion is superficial damage not extending beyond the dermis. If the wound changes shape significantly when pulling on the surrounding skin, a full-thickness skin wound has occurred – not an abrasion.

Most abrasions are a result of road traffic accidents (Figure 2.4), often associated with more severe multiple injuries. Even single wounds generally involve areas with variable damage, with a combination of graze, abrasion and avulsion. Occasionally abrasions are seen on footpads following excessive exercise on a rough surface.

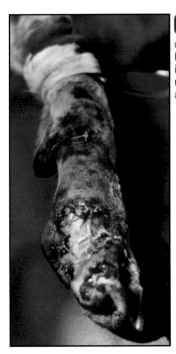

2.4 Abraded nail and surgically closed traumatic laceration above it, the initial trauma being the result of a road traffic accident.

Although abrasions can be managed by surgical debridement and primary closure, epidermal healing can easily be achieved using open wound management techniques (see Chapter 4).

Complications

Abrasions are generally heavily contaminated with debris, devitalized tissue and bacteria. Further abrasion may occur from accumulation of debris within the rough wound surface, leading to deeper contamination with foreign material. In severe abrasions there may be ongoing tissue necrosis due to damage to deeper dermal structures, resulting in the abrasion being reclassified as an avulsion (see below).

Degloving and avulsion wounds

These injuries frequently occur together as a result of severe trauma following road traffic accidents or animal fights. They often require similar treatment regimes and have similar complications.

Degloving describes how skin and deeper tissues can be torn from an extremity, just as a glove is removed from the hand. The process of degloving may be either mechanical or physiological.

Mechanical degloving occurs when the skin is pulled from its subdermal attachments until the skin tears and is frequently missing altogether, exposing the deeper tissues. Most commonly this is the result of road traffic accidents where the skin of an extremity becomes trapped under a wheel (Figure 2.5). In cats degloving commonly involves the tail and can be associated with a dislocation of the coccygeal vertebrae and stretching of the coccygeal nerves; the tail may ultimately require amputation. Physiological degloving occurs when skin suffers damage to its vascularity and subsequently necroses and sloughs.

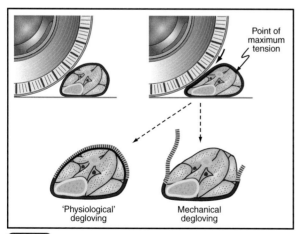

2.5 Mechanical and physiological degloving.

Avulsion injuries are characterized by the separation of tissue from their deeper attachments (Figure 2.6) and usually include muscle. Examples include:

- Large skin avulsions due to dog fights, especially those involving badgers or foxes
- Avulsion of the mandibular skin and muscle with concurrent mandibular symphyseal separation following road traffic accidents in cats. Reattaching avulsed tissue can be challenging when the mandible has little or no residual soft tissue coverage
- Avulsion of auricular cartilage detached from the skull despite intact skin.

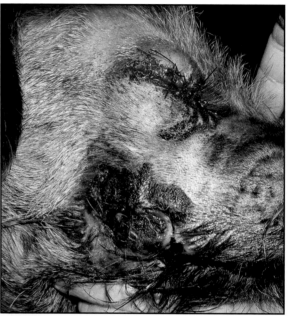

2.6 This Border Terrier had been dragged by a car. The skin has been severely contused and there was underling avulsion of the mucosa from the dental arcade. The dog had also suffered a proptosis and the eyelids have been temporarily sutured closed; unfortunately, the eye subsequently underwent enucleation.

Complications

Concurrent injuries usually require attention before wound reconstruction can be performed. Although degloving and avulsion injuries may be initially free of bacterial contamination, without appropriate wound management rapid colonization and infection of necrotic tissue will occur. The veterinary surgeon needs a good understanding of open wound management techniques and the principles of surgical decision-making when managing these wounds. as defects are often extensive and complex (see Chapters 3 and 4). As adjacent skin is at a premium in wounds involving the extremities, remaining degloved skin should be preserved where possible.

Shearing injuries

Shearing injuries have a similar aetiology to degloving wounds and are almost always the result of road traffic accidents. They usually involve loss of deeper tissues, including skin, tendons, muscle and sometimes bone, and frequently expose the joints of the distal limb (Figure 2.7).

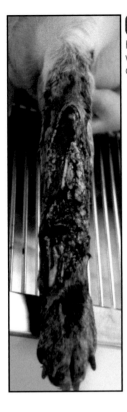

2.7 A badly sheared leg. There is loss of many layers of soft tissue and bone, with joint exposure and severe contamination.

Complications

These wounds are heavily contaminated with bacteria and debris and are extremely prone to infection. They will always involve open wound care if any attempt to salvage the limb is to be made (see Chapter 4).

The involvement of joints and their supporting soft tissue structures such as ligaments or tendons necessitates concurrent orthopaedic treatment. Severely damaged open joints may require arthrodesis. Use of external skeletal fixation for orthopaedic injuries allows easier management of soft tissue deficits. Surgical procedures are detailed in the *BSAVA Manual of Canine and Feline Fracture Management and Repair* and the *BSAVA Manual of Canine and Feline Musculoskeletal Disorders*.

Puncture wounds

A puncture wound is caused by any sharp object that pierces the skin to create a relatively small deficit or hole.

- Bites from other animals are the most commonly seen puncture wounds. Cat bites usually result in a very small puncture and the wound may go initially undetected. Dog bites may be multiple, and can involve more serious superficial and deep tissue damage. Further information on bite wounds is given in Chapter 11.
- Oropharyngeal penetration injuries occur during stick retrieval, when dogs 'run on to' a stick which is lodged in the ground at an angle. The stick may cause a wound to any of the anatomical structures of the oropharynx, most commonly the base of the tongue (see Chapter 11).

- Impalement on a sharp object, usually as the result of slipping and falling from a height (cats) or jumping over a hurdle and landing on an unseen hazard on the other side (dogs). Sometimes there will be full perforation, with both an entrance and an exit wound.
- Other puncture wounds have more specialized aetiologies, such as snake/insect bites, firearm wounds or porcupine quills, with their own presentation and complication characteristics.

Complications

The small, injection-like punctures of most cat (and some dog) bite wounds usually heal rapidly but the inoculation of bacteria into an essentially closed space results in the development of infection and abscessation which will often break through the skin a few days later (see Figure 2.8). The hypoxic environment favours bacteria such as *Pasteurella multocida* (particularly in cats), *P. canis* or *Clostridium* spp. Dogs diagnosed with tetanus may have a recent history of a puncture wound. Severe puncture wounds with associated haematoma, devitalized and/or contused tissues are prone to infection involving endogenous or exogenous *Staphylococcus* and *Streptococcus* species.

2.8 A typical puncture mark caused by a cat bite. The cat has been treated with antibiotics for a *Pasteurella multocida* infection and the wound is healing by second intention.

In so-called 'big dog/little dog' confrontations the damage can be very extensive, involving puncture, crushing and avulsion injuries, as well as contusion due to shaking of the victim. There may be multiple bite wounds, which may penetrate body cavities. Body wall ruptures, damage to internal organs, and concurrent orthopaedic injuries are possible. Rarely will such cases be simple to treat and the prognosis is likely to be poor unless the patient can be stabilized rapidly.

Stick injuries may present immediately after the incident, allowing prompt and thorough treatment with a high cure rate. Many cases are either not presented acutely or are not surgically explored, however, and so present later as chronic wounds due to foreign material or bacteria being retained in the wound. This leads to formation of a cervical or pharyngeal swelling and/or draining sinus tract. Failure to resolve clinical signs occurs in nearly 40% of dogs presented with chronic wounds.

Snake and arthropod bites and stings

Snake and insect or spider bites are forms of puncture wound but may have particular complications as a result of inoculation of the victim with chemical substances or microorganisms. Snake bites are uncommon in the UK and usually involve non-venomous snakes. The only indigenous venomous snake is the adder *Vipera berus.* Adder bites are most common in the summer, occuring as a result of dogs surprising an adder in long grass or heathland. Fatalities are rare but envenomation may cause significant morbidity from pain and swelling. Dangerous bites may occur from non-indigenous species kept as pets.

In Europe there are few species of insect likely to cause significant wounding, although the local effects may cause secondary self-trauma. The exception is idiosyncratic anaphylactic reactions causing swelling and/or blistering.

There are very few dangerous native spiders in the UK, although venomous imported spiders may be kept as pets. There are two main actions of spider venom – neurotoxicosis and necrosis – although most spider bites do not cause envenomation. The spider responsible for any serious bite needs early and prompt identification to allow for treatment.

Tick bites may lead to secondary infection or granulomas if incomplete removal has left mouthparts beneath the skin. Moreover they can transmit diseases such as Lyme disease.

Complications

Fortunately, death from snake or spider bite is very rare in the UK. Complications from snake or spider venom include:

- Local effects: oedema; pain; compartment syndrome; tissue necrosis leading to open wound formation
- Systemic effects: arrhythmia; hypotension; nausea/vomiting; organ failure; neurotoxicity.

Firearm injuries

In the UK high-powered gunshot injuries are relatively uncommon in dogs and cats; gunshot wounds are seen more frequently in the USA. Bullets and cartridges (Figure 2.9) vary in calibre (diameter), mass, composition, shape and velocity:

Low velocity	shotguns, airguns, handguns	<300 m/s
Medium velocity	hunting rifles	300–800 m/s
High velocity	military air rifles	>1000 m/s

Ballistic injuries vary depending on these variables and the degree of fragmentation created within a wound.

High-velocity bullets (>1000 m/s) have a huge amount of energy, and cause extensive damage

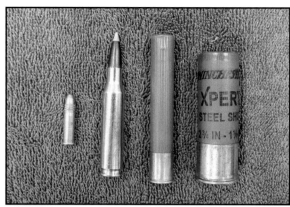

2.9 Cartridges for (left to right): .22 calibre rimfire rifle; 7 mm 08 calibre centre fire rifle; .410 bore shotgun; 12 gauge shotgun. (Courtesy of J Niles)

through cavitation and shock waves leading to stretching and compression of tissues. A bullet capable of mushrooming or fragmentation is more destructive. Cavity size may be 30–40 times the diameter of the bullet, with large amounts of dead and devitalized, contaminated tissue. Once the bullet has passed through the animal the cavity will collapse and, due to the subatmospheric pressure, will suck air, debris, hair and bacteria into the wound.

Low-velocity handgun bullets (200–300 m/s) are relatively heavy, have relatively low kinetic energy and tend to be used at a range of <100 m. They bore a hole through tissue and only damage those tissues with which they are in direct contact. Damage is only life-threatening when vital tissues are in their path. This path can be very unpredictable, with no relationship between entry and exit holes, as they may be deflected by organs such as the liver or spleen.

Shotgun injuries in working gundogs are usually an incidental finding. Shot patterns typically expand from the gun muzzle in a cone-like configuration. When the shotgun is outside the effective range (30–40 m) the pellets only enter the subcutaneous and deep fascial layers, where they cause little or no harm. Occasionally dogs are shot at close range, where the gun generates a significant amount of kinetic energy and can cause much more severe tissue destruction.

All penetrating injuries of this type are contaminated. Dense tissues such as bone absorb a greater amount of kinetic energy from the projectile and fragment, causing further damage to adjacent soft tissues. Tissue with a greater elastic component such as skin and lung can absorb a proportion of the kinetic energy and damage is less extensive.

Complications

Animals presented with gunshot wounds may have severe life-threatening injuries.

Tissue injury:

- The degree of soft tissue injury can vary greatly between wounds. Thorough exploration of any wound is necessary to identify any more serious internal injury.

- Wounds penetrating the abdominal or thoracic cavities carry their own special requirements (see Chapter 11).
- Treatment of heavily contaminated orthopaedic wounds can be very challenging. External skeletal fixation can be useful to stabilize long bones and joints whilst treating soft tissue wounds.

Contamination: The level of contamination of a gunshot wound will be affected by many variables:

- Velocity of missile
- Penetration of internal viscera such as the gastrointestinal tract
- Level of tissue damage.

Infection: The degree of infection can vary at presentation, given that there may be a delay between injury and treatment. Some wounds will have deep and well established infection whilst in others prompt and effective treatment can dramatically reduce both the level of contamination and risk of persistent infection.

Lead poisoning: This is not generally a concern in gunshot injuries given that the levels are low and systemic absorption is poor. The exception to this may be where fragments are within a joint and lead absorption may be enhanced by synovial fluid. In such cases, joint lavage is a sensible precaution.

Burns

A burn is the damage to the skin caused by an extreme of temperature (hot or cold) or by contact with a chemical substance, electricity or radiation.

Classification as first-, second- and third-degree burns has been replaced by the terms partial-thickness and full-thickness burns, depending upon the amount of dermis involved (Figure 2.10). Partial-thickness burns are further classified as superficial or deep. A combination of partial- and full-thickness damage is seen in most burn wounds. Judging both the depth of burn and particularly the extent of the damage makes the assessment of a patient with burns more accurate. Burns can be assessed depending on overall severity,

where partial-thickness burns of <15% of the total body surface area (TBSA) require minimal treatment and deep partial or full-thickness burns of >15% TBSA require emergency treatment and extensive surgical wound management.

Thermal burns

The most common thermal burn is caused by dry or wet heat. The extent of the injury depends on the temperature and tissue contact time. Some patients may have increased susceptibility to thermal damage (Figure 2.11). Hypothermic burns are unusual in the UK as they require extreme drops in temperature.

Inability to move away from the heat source
Inability to sense the heat source (neurological dysfunction)
Dehydration
Poor peripheral perfusion
Less hair covering than usual
Concurrent disease (e.g. Cushing's syndrome)
Concurrent medication (long-term corticosteroid use resulting in thinner than normal skin)

2.11 Patient factors predisposing to thermal injury.

Dry burns

Dry burns involve contact with a heat source when the animal is either unaware of the heat or unable to escape it quickly enough. Examples:

- Iatrogenic damage from heat pads in the anaesthetized or recumbent patient
- A hot exhaust pipe in a road traffic accident (Figure 2.12)
- Jumping on to hot surfaces, causing burns to footpads.

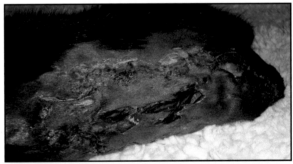

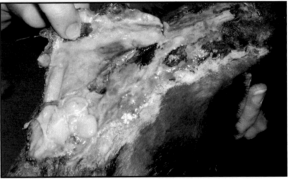

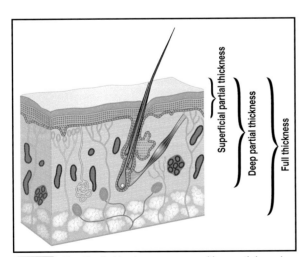

2.10 Depth of skin damage caused by partial- and full-thickness burns.

2.12 A cat with a broken pelvis following a road traffic accident that 5 days post-injury developed a large skin wound due to being trapped by a hot exhaust pipe.

Wet burns

Wet burns are usually scalds from contact with hot liquid. Classically, a dorsal pattern is seen when hot liquid is dropped on to a passing animal. Ventral burns are usually the consequence of an animal being lowered, or jumping, into the liquid. Deliberate application of a flammable substance, which is then ignited by a flame, has been described in cruelty cases (see Figure 2.15).

Chemical burns

There are many caustic liquids that can cause chemical burns. The damage may be to the skin or to the oropharynx/oesophagus in cases of oral contact or swallowing. Acidic corrosives cause pain, which generally restricts exposure; alkaline liquids (pH>11) do not, resulting in prolonged contact times and more severe wounds. This means that damage caused by acidic liquids can generally be assessed soon after exposure, whereas damage from alkaline products may not fully develop for many hours.

Possible treatment:

- Emesis – contraindicated due to risk of stomach perforation
- Neutralizing solutions – contraindicated as cause an exothermic reaction resulting in thermal damage
- Inactivated charcoal – of no benefit
- Dilution and supportive treatment.

Electrical burns

Electrical burns typically result from contact with a low voltage source, usually when a puppy or kitten chews an electric cable. Rarely, an animal will suffer a flash burn from a high voltage source (e.g. railway line) as the electricity arcs to earth through the animal's body.

Radiation burns

With increasing access to radiation facilities in the UK, veterinary surgeons may encounter oncological patients with radiation burns. Burns usually result from exposure to doses above 40 Gy. Different tissues have differing tolerance levels to radiation injury; hair will often grow back a different colour.

Complications

The problems associated with burns in small animals are poorly understood. In human patients the 'rule of nines' is used to measure the percentage of affected skin and this can be extrapolated to give a rough estimate in veterinary patients (Figure 2.13). In general this overestimates the burn area affected but is useful in giving a rapid initial assessment to identify patients where euthanasia may be advisable (burns of >50% TBSA).

Metabolic complications

Animals are more resistant to the life-threatening metabolic changes seen in human patients.

- Increased vascular permeability will result in loss of fluid, electrolytes and albumin into the tissues.
- In the early stages hyperkalaemia can be the result of red blood cell damage but will generally resolve with diuresis.
- Hypokalaemia subsequently develops due to increased renal potassium excretion and potassium supplementation may be required (for further details on fluid therapy and potassium supplementation see the *BSAVA Manual of Canine and Feline Emergency and Critical Care*).
- Albumin loss in the first few days can be such that colloids may be required to maintain intravascular volume and decrease ongoing extravasation.

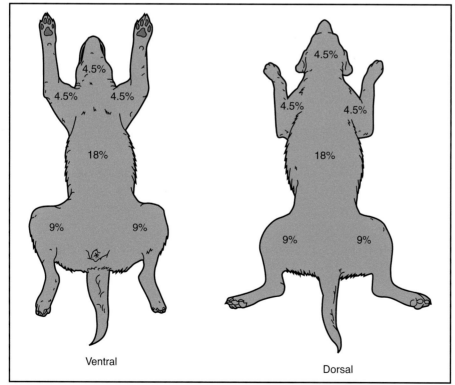

2.13 The 'rule of nines' allows an estimate of percentage total body surface area affected by burns.

Ventral

Dorsal

- Red blood cells are lost directly through thermal damage and prematurely removed from the circulation as a result of cell membrane damage. Concurrent fluid loss in the early stages means that anaemia may not be documented for several days until hypovolaemia has resolved. Reduced erythropoietin levels in severe burns may affect the patient's ability to regenerate erythrocytes.
- Other electrolyte changes may include hypernatraemia, hypophosphataemia and hypocalcaemia.

> **WARNING**
> **It is essential to monitor electrolytes, especially potassium, regularly.**

Some patients may be markedly hypovolaemic on presentation and require aggressive fluid therapy (see also Chapter 11). Constant and careful monitoring of fluid status by clinical examination is of paramount importance, and may be more accurate than the use of formulae adapted from the human field that predict fluid requirements based on the percentage of TBSA affected (Figure 2.14). Animals with minor burns may not be presented until several days later and be stable without receiving intensive care.

---

1. Calculate percentage of total body surface area affected (%TBSA) using the 'rule of nines' (see Figure 2.13).

2. Estimate volume of fluid required in ml = %TBSA x bodyweight (kg) x 4.

3. Give half of calculated volume in the first 8 hours.

4. Give remaining half over the subsequent 16 hours.

Example:

For a 20 kg dog with 25% burns:

%TBSA x bodyweight x 4 = 25 x 20 x 4 = 2000 ml

Give 1000 ml in first 8 hours = 125 ml/h
Give 1000 mls over next 16 hours = 62.5 ml/h

2.14 How to calculate the fluid requirements for burn patients in the first 24 hours.

Inhalation injury

- Inhalation of hot air can lead to dramatic upper respiratory tract oedema requiring urgent treatment. Fortunately this rarely extends beyond the upper respiratory tract due to efficient heat exchange within the nose, pharynx and larynx.
- Smoke inhalation may result in lower respiratory tract mucosal damage, leading to oedema, bronchospasm, obstruction by necrotic mucosa and secondary bacterial infection. The severity depends upon the substance, extent and duration of toxin exposure. Such injuries are unlikely to be seen at initial presentation and patients that do not develop complications within the first 24 hours are likely to make an uncomplicated recovery.
- Inhalation of carbon monoxide will cause severe respiratory compromise due to the high affinity of carbon monoxide for haemoglobin. Affected patients have a characteristic cherry red mucosa.

Patients suspected to be vulnerable to late onset respiratory compromise will benefit from close monitoring: repeated auscultation; thoracic radiography; pulse oximetry and arterial blood gas analysis. Judicious use of fluids must be implemented to avoid iatrogenic pulmonary oedema, and supplemental oxygen is vital. For further details see the *BSAVA Manual of Canine and Feline Emergency and Critical Care*.

Infection

Burns are highly susceptible to secondary infection, although opinion is divided about the use of prophylactic antibiotics. Systemic antibiotics are best confined to cases with confirmed culture and sensitivity results. Topical 1% silver sulfadiazine ointment is most commonly used to prevent bacterial colonization due to its broad spectrum of activity (UK veterinary surgeons are reminded that its use should comply with the cascade). Septicaemia is a potentially life-threatening complication requiring aggressive antibiotic treatment.

Nutritional deficiency

Early consideration should be given to the nutritional requirements of burns patients, who may have an increased calorific requirement and/or an inability to eat.

Scars, eschars and contractures

Scar formation is only seen in burns deep to the epidermis. Full-thickness burns that can be easily excised and reconstructed at an early stage will avoid most complications; however, those burns that require prolonged medical management may result in eschar and/or contracture formation, severely impairing normal function. In most cases they will require surgical intervention to allow for a return to normal function (Figure 2.15). Eschars may be restrictive to breathing when they form over the thorax, or can lead to vascular compromise when they form circumferentially on an extremity, and will need early surgery.

Complications of specific burns

The most commonly seen electrical burn is that caused by a juvenile chewing through an unearthed cable. The resultant damage can be very extensive and complex to reconstruct. The injuries have their own particular complications since the tissues are immature and the patient is still growing, making even minor scar tissue potentially serious.

Oncology patients suffering from radiation burns may have a multitude of complicating factors tending to delay or prevent healing.

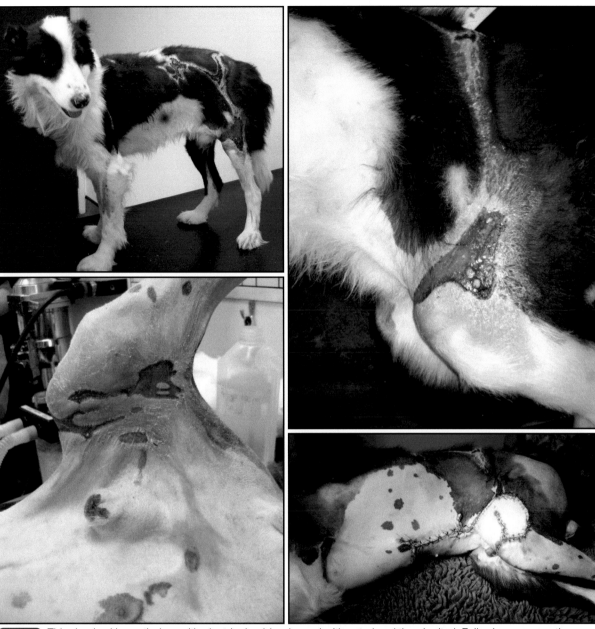

2.15 This dog had been tied up with electrical cable, doused with petrol and then ignited. Following conservative management, his injuries showed marked contraction and the prepuce had deviated abaxially. A caudal superficial epigastric axial pattern flap was created to release the contraction.

Pressure sores

Pressure sores (decubital ulcers) are typically found on the elbows and hocks of recumbent patients or giant breed dogs. They can be open or closed wounds and can be graded for severity according to the depth of damage. They are best avoided by meticulous attention to nursing. Once a pressure sore has developed, its treatment will vary according to severity. Pressure sores can be treated medically or surgically.

- Open sores are prone to infection and in very deep sores the infection can involve bones and joints.
- Hygromas (false bursas) are best treated medically but can become infected; surgical intervention should only be considered as a last resort, however.
- Chronic wounds will usually require surgical debridement and strict attention to bandaging technique after surgery.

Cast- and bandage-related wounds

Unfortunately iatrogenic wounds are not uncommon and are usually the result of:

- Ischaemic injury due to overtight application of bandaging
- Inadequate padding of vulnerable areas
- Excessive exercise, allowing bandage slippage
- Wet or dirty bandages, with a higher risk of bacterial strikethrough and infection.

If a bandage or cast is applied to a swollen limb, it will need replacing more quickly as the swelling dissipates resulting in a dressing that can move and damage the underlying skin. The frequency of bandage changing must be altered to suit the type of wound and patient.

Minor wounds involve skin damage only and have few complications. They can be managed with more careful ongoing bandaging using appropriately protective padding over the new defect.

More serious wounds may result in the loss of digits and even limbs, and require surgical debridement and reconstruction. Infection can also be a complicating factor.

Acknowledgement

Additional information on burns and firearm injuries was provided by Jacqui Niles.

References and further reading

Beardsley SL and Schrader SC (1995) Treatment of dogs with wounds of the limbs caused by shearing forces: 98 cases (1975–1993). *Journal of the American Veterinary Medical Association* **207**, 1071–1075

Fullington RJ and Otto CM (1997) Characteristics and management of gunshot wounds in dogs and cats: 84 cases (1986–1995). *Journal of the American Veterinary Medical Association* **210**, 658–662

Griffiths LG, Tiruneh R, Sullivan M and Reid SW (2000) Oropharyngeal penetrating injuries in 50 dogs: a retrospective study. *Veterinary Surgery* **29**, 383–388

Harborne DJ (1993) Emergency treatment of adder bites: case reports and literature review. *Archives of Emergency Medicine* **10**, 239–243

Johnson MD, Magnusson KD, Shmon CL and Waldner C (2006) Porcupine quill injuries in dogs: a retrospective of 296 cases (1998–2002). *Canadian Veterinary Journal* **47**, 677–682

Schultz GR, Sibbald G and Falnaga V (2003) Wound bed preparation: a systematic approach to wound management. *Wound Repair and Regeneration* **11**, S1–S28

Shamir MH, Leisner S, Klement E, Gonen E and Johnston DE (2002) Dog bite wounds in dogs and cats: a retrospective study of 196 cases. *Journal of Veterinary Medical and Physiology; Pathology and Clinical Medicine* **49**, 107–112

3

Decision-making in wound closure

John Williams

'The end for which the physician is working is that the features should fulfil their offices according to nature's decree.'

Gaspare Tagliacozzi, 1597

Introduction

Wound closure and reconstruction should aim to return the patient to normal function as soon as possible. To achieve this aim, the key questions in decision-making are when and how a particular wound should be closed. To answer these, the veterinary surgeon must take into account a number of factors such as the overall condition of the patient, how the wound was caused, and the degree of trauma at the site of the wound. Failure to take such factors into account may not only lead to local wound complications and dehiscence but, with severe trauma, the consequences to the patient could be catastrophic. Essentially there are two key areas of management: the whole patient; and the local wound environment.

Assessment and stabilization

Whole patient evaluation

With any severe localized trauma it is all too easy to concentrate on the wound and to forget other body systems. It is essential on presentation to evaluate the injured patient fully to ensure that there are no life-threatening injuries.

The veterinary surgeon should develop a routine for rapid and accurate evaluation of the trauma patient, which allows full assessment of vital parameters and the institution of rapid life-preserving measures when required. **With all trauma patients the most important step is to determine that there is a patent airway and that the cardiorespiratory system is functional; all other body systems are secondary to this.** It is useful to use charts or plans to ensure that no systems are missed. Figure 3.1 gives general guidelines as to which types of trauma must be dealt with immediately and which may be safely left.

In addition to broad-sweep assessment it is useful to have an organized rapid system for evaluation of the patient. An example of such a system is given in Figure 3.2 (greater detail is to be found in the *BSAVA Manual of Canine and Feline Emergency and Critical Care*).

Level of injury	Must act	Examples
Very severe or life-threatening	Within MINUTES	Cardiac arrest Airway obstruction Respiratory arrest Rapid arterial/venous haemorrhage
Severe	Within FIRST hour	Hypovolaemia Shock Penetrating wounds to thorax or abdomen Loss of consciousness Respiratory distress Spinal trauma Neurological deficits
Serious	Within first few hours	Multiple deep lacerations Blunt trauma Moderate degree of shock Open fractures Septicaemia
Major	Within 24 hours	Fractures Deep puncture wounds

3.1 Triage organization.

A	Airway	P	Pelvis
C	Cardiovascular	L	Limbs
R	Respiratory	A	Arteries
A	Abdomen	N	Nerves
S	Spine		
H	Head		

3.2 A CRASH PLAN.

WARNING
It must be remembered that any injured patient may destabilize rapidly and should be assessed at regular intervals.

In evaluating a patient following trauma, consideration should be given, where appropriate, to radiography of not only the affected part (e.g. pelvis or distal limb) but also of the thorax or abdomen to look for evidence of air or fluid. Fractures of limbs will of necessity require management, and the surgeon must prioritize what needs to be dealt with first. External fixators help considerably in the management of fractures associated with open wounds (see *BSAVA*

Manual of Small Animal Fracture Repair and Management) as they can be applied early on, following presentation, and allow any open wound to be managed appropriately. A full discussion on trauma management is outside the scope of this chapter and readers are referred to the *BSAVA Manual of Canine and Feline Emergency and Critical Care*.

It is inevitable that in some situations, such as a severe wound of a distal extremity, wound management and return to normal function may not be possible; in such situations the veterinary surgeon should consider the possibility of limb amputation or, in some extreme situations, euthanasia. Financial constraints must also be considered, as treatment of traumatic wounds in particular can be very expensive. It is essential not to lose sight of the fact that despite advances in wound care and reconstruction, we must provide the patient with an adequate quality of life.

Pain control and sedation
In the initial period it is important to remember that traumatized patients will be suffering pain and this must be addressed. Analgesic agents include the opioids, non-steroidal anti-inflammatory drugs (NSAIDs) and local anaesthetics (see *BSAVA Manual of Anaesthesia and Analgesia* and the *BSAVA Small Animal Formulary* for details). Opioids, particularly pure µ agonists such as morphine or methadone, are the cornerstone of analgesic regimens in the trauma patient despite their potential side effects of respiratory depression, bradycardia, altered mental state and vomiting. In general, patients in pain are less likely to exhibit these side effects. NSAIDs are valuable as analgesics but must be administered with care in traumatized and hypovolaemic patients due to their potential adverse effects on renal and gastrointestinal function. Local and regional anaesthetic techniques have the advantage of diminished systemic effects, whilst providing total local analgesia. Either lidocaine or bupivacaine (longer acting) can be used. Detailed descriptions of these techniques can be found in many texts including the *BSAVA Manual of Canine and Feline Anaesthesia and Analgesia*.

Fractious patients, in pain, frequently require sedation or general anaesthesia prior to thorough evaluation of the wound. Sedatives can be used alone or in combination with analgesics, either solely to aid in calming and reducing pain in the trauma patient or as a premedicant prior to proposed general anaesthesia. A detailed discussion of sedative and anaesthetic protocols for the traumatized patient is outside the scope of this manual and the reader is referred to the *BSAVA Manual of Canine and Feline Emergency and Critical Care* and the *BSAVA Manual of Canine and Feline Anaesthesia and Analgesia*.

Evaluating the local wound
The likelihood of success in deciding when to close a traumatic wound depends on a number of factors:

- Degree and type of bacterial contamination
- Degree of contamination with foreign material
- Degree of tissue ischaemia
- Time from trauma to presentation

- Type of wound (see Chapter 2)
- Local blood supply
- Amount of local tissue loss.

There are no absolute rules as to the timing of traumatic wound closure, as each wound is different. It is important to remember, however, that contaminated wounds (Figure 3.3) should not be closed primarily and in such situations appropriate open wound management should be used. (See Chapter 4 for further details.)

> **WARNING**
> **Contaminated wounds should never be closed primarily. If the veterinary surgeon has any doubt as to the degree of contamination, it is safer to deal with the wound as an open wound.**

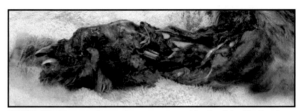

3.3 Contaminated open wound in the hindlimb of a German Shepherd Dog following a collision with a train. (© CSH Sale)

Wound classification
Surgical and traumatic wounds have long been classified according to the system developed by the American College of Surgeons in 1964 (Figure 3.4).

Classification	Criteria
Clean elective	Non-emergency, non-traumatic No acute inflammation Respiratory, gastrointestinal and genitourinary tracts not entered No break in surgical aseptic technique
Clean–contaminated	Urgent or emergency case that is otherwise clean Elective opening of respiratory, gastrointestinal or genitourinary tract with minimal spillage (not encountering infection) Minor break in surgical aseptic technique
Contaminated	Non-purulent inflammation Gross spillage from gastrointestinal tract Entry into genitourinary tract in the presence of infection Major break in surgical aseptic technique Traumatic wound <4 hours old [a] Chronic open wounds
Dirty	Purulent inflammation (e.g. abscess) Preoperative perforation of respiratory, gastrointestinal or genitourinary tract Traumatic wound >4 hours old [a] or with gross foreign material present or with marked evidence of devitalized tissue

3.4 Classification of operative wounds based on degree of microbial contamination. (Adapted from Berard and Gandon, 1964). [a] It should be noted that 4 hours does not constitute the 'golden period' where closure can be achieved after traumatic wounding. The timing of closure depends on a number of key factors that must be considered (see text).

This system allows a straightforward assessment of wound contamination or potential contamination. By this system, most traumatic wounds at the time of presentation will either be *contaminated* or *dirty*. Aggressive wound lavage and debridement (see Chapter 4) will allow conversion of such wounds to a *clean–contaminated* state, which will allow closure. It is this conversion that is key to the success of traumatic wound management. It may occur on the day of presentation, or many days later, depending on the degree of trauma and contamination.

Wound ischaemia/devitalization

Although the accepted wound contamination criteria are valuable, they do not give the full picture in assessing a wound; the veterinary surgeon must also take into account the degree of vascular injury to the site. The type of trauma encountered will influence the degree of damage to the tissues. With high-velocity gunshot wounds (fortunately rare) (Figure 3.5), crush injuries and bite wounds, vascular injury will extend well beyond what can be seen grossly as the margins of the wound. Given this caveat, it may in fact be difficult to assess tissue viability fully at the time of presentation. If there is any doubt about the viability of tissue, it is best to treat it as an open wound initially (see Chapter 4).

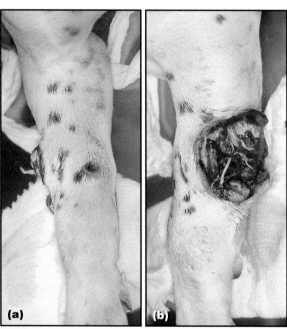

(a) **(b)**

3.5 Firearm wound. A high-velocity ballistic wound involving the forelimb of a dog that was shot by a 0.223 calibre military weapon. **(a)** The entry wound is small, round and regular with little indication of the underlying trauma. **(b)** The size of the exit wound emphasizes the conical shape of the wound caused by the shockwave of the impacting ballistic. The distal two-thirds of the radius and ulna had been removed by the shockwave through the exit wound. (© RAS White)

The veterinary surgeon must also assess damage to deeper tissues and balance the risks of open wound management against those of more immediate closure.

- Open thoracic wounds need to be closed as soon as is practical.
- Open fractures, which are frequently associated with extensive soft tissue loss, may develop osteomyelitis and result in poor bone healing. Ideally, prolonged open wound management is to be avoided. Aggressive lavage and surgical debridement (see Chapter 4) should be carried out, with early reconstruction of the wound using well vascularized tissues, within 72 hours if possible. However this may not always be feasible; the use of an external fixator will help with fracture stabilization and wound management (Figure 3.6).

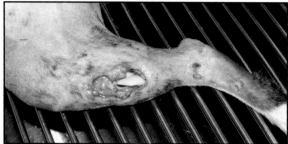
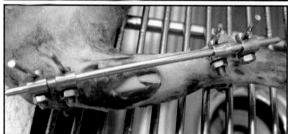

3.6 An open fracture managed by early application of an external fixator and continued open wound management. (© CSH Sale)

The role of systemic antibiotics

> **WARNING**
> **Antibiotics are not a substitute for effective wound lavage and debridement.**

Antibiotics, if used, must be chosen based on clinical judgement and scientific surgical principles; they are NOT a substitute for wound lavage and debridement, and their use is not without controversy. In hospitalized patients it can be argued that since the wound is constantly exposed to bacterial contaminants, the use of systemic antibiotics may lead to the establishment of nosocomial or antibiotic-resistant organisms. In such a scenario antibiotics are best used to manage established or developing wound infection. However, in human trauma cases it is advocated that antibiotic prophylaxis is used in all cases where the wound is classified as *clean–contaminated* or *contaminated,* and that ongoing specific targeted antibiotic therapy should be considered where the wound is classified as *dirty* or where there are early clinical signs consistent with infection (Leaper, 2006).

It must be remembered that intravenous systemic antibiotics only prevent bacterial multiplication for up to 3 hours and that they have their maximal effect at about 1 hour. Any systemic antibiotic should be bactericidal and directed toward the most likely wound contaminants:

- Coagulase-positive staphylococci
- *Escherichia coli*
- *Pasteurella* spp.

Where infection is already established, the choice should be based on the results of bacteriological culture and *in vitro* antibiotic sensitivity testing. The author cultures both tissue and fluid from the deep part of the wound, prior to lavage.

Timing of wound closure

The four options for closing a wound (Figure 3.7)

are:

- Primary closure
- Delayed primary closure (closed after 48–72 hours, before granulation tissue develops)
- Secondary closure (closed after granulation tissue develops, 5–7 days)
- Second intention healing (contraction and epithelialization).

Which option is most appropriate?

The degree of contamination and of tissue viability play a major role in this decision-making process. To be able to close a traumatic wound primarily it must be possible to convert it from a *contaminated* to a *clean–contaminated* wound, and there can be no evidence of tissue necrosis or foreign debris.

It is also important not to manage an open wound for an excessive period. The role of open wound management is to create an environment that will allow wound closure and return to function. There is no merit in dressing a wound for months on end with no clear plan as to how to reconstruct the wound. Such action frequently leads to contracture or formation of exuberant granulation tissue with tissue that is covered by thin friable epithelium (Figure 3.8) and may prove to be more expensive than early surgical reconstruction.

Closure option	Wound classification	Wound management
Primary closure	Clean wound	Immediate closure without tension. May require an appropriate flap or grafting technique
Delayed primary closure	Clean–contaminated or contaminated wounds, or where there is questionable tissue viability or oedema, or skin tension is likely if primary closure is attempted	Lavage and debridement of open wound. Appropriate dressing used. Closure performed 2–3 days after wounding. May require an appropriate flap or grafting technique
Secondary closure	Contaminated or dirty wounds	Lavage and debridement of open wound. Appropriate dressing used. Closure carried out 5–7 days after wounding. May require an appropriate flap or grafting technique
Second intention healing	Wound unsuitable for surgical closure technique: extensive contamination and devitalization. **Do not consider over a joint surface as it may lead to joint contracture**	Lavage and debridement of open wound. Appropriate dressing used. Allowed to heal by granulation, contraction and epithelialization

3.7 Closure options for traumatic wounds.

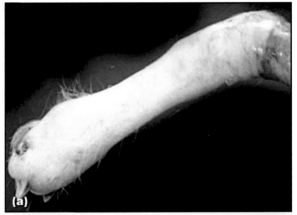

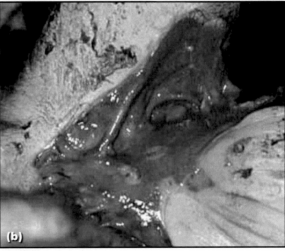

3.8 **(a)** Thin hairless skin of a chronically managed wound on a cat's leg. **(b)** Chronic wound contraction in the inguinal area of a cat.

Early wound reconstruction and closure should be considered:

- If vital tissues are exposed
- Where reconstruction of the tissue is required for structural support, e.g. footpads
- Where wounds are located over the flexor surface of a joint and prolonged open wound management may lead to contracture
- For open wounds over tendons, as scar tissue may form which will prevent the normal gliding action of the tendons
- For orofacial wounds, where the vascular supply is particularly rich and early return to function is often a requirement (e.g. eyelids).

Basic closure techniques

Methods for wound lavage and debridement are described in Chapter 4. Once the decision has been made to close a wound, the surgeon needs to decide on the optimal and simplest method of closing that wound.

Surgical principles

As with all surgery, wound reconstruction relies heavily on the basic tenets which were put forward by Halstead:

- Gentle tissue handling
- Accurate haemostasis
- Preservation of local blood supply
- Aseptic technique
- Close tissues without tension
- Careful approximation of tissues
- Ensure no dead space

These should be closely adhered to. Performing surgery without regard to the surviving tissues will inevitably lead to failure. As with all surgery it is important that tissues do not dry out under hot theatre lights and that correct instrumentation is used.

Instrumentation and tissue handling

Instruments used to handle delicate tissues such as the skin and subcutaneous tissue should cause minimal trauma. Coarse rat-toothed forceps and Allis tissue forceps have no role to play in reconstructive surgery. Skin edges should be handled as little as possible and fine instruments such as skin hooks, Debakey forceps, or fine-toothed Adson forceps or Adson–Brown forceps are least traumatic (see Chapter 4). Alternatively, fine monofilament nylon or polypropylene stay sutures (1.5 or 2 metric; 4/0 or 3/0 USP) can be used.

All incisions should preferably be carried out with a scalpel blade and not scissors, as the latter crushes and tears tissues. When incising the skin it should be done vertically and not at an angle to the surface; this makes for better apposition when closing the wound. Suture material should be fine gauge (1.5 or 2 metric; 4/0 or 3/0 USP) and monofilament with swaged-on reverse cutting or taper point needles. Needle-holders are a matter of personal preference, but should be fine-tipped so as not to damage the needle and should lock to allow accurate placement, for example Debakey or Mayo pattern.

Tissues must be handled gently to prevent further vascular injury and an increased inflammatory response. Control of haemorrhage reduces the risk of systemic complications secondary to hypovolaemia, reduces the risk of postoperative infection, and diminishes the incidence of haematoma and seroma formation. Accurate identification of tissue layers and precise apposition of tissues reduces the incidence of dehiscence, and improves the quality and cosmetic result of the reconstruction. All wound edges, following surgical debridement, should be incised vertically, to allow true apposition with minimal scar formation. Dead space is common following wound reconstruction, and should be managed by suture apposition of deep tissue layers (Figure 3.9) or through the use of passive or active drains (see Chapter 5).

Choice of technique

When deciding which reconstructive closure technique to use, the aim is to obtain rapid wound closure with the simplest technique possible and with minimal compromise of function, patient morbidity and cost. This is a very well established principle in human surgery, where plastic surgeons refer to the 'reconstructive ladder'. The more extensive or difficult a wound is, the higher up the ladder the surgeon has to climb to find an appropriate technique. Such a ladder is readily adapted to veterinary use (Figure 3.10) and helps in the decision-making process, though individual surgeons may have personal preferences that will sway them more towards one technique than another.

> **WARNING**
> **The surgeon must always remember that although wound reconstruction is often an exciting surgical challenge, the technique chosen should be for the benefit of the patient and not the surgeon.**

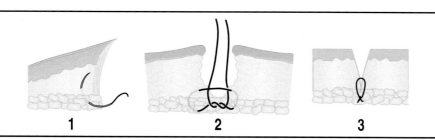

3.9 Suture apposition of deep tissue layers using buried absorbable suture material. Note that the knot is placed deep in the tissue.

1   2   3

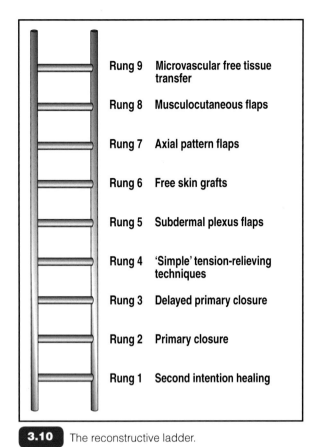

3.10   The reconstructive ladder.

Rung 9	Microvascular free tissue transfer
Rung 8	Musculocutaneous flaps
Rung 7	Axial pattern flaps
Rung 6	Free skin grafts
Rung 5	Subdermal plexus flaps
Rung 4	'Simple' tension-relieving techniques
Rung 3	Delayed primary closure
Rung 2	Primary closure
Rung 1	Second intention healing

Primary closure

The cardinal rule of wound reconstruction is to avoid excessive wound tension. Wounds with an adequate amount of elastic surrounding skin can be closed using direct skin mobilization. Appositional suturing techniques should be used to minimize tension on the wound.

Suturing

Suturing all surgical wounds should be done accurately and atraumatically using fine suture materials and this is especially true for skin. Inaccurate suture placement will lead to a ragged wound edge and a poor looking scar. All needles should be swaged on, and suture gauge range from 3 metric (2/0 USP) for the largest dogs to 1.5 metric (4/0 USP). Absorbable monofilament suture material, such as polydioxanone or polyglyconate, is used in subcuticular tissues; whereas non-absorbable monofilament suture material, such as monofilament nylon or poly-propylene, is used in the skin.

Some tension on a wound can be reduced by the use of subcutaneous or intradermal continuous sutures. Monofilament absorbable suture material should be used, so that there is minimal tissue drag. Such a suture should always be placed when skin staples (see below) are used. The start knot should be buried. The suture material is passed through the tissue parallel to the wound surface. The end knot is best tied as an Aberdeen (chain stitch) knot (Figure 3.11); this is known to be as secure as a square knot at the end of a continuous suture but produces a smaller knot (Richey and Roe, 2005).

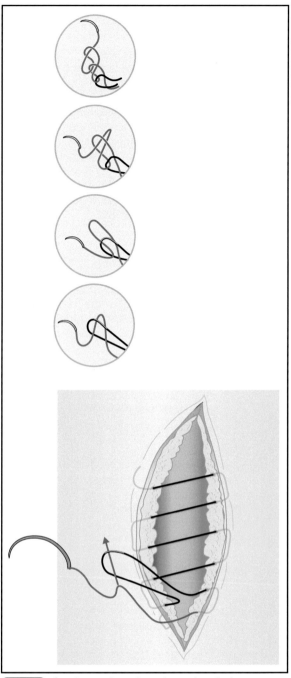

3.11   Continuous intradermal or subcuticular suture, showing an Aberdeen knot.

Correct placement of skin sutures is important so that optimal healing will occur: they should be placed some 3–5 mm from wound edges and spaced at intervals of about 5 mm (Figure 3.12) so that tension is spread evenly and there is minimal interference with local blood supply. In practice the spacing between sutures will vary with the length of wound and gauge of suture used. It is also useful to take a wider bite at the deep part of the wound; this helps to slightly evert the wound edges, which helps to create a flatter scar when the sutures are removed (Figure 3.13). The bite taken is important in creating accurate apposition; the suture can be adjusted to even out slight discrepancies in the wound edge apposition (Figure 3.14).

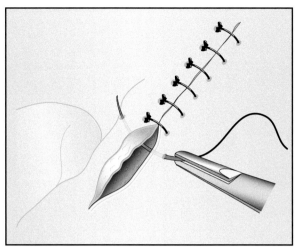

3.12 Simple interrupted sutures, placed 3–5 mm from wound edges and spaced at intervals of about 5 mm.

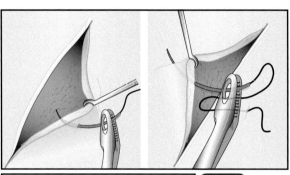

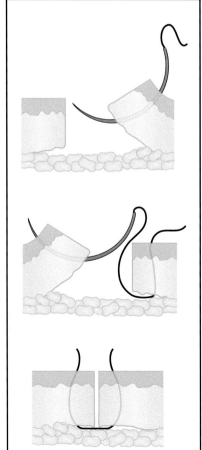

3.13 Creating slight eversion of the wound edge by a combination of instrument (skin hook (illustrated above) or fine thumb forceps) and ensuring a wider bite at the deeper part of the wound. Note the curved path taken by the needle on passing through the wound edges.

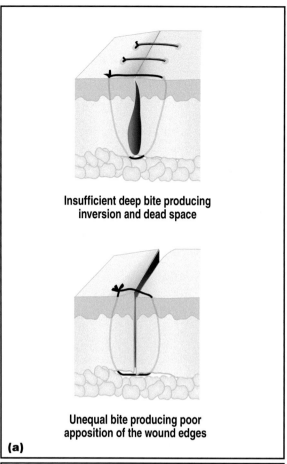

Insufficient deep bite producing inversion and dead space

Unequal bite producing poor apposition of the wound edges

(a)

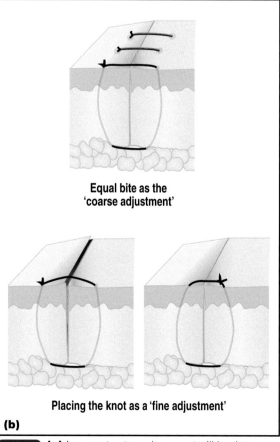

Equal bite as the 'coarse adjustment'

Placing the knot as a 'fine adjustment'

(b)

3.14 **(a)** Incorrect suture placement will lead to poorer wound healing. **(b)** Adjustment of the suture allows more accurate wound apposition.

Sutures should not be tied too tightly as, in addition to causing discomfort, this will disrupt local blood supply and lead to delayed healing. Skin sutures should allow for slight oedema of the skin, which will occur during healing. If a suture loop is tight initially then the suture will cut into the skin as wound oedema occurs, causing irritation and compromising the local circulation.

For long wounds the use of a simple continuous or a Ford interlocking suture pattern (Figure 3.15) can be considered; these help to spread tension evenly across the wound and reduce the risk of tying many individual knots too loosely. When continuous patterns are used it is essential that the knots at either end are tied securely with an adequate number of throws. For all continuous suture patterns it is necessary to add extra throws for security.

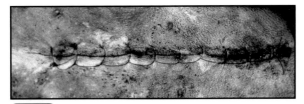

3.15 Ford interlocking (continuous) suture pattern.

Where there is slight tension at a wound edge it can be relieved by the use of subcuticular absorbable suture patterns (see below) or by judicious interspersing with tension-relieving suture patterns (Figures 3.16, 3.17 and 3.18). Care must be taken when using tension-relieving sutures, as it is all too easy to overtighten these, especially mattress sutures, which can lead to large areas of skin becoming devitalized.

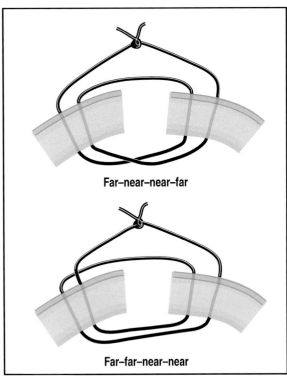

Far–near–near–far

Far–far–near–near

3.16 Tension-relieving sutures.

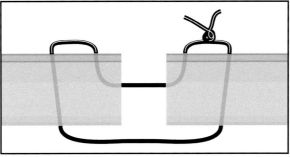

3.17 Vertical mattress suture. These are placed at a distance from the wound margin so there is less tendency to reduce circulation. They are generally used in combination with simple interrupted sutures.

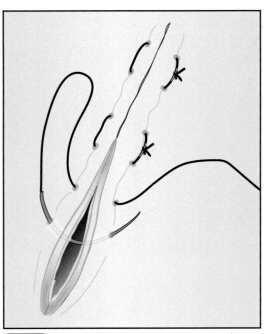

3.18 Horizontal mattress suture pattern. If not placed correctly, this will lead to marked eversion of the wound edges and damage to the local blood supply.

> **WARNING**
> **Tension-relieving sutures should not be used when there is moderate to severe skin tension; in such cases other reconstructive techniques are more appropriate.**

When suturing any wound where a flap has been created or the shape of the wound is irregular, 'corners' often occur that need special attention in technique. To prevent either necrosis of the point of the corner or an unsightly bunching of the skin, a 'three-point' suture can be used (Figure 3.19). This is essentially a modification of horizontal mattress sutures, with part of the suture buried in the flap corner. The key points to making this suture successful are:

- The suture material must leave and enter the knot end of the wound at the same level at which it is placed in the flap corner
- The suture material should emerge so that the knot is placed some distance from the wound edge.

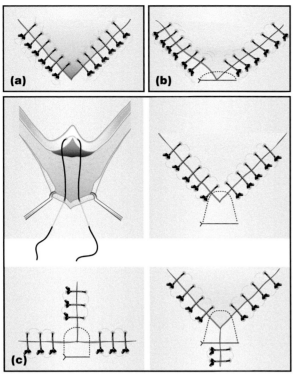

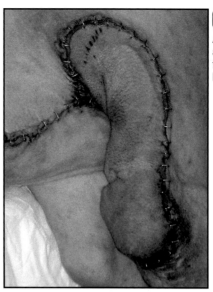

3.21 A stapled axillary fold flap. (© Alison L. Moores)

3.19 Suturing corners. **(a)** Flap tip necrosis due to suture strangulation. **(b)** Bunching of the flap tip from incorrect suture placement. **(c)** The three-point suture technique. The dotted lines show the intradermal portion of the suture.

Skin staples

Skin staples are a fast and cost-efficient way of closing wounds and have a particular appeal for primary closure of wounds in the trauma patient or for large wound reconstructions. As with all wounds, it is important to remember the principles of wound management before reaching for the staple gun. As noted above, wound edges are best apposed with intradermal or subcuticular sutures before applying the staples. Staples are relatively atraumatic and, when placed accurately, provide a good cosmetic closure of the wound (Figures 3.20 and 3.21). Staples are best removed using a staple remover (Figure 3.22), although if one is unavailable the points can be spread apart using a pair of Mosquito forceps.

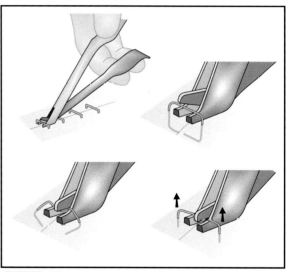

3.22 The staple remover bends staples in the middle to release them from the skin.

Tissue glue

Tissue glues would appear to provide another simple and rapid method for wound closure, though for any long wounds it is advisable to place intradermal or subcuticular sutures as well. *N*-Butyl-2-cyanoacrylate was developed in the 1970s, producing negligible tissue toxicity with good bonding strength and good cosmetic results. 2-Octylcyanoacrylate is the latest development in cyanoacrylate technology and has lower toxicity and almost four times the strength of *N*-butyl-2-cyanoacrylate. It reaches maximum bonding strength within 2½ minutes and is equivalent in strength to healed tissue at 7 days post repair. Tissue glues must be used with great care in traumatic wounds as their use has been associated with increased tissue toxicity, granuloma formation, ongoing wound infections and delayed healing if the wound edges are separated. There is also very poor adhesion on excessively moist surfaces.

Delayed primary closure

Wound contraction is seen in healing open wounds in 5–9 days and results in a centripetal reduction in the

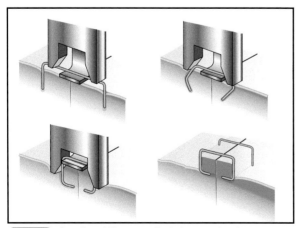

3.20 Stapling. When applied, the staple closes to evert the wound edges slightly and also allows some space for drainage of wound oedema.

size of the wound. The process of wound contraction stops when the wound margins contact each other or when tension from the skin adjacent to the wound is equal to, or greater than, the contractile forces generated by myofibroblasts within the granulation tissue (see Chapter 1). In dogs and cats, wound contraction is more rapid on the trunk than the extremities because of the larger amount of skin available and its inherent elasticity. By definition, delayed primary closure is performed *prior to* the appearance of granulation tissue within the wound.

It is essential that when delayed primary closure, secondary closure or second intention healing is chosen, the wound undergoes adequate debridement and open wound management, since wound contraction is facilitated by:

- A moist wound bed
- Adequate debridement
- Control of wound infection.

Inadequate debridement is the most common reason for delayed wound healing and persistent wound infection. Wound contraction is delayed by:

- Wound infection
- Desiccation
- Exposed bone
- Exuberant granulation tissue.

The normal process of wound contraction can be facilitated by:

- Presuturing lesions prior to excision
- Placement of tension sutures
- Using skin-stretching devices across open wounds.

Closure of large trunk wounds, or smaller wounds of the extremities, may be difficult without excessive tension. The elastic properties of skin can be used to advantage in these situations. Presuturing of wounds (Figure 3.23), through the placement of several mattress sutures adjacent to the area of excision, can be used to mobilize skin for subsequent wound reconstruction in planned excisions. In traumatic wounds, intradermal tension sutures can be placed along the wound edges. The continuous intradermal suture is tightened on a daily basis, facilitating contraction of the wound margins. This process of 'enhanced contraction' will greatly reduce the length of time required to achieve closure of large cutaneous deficits. Alternatively an external skin-stretching device can be used (Pavletic, 2000). Such techniques have little advantage if a local flap can be used, and may lead to longer and more expensive treatment.

Secondary closure

This is done following open wound treatment that extends beyond 5 days, allowing complete debridement and management of an infected wound before closure. By definition, secondary closure is performed *after* the appearance of granulation tissue in the wound.

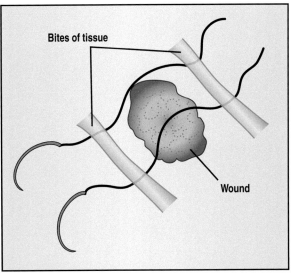

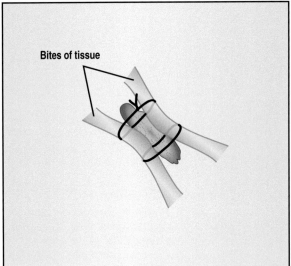

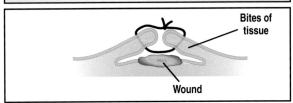

3.23 Presuturing a wound by placement of mattress sutures.

Second intention healing

This is defined as wound healing by granulation, contraction and re-epithelialization. Second intention healing is generally reserved for wounds located in areas with abundant surrounding skin, or for smaller wounds located on the extremities.

Reconstructive techniques

If simple tension-relieving techniques do not result in closure, or appear to place undue tension on the wound, more advanced reconstructive techniques, such as subdermal plexus flaps, axial pattern skin flaps or free skin grafts, should be considered. Once debridement and preparation are complete, surgical reconstruction can be planned. Reconstructive techniques should be used to achieve early coverage of vital structures, promoting an early return to function. The various reconstructive techniques are discussed in greater depth in later chapters.

Axial pattern skin flaps

Axial pattern flap circulation depends on preserving a direct cutaneous artery to the area of skin in question. The flap will survive based only on the vascular attachment. These flaps can be created to be longer than subdermal plexus flaps; therefore, their range of use and their ability to manage large defects, particularly of the extremities, by immediate closure is a great advantage. In addition, axial pattern flaps provide full-thickness skin and can be combined in some regions with muscle, resulting in musculocutaneous composite flaps. The major disadvantage of axial pattern flaps is that flap designs are restricted to the sites with a well defined and robust direct cutaneous artery. (See Chapter 7 for further details.)

Skin grafts

Free skin grafts in dogs and cats are usually of full thickness. They may be applied immediately to clean wound beds with a good blood supply, such as regions of the face or on muscular surfaces, or on to mature granulation tissue. Variations of free skin grafts include sieve, punch, meshed and strip grafts. (See Chapter 8 for more details.)

Pedicled muscle flaps

These flaps are used to provide vascularized soft tissue coverage of vital structures and for padding of bony prominences such as the elbow. For example, cranial sartorius muscle flaps can be used to close caudal abdominal wall defects or to cover exposed bone after disarticulated pelvic limb amputations. Musculocutaneous flaps supplied by the thoracodorsal artery and vein, including cutaneous trunci muscle and a portion of the latissimus dorsi muscle, can be used to cover defects involving the elbow in dogs or cats. Pedicled muscle flaps are also useful for covering exposed bone or joints after traumatic exposure with skin loss (see Chapter 9).

Microvascular free tissue transfer

Free flap transfer using microvascular anastomosis to restore circulation after temporary interruption of blood supply provides a technically difficult but very useful method of covering difficult architectural defects by primary repair. Cutaneous, musculocutaneous and muscle flaps can be harvested from distant sites, moved directly to recipient areas, and sutured in place after vascular anastomosis. (See Chapter 10 for more details.)

Orthopaedic injuries

Joint trauma

Any injuries associated with joint trauma must be debrided carefully, with debris, clots and cartilage fragments removed, and the joint must be lavaged thoroughly. Large fragments that have soft tissue attachments can be rigidly stabilized and, where possible, the surrounding ligaments and joint capsule sutured using monofilament absorbable suture material. The joint should be covered by well vascularized soft tissue, if possible, and stabilized. Stabilization may be accomplished using external coaptation (e.g. a half cast that can be changed daily) or preferably by use of an external fixator. Stabilization is especially important if the joint surface cannot be covered with vascularized tissue.

Fractures

Wounds associated with orthopaedic injury are sufficiently painful that stabilization of the injury by internal or external fixation is essential to decrease discomfort. Clearly the surgeon must prioritize what needs to be dealt with first – the fracture or the wound. The use of external fixators can help in this decision-making, as placing of such apparatus will allow further wound management. As stated above, coverage of open fractures with well vascularized tissue will frequently facilitate fracture repair.

Basic principles of reconstructive oncological surgery

Many major advances in reconstructive surgery have been in response to the development of aggressive veterinary oncological surgery. A greater understanding of the biology of tumours, in particular the sarcomas, has moved the surgeon away from simple 'lumpectomies' to radical excisions. Such deficits have meant that the surgeon must not only plan to excise a tumour with adequate margins but also plan how to close the resultant wound.

In evaluating a patient with a solid tumour it is necessary to stage the patient according to the TNM classification system:

- T – primary tumour
- N – regional lymph nodes
- M – distant metastasis.

Such staging allows the veterinary surgeon to know the full extent and type of the primary tumour, together with knowledge as to whether it has spread within the patient; such information is essential to allow a prognosis to be given. This gives the surgeon and the client the maximum amount of information possible in order that an informed judgement can be made on management.

The minimum database available for an oncological case should be:

- Histology of the primary tumour
- Size and full extent of the primary tumour
- Evaluation of local draining lymph nodes for metastatic spread
- Radiographic evaluation of the thorax for evidence of metastasis
- With certain tumour types it may be valuable to assess other organs and body systems with radiography, ultrasonography, MRI or CT scans.

For further details on tumour staging, the reader is referred to the *BSAVA Manual of Canine and Feline Oncology*.

Careful planning is the cornerstone of successful oncological surgery, with appropriate biopsy samples taken that do not interfere with the eventual surgical procedure. The surgeon should also work closely with medical oncologists so that appropriate multimodal treatment can be instituted where required. This may include pre- or postoperative chemotherapy and/or radiotherapy. If such management is planned, it is essential that the timing of surgery is such that adjunctive therapy should have a minimal effect on wound healing. Planning combination therapy will also help decide whether the surgeon is attempting complete (radical excision) or cytoreductive surgery prior to reconstruction of the wound. Cytoreductive surgery should not be attempted unless there is follow-up therapy to control the remaining tumour deposits or the client is fully aware that surgery is purely palliative.

Planning management and reconstruction

Successful reconstruction of any wound relies on careful planning using the 'reconstructive ladder' (see above). It is probably best if the surgeon has more than one plan in mind. One of the leading human plastic and reconstructive surgeons of the twentieth century, Sir Harold Gillies, was quoted as saying 'never do today what can best be done tomorrow'. It is not infrequent to find that the initial plan may not work, due to poor local or distant blood supply or, in the case of oncological surgery, because the original excision is larger than anticipated. The most successful reconstructions tend to be those where the surgeon has more than one plan in mind at the outset and is able to alter his/her strategy as required.

An overview of planning wound reconstruction is given in Figure 3.24.

References and further reading

Berard F and Gandon J (1964) Postoperative wound infections: the influence of ultraviolet irradiation of the operating room and of various other factors. *Annals of Surgery* **160** (Suppl. 1), 1–192

Leaper DJ (2006) Traumatic and surgical wounds. *British Medical Journal* **332**, 532–535

McGregor AD and McGregor I (2000) *Fundamental Techniques of Plastic Surgery and their Surgical Applications, 10th edition.* Churchill Livingstone, Edinburgh

Pavletic MM (1999) *Atlas of Small Animal Reconstructive Surgery, 2nd edition.* WB Saunders, Philadelphia

Pavletic MM (2000) Use of an external skin-stretching device for wound closure in dogs and cats. *Journal of the American Veterinary Medical Association* **217**, 350–354

Richey ML and Roe SC (2005) Assessment of knot security in continuous intradermal wound closures. *Journal of Surgical Research* **123**, 284–288

Trout N J (2003) Principles of plastic and reconstructive surgery. In: *Textbook of Small Animal Surgery, 3rd edition*, ed. D Slatter, pp.274–292. WB Saunders, Philadelphia

Websites

Plastic and Reconstructive Surgery Essentials for Students: http://www.plasticsurgery.org/medical_professionals/publications/Plastic-and-Reconstructive-Surgery-Essentials-for-Students.cfm

- Note wound size and location
- Identify vital local structures, e.g. blood vessels and nerves
- Assess where loose skin is available for reconstruction
    - Skin may not be available on one or more sides of the wound: adjacent to openings such as the anus; in areas where skin is tightly adherent to underlying muscle such as the proximal thigh; or where use of tissue will distort adjacent structures such as the eyelids, prepuce or anus
- Confirm that the donor site can be closed or, if it cannot, that healing by second intention is a viable option
- Choose the simplest effective technique available (see Figure 3.10)
- Have several options available for wound closure in case the chosen technique will not close the wound or more than one reconstruction technique needs to be used
- Use a surgical marking pen to outline any flaps to be used
- Ensure that, whatever techniques are considered, hair is clipped from a wide area: this may involve clipping the whole flank and going beyond the midline both ventrally and dorsally
- Once in the operating theatre, patients should be positioned in such a way as to maximize the amount of free skin available to the surgeon.

3.24 Overview of planning wound reconstruction.

4

Management of open wounds

Davina Anderson

Introduction

Open wound management in small animals is a common event in veterinary practice. It is economically significant and can cause considerable distress and pain to the animal. The aim of wound management is to provide conditions that allow for optimal wound healing or to prepare the wound for definitive closure by reconstructive techniques. However, every wound is unique and this problem is reflected in the paucity of published studies analysing the effectiveness of wound dressing products in the management of small animal wounds. Wounds must be properly evaluated at the first presentation (see Chapter 3) in order to plan a treatment protocol and to give the owner an indication of the expected duration of treatment and ultimately the prognosis. This chapter considers how to manage open wounds and how to use dressings and bandages to optimize the healing process.

Principles of wound management

- **Control and identify infection**
- **Manage contamination and necrosis**
- **Contain ongoing deterioration**
- **Prevent further damage**

These four principles are used to determine what is required to manage the wound. In the early stages, control of infection (including lavage) and debridement are the most important goals. As the wound starts to granulate, the priority is to prevent damage to the wound surface, including prevention of desiccation.

> **PRACTICAL TIP**
> Be prepared to anaesthetize the animal for wound inspection and management. A light short general anaesthetic is safer than deep sedation and recovery will be better.

Wound lavage

Wound lavage is the single most important aspect of open wound management. Lavage can be used to:

- Rehydrate necrotic tissue
- Reduce bacterial contamination or foreign material

- Remove toxins, cytokines, debris and bacteria associated with infected wounds.

Lavage also helps remove remnants of wound dressings. It should be carried out at *every* dressing change and not just when the wound is first presented in the clinic. Fluid used for lavage should be isotonic and non-toxic to the cells. The key principle is to use *large volumes* so that the bacteria and contaminants are at the very least *diluted,* even if they are not completely removed.

Solutions

Historically, lavage solutions have included antiseptic solutions and reducing agents (hydrogen peroxide, chlorhexidine, povidone–iodine) but there is no evidence that these solutions are better than an adequate volume of isotonic fluid and, in fact, they may be more harmful. It is unlikely that the antiseptic agents are in contact with the bacteria for long enough to contribute to control of infection in the wound. Tap water has been used to lavage wounds; although this is probably better than concentrated antiseptic solutions, it is hypotonic and usually too alkaline for body tissues.

Isotonic fluids are considered the best choice, as they are non-toxic and do not cause cell rupture or electrolyte imbalance. They may also be better if they have buffering ability, so there is some evidence that lactated Ringer's (Hartmann's) solution may be better than 0.9% saline. TrisEDTA is an isotonic solution that has been used for wound lavage, and there is some evidence that it may have useful antibacterial effects by enlarging pore size in antibiotic-resistant Gram-negative bacteria, thereby increasing bacterial kill rates. There may be some advantages in using this for topical wound application but there is no evidence that it is of specific use for lavage (when most of the fluid is allowed to wash off).

Technique

Large volume is the key. A giving set attached to a bag of sterile fluids allows constant and rapid delivery of fluids on to a wound (Figure 4.1).

> **PRACTICAL TIP**
> Be prepared for large volumes of fluid – large wounds may need 3 litre fluid bags.

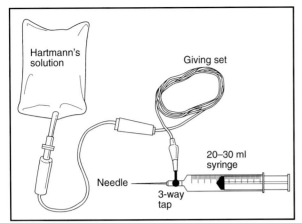

4.1 Wound lavage is best carried out using sterile isotonic fluids. A bag of intravenous fluids is attached to a three-way tap via the giving line. The fluids are drawn into a 20 ml syringe and the wound is lavaged with an 18 gauge needle. The fluids should not be re-used for another case; it is important to keep all items used for wound management dedicated to one case only.

The pressure at which fluid should be delivered on to a wound is controversial: high pressures dislodge surface particles but may drive some bacteria into deeper tissue planes; low pressures may not be sufficient to move material out of the wound. Suggested lavage fluid pressures are 6–8 psi, which is probably about the pressure delivered by a 20–30 ml syringe with an 18 gauge needle (Figure 4.2). The appropriate force is created by pushing gently but firmly on the plunger and creating a steady stream of fluid. Lavage should be a gentle non-painful process and sedation is not necessary.

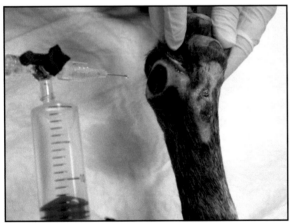

4.2 Wound lavage carried out with a 20 ml syringe and hypodermic needle. The spray is at an appropriate pressure to dislodge debris and necrotic material without driving them further into the tissues.

PRACTICAL TIP
Closely inspect the loose areolar tissue in a wound during lavage. Too high a pressure will force bubbles of fluid into the areolar tissue and these will be evident early on.

Wound lavage should be considered an essential part of assessing a wound, as well as part of its treatment. During wound lavage, the practitioner can see how much exudate or necrotic material is removed and how much the wound improves as it is cleaned. All wounds should be lavaged at every assessment and inspection, as it is impossible to make a decision until the wound has been thoroughly cleaned.

Wound debridement

Following copious lavage, the wound is reinspected for remaining debris, contamination or necrotic tissue. The next step is to remove this material, the aim being to minimize infection and promote healing. Debridement may be achieved globally throughout a wound or locally in specific areas and the technique used will dictate to some extent how much of the non-viable tissue is removed and how much of the healthy tissue is accidentally damaged. With a heavily contaminated wound it may be necessary to carry out repeated lavage and debridement over several days. The wound should be managed as an open wound in between these repeated surgical procedures.

Surgical debridement
This is the gold standard: sharp dissection is used to meticulously remove all the contaminated, necrotic or devitalized tissue seen in a wound, whilst identifying and preserving normal tissue and essential structures. Strict aseptic technique should be employed.

Patient preparation
In many instances general anaesthesia should be used to allow for proper preparation of the patient and a thorough evaluation of the wound. A wide area should be clipped around the wound with a No. 40 clipper blade; the wound can be packed with sterile aqueous jelly or saline-soaked swabs (Figure 4.3) to prevent clipped hair from contaminating the wound. The jelly is rinsed off with sterile water or wiped out using sterile surgical swabs (sponges) after clipping. Normal dilutions of antiseptic agents should be used to prepare the adjacent skin, but skin preparations containing alcohol should be avoided. Similarly, detergent-based antiseptic solutions should not be

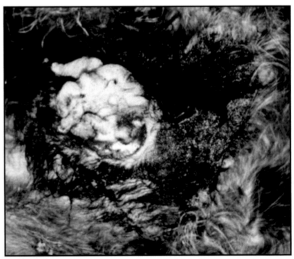

4.3 Wound packed with sterile saline-soaked swabs (sponges).

used, as they may delay the healing process. Detergents should never be used in conjunction with povidone–iodine as they may combine to form surfactants that damage tissue and enhance infection. The value of povidone–iodine as an antiseptic solution in traumatic wounds is extremely limited, as it is deactivated by soil particles. Antiseptic preparations are not applied to the open wound.

PRACTICAL TIP
Lavage should be carried out *after* clipping of the hair but *before* skin preparation.

Instrumentation

Surgical debridement is a procedure for which fine instruments should be used. Ideally, a surgical kit for debridement should include at least sharp Metzenbaum scissors (straight and curved on flat), Adson toothed thumb forceps, Adson–Brown thumb forceps, Debakey thumb forceps, skin hooks and a number 4 scalpel handle with No.11 and No.15 blades (Figure 4.4). It is also beneficial to have sterile saline or lactated Ringer's solution available for further lavage of the wound during the debridement process. A good light source is essential so that any debris and potentially ischaemic tissue can be seen; magnifying loupes can also be useful.

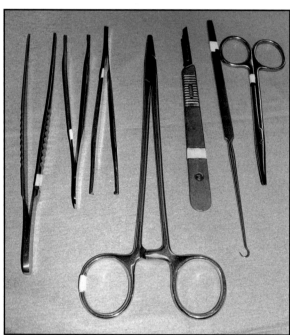

4.4 Surgical instrumentation suitable for wound debridement. Left to right: Debakey thumb forceps; Adson–Brown thumb forceps; fine-toothed Adson thumb forceps; Debakey needle-holder; scalpel handle with No.15 blade; skin hook; short Metzenbaum scissors. (Courtesy of L Hopley)

Layered debridement

Layered debridement is the commonest technique and is best carried out with a scalpel blade, which can be used to cut away tiny pieces of contaminated or necrotic material. It begins by excising devitalized tissue and removing any debris at the surface of the

wound, before progressing to the deeper tissues (Figure 4.5). Tissue is cut back to clean surfaces or to viable tissue. If in doubt about the vitality of an area of tissue, it should be excised. Although the presence of haemorrhage (Figure 4.6) can be used as an indicator of viable tissue, lack of haemorrhage should not be used as the only parameter to assess tissue viability, as it may be temporarily absent from tissues due to vasospasm or hypotension. Furthermore, necrosis can occur later on in tissue that is actively bleeding.

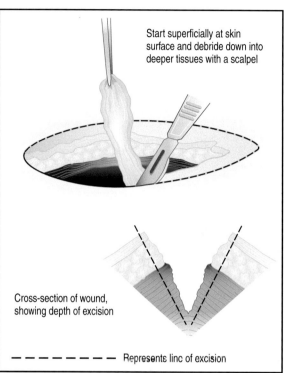

Start superficially at skin surface and debride down into deeper tissues with a scalpel

Cross-section of wound, showing depth of excision

— — — — — — Represents line of excision

4.5 Layered debridement is used to remove contaminated or necrotic material in a wound, gradually in layers, until clean tissue is reached. Instruments and gloves should be changed after each layer so as to convert the contaminated wound into a clean wound as far as possible.

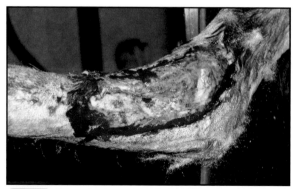

4.6 Wound edges debrided until haemorrhage occurs.

Caution may be necessary in areas where there is huge tissue loss or where reconstruction will be difficult (e.g. the distal limb). Keeping as much tissue as possible is of vital importance for large deficits where skin, subcutaneous tissue and muscle should be preserved in order to allow closure. In these cases, debridement should be conservative and the wound re-inspected after open management for 1–2 days. Tissue that is clearly non-viable should be removed at the earliest opportunity, as it is likely to increase the risk of further skin loss due to thrombosis of vessels. If open management is not an option, e.g. closure of a large wound that is communicating with the thoracic cavity, debridement is less cautious.

The contaminated material removed is kept separate from the rest of the instruments on the surgical trolley and once the debridement procedure is complete the surgeon should change gloves and start closure with clean drapes and instruments.

En-bloc debridement

En-bloc debridement is the complete wide local excision of a contaminated wound followed by primary closure of the resultant clean deficit. It is occasionally used as a technique to convert a dirty wound into one suitable for primary closure. The technique is rarely used in veterinary patients except where there is sufficient skin available for reconstruction (e.g. trunk,

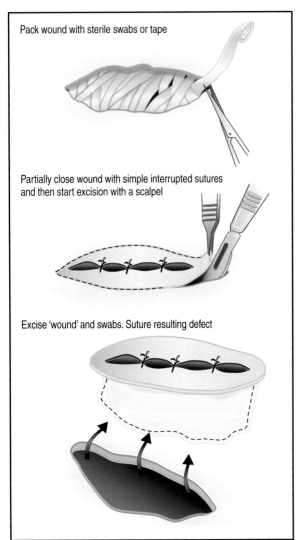

Pack wound with sterile swabs or tape

Partially close wound with simple interrupted sutures and then start excision with a scalpel

Excise 'wound' and swabs. Suture resulting defect

4.7 *En-bloc* debridement involves closing a contaminated wound so as to seal the dirty surface off from the surgical procedure. The wound is then removed in one piece, leaving only sterile tissue exposed for primary closure.

proximal limbs). The major advantage of this technique is that it allows for primary wound closure and therefore may reduce time and cost in management of an open wound. It must be remembered, however, that if it is used inappropriately or performed badly it may lead to wound infection – and increased time and cost!

The wound is packed with sterile swabs and sutured closed, and the area is then clipped and prepared for surgery. The whole wound is then removed *en bloc* (rather like a tumour) and the defect reconstructed as a completely sterile procedure (Figure 4.7).

Non-surgical debridement

Non-surgical debridement is the procedure used regularly throughout the early period of management of a wound through the use of dressings and bandaging. It is useful for removing contamination that cannot effectively be removed using lavage or surgical debridement, or in cases where surgical debridement is not immediately possible. Adherent dressings are very effective at debriding but are non-specific, so delicate structures or healing areas of the wound will be damaged indiscriminately. More modern dressings may be used to debride areas of the wound actively whilst protecting the environment of the healing parts. Hydrogels are used to rehydrate necrotic tissue while absorbing and trapping exudate, loose necrotic cellular material and inflammatory mediators and cytotoxins. Hydrocolloids also have some debriding activity, as do honey and sugar as topical agents (see later).

Systemic treatments

Antibiotics

At the time of presentation, most wounds are contaminated or infected, and the use of systemic broad-spectrum antibiotics should be considered. Contamination of the traumatized tissue can be treated with antibiotics to reduce bacterial numbers, but systemic antibiotics cannot prevent or treat infection as effectively as adequate lavage and debridement, particularly where the wound is contaminated or infected with multiple-drug-resistant bacteria.

> **WARNING**
> **Antibiotic use alone, without effective lavage and debridement, is inadequate for the treatment of open wounds.**

Ideally, an antibiotic is chosen based on the results of culture and sensitivity testing. However, these are not often available at presentation and the choice has to be based on the most likely contaminants (coagulase-positive staphylococci or *Escherichia coli*). A Gram stain of a direct smear from the wound can give an indication of the likely bacteria and provide objective data on which to base antibiotic choice pending culture results. Broad-spectrum antibiotics such as clavulanic acid-potentiated amoxicillin, second-generation cephalosporins or fluoroquinolones are not unreasonable choices; the veterinary surgeon should choose a preferred antibiotic that is a regular

Management of open wounds

first-line choice and use it judiciously. When a wound is adequately debrided and lavaged, continued antibiotic therapy beyond 24 hours after presentation is rarely justified unless there is still contaminated or necrotic tissue left *in situ*, devitalized tissue or deep penetrating wounds. Continued use of antibiotics when the wound is granulating, or change of antibiotic without objective data to support the decision, may predispose to nosocomial infections with multiple-drug-resistant organisms such as pseudomonads, *Klebsiella* and methicillin-resistant staphylococci (see Chapter 3).

Chronic wounds should have samples cultured and the sensitivity pattern of isolates determined before antibiotic treatment is started. Tissue from the deep part of the wound will be more reliable for culture than fluid or surface swab samples.

Analgesics

> **PRACTICAL TIP**
> **The most important systemic treatment for the ongoing care of a wound is adequate analgesia.**

Wounds are painful. If an animal is in pain, it is more likely to interfere with the wound and actively remove dressings or to be restless and overactive, dislodging dressings. Adequate opiate analgesia should always be used at dressing changes, and the animal should be given non-steroidal anti-inflammatory drugs for daily analgesia. Local anaesthetic gels may help during inspection of a wound. When animals are sedated for dressing changes using alpha-agonists, it must be remembered that reversal of the sedation will also reverse the analgesia, so another analgesic will need to be given at the same time. Animals with very painful injuries may be given 'at home' supplements for analgesia, using codeine or oral buprenorphine or morphine preparations.

Bandages and dressings

Bandages are used in open wound management in order to provide an optimal environment for granulation, contraction and epithelialization. Bandages may fulfil a number of functions (Figure 4.8). Correctly applied, they can be used to enhance wound healing by delivering topical products, absorbing exudate or debriding the wound.

Protect the wound from contamination by the environment
Prevent interference from the patient
Prevent further tissue damage from desiccation
Provide a moist environment for optimal wound healing
Provide warmth (faster rate of healing)
Provide pain relief
Immobilize skin edges
Provide pressure to close dead space or reduce swelling or haemorrhage
Deliver topical agents to control wound healing
Absorb exudate
Debride wounds using specific products
Stabilize concurrent orthopaedic injuries

4.8 Functions of a bandage.

Bandages are classically constructed in three layers:

* The *primary layer* is the material applied directly to the wound itself
* The *secondary layer* is often absorbent; it essentially holds the primary layer in place and applies light pressure to provide structure to the bandage
* The *tertiary layer* is the outer layer and usually protects the secondary layer from the patient, environment and trauma as the animal moves around.

Traditionally, wounds have been dressed with antiseptics, antibiotics or products to 'dry the wound'. However, it has been known since 1952 that moist wounds heal much more quickly and there is no rationale for exposure and desiccation of wound surfaces. Wound dressings and medications should, above all else, 'do no harm'. Thus, they should fulfil certain basic criteria such as being non-toxic and non-irritant (Figure 4.9).

Non-toxic
Non-irritant
Non-allergenic
Absorbent
Sterile
Cost-effective
Allow gaseous exchange (oxygen, carbon dioxide)
Vapour-permeable
Provide thermal insulation
Maintain a moist environment
Promote wound healing

4.9 Ideal characteristics of dressings.

The dressings and topical products described in this chapter merely 'scratch the surface' of the variety of dressings available on the human market. There are whole ranges of products designed to treat specific injuries and wounds in people that are not discussed here (see Further reading for more information). Dressings that have been approved for use as medical devices in the human field are available for use in veterinary practice, without special licence. However, those dressings that are classified as pharmaceuticals can only be used at the clinical discretion of the veterinary surgeon under the 'cascade' system.

Topical medications

These are products that are put into the wound to promote healing. Wound powders are generally not a good idea as they are largely irritant and leave foreign material in the wound that has to be removed before healing can commence. Antibiotics and antiseptics are rarely used as they are also irritant, may inhibit the proliferation of cells and are usually diluted by the wound exudate to a point where they are no longer at effective concentrations.

Antiseptics

If a wound is dressed with antiseptic agents, then it is important that the correct concentration is used (chlorhexidine 0.05%; povidone–iodine 1%); otherwise they may be toxic to the cells in the wound. Chlorhexidine may be of benefit, as it binds to the surrounding skin and has residual antibacterial activity, but both agents will be washed out of the wound by the exudate. Povidone–iodine is inactivated by pus, debris and blood. Other antiseptic ointments or dressings inhibit wound healing due to cytotoxicity.

Antibiotics

Topical antibiotics are unlikely to be of any practical use in the management of infection as they are diluted by the exudate and therapeutic levels are not sustained. Systemic antibiotics are only indicated if there are signs of infection. Generally, infection is best controlled by lavage and debridement (see above) rather than by use of antibiotics.

Hydrogels and hydroactive products

These are available commercially as sheets or in tubes of paste that are put into a wound. Their action will be considered later in the section on dressings.

Honey and sugar pastes

The use of honey or sugar pastes in wound management is centuries old. Sugar pastes for clinical use are made up using caster and icing sugar (additive-free) dissolved in hydrogen peroxide and polyethylene glycol 400. The paste has a low pH and is bacteriostatic; it is also able to debride wounds by drawing fluid through the tissues due to its high osmotic pressure. The sugar competes with bacteria for water. It should be confined to use in necrotic wounds and can sting on application.

Preparations of honey made from specific pathogen-free bees are available for clinical use. Manuka honey is said to be more potent than other honeys, due to growth factors. The high osmotic potential debrides wounds and draws exudate out of the wound bed. Honey is also anti-inflammatory and promotes rapid formation of granulation tissue. Excessive exudate will dilute the honey and reduce its osmotic effects, but as honey also contains antibacterial products it will still control infection. Anecdotal reports using honey for treatment of chilblains also report it to be analgesic.

Enzymatic debriding agents

Commercial preparations of collagenolytic enzymes are available that can be applied to wounds to debride necrotic tissue selectively and leave healthy tissue unaffected. The enzymes used act on collagen, protein, fibrin, elastin and/or nucleoproteins. They are relatively expensive but are a human prescription-only medicine and only rarely used in veterinary medicine; they would need to be prescribed under the cascade, which would be difficult to justify.

Organic acids

Proprietary veterinary products containing mild acidic agents such as benzoic acid, malic acid, salicylic acid, boric acid and propylene glycol are readily available as wound cleansing and debriding agents. They are primarily debriding agents and achieve separation of necrotic tissue from the wound through causing differential swelling of healthy and necrotic tissue. It is important to remember that they are appropriate only in the management of grossly necrotic wounds and that the autolysis and low pH will cause damage to healthy tissue. The availability of more physiological and safer agents, such as the hydrogels, makes the use of organic acids difficult to justify.

Larvae

Maggots are the ultimate wound-debriding agents. The first-stage larvae have underdeveloped mouthparts and feed on liquid protein, i.e. exudate and necrotic or infected tissue. Once they develop into second-stage larvae, the mouthparts can potentially damage intact skin, but they will still only feed on dead cells, exudate, secretions and debris, and live tissue is left alone. *Lucilia sericata* is usually the species used to produce sterile stage-one maggots for surgical use.

Larvae are available for purchase for clinical use and can be ordered for next day delivery. Maggots may be supplied in a little absorbent gauze 'bag' that is applied to the wound directly, with the maggots confined to the bag; wound cleansing is then achieved remotely by the maggots' enzymatic secretions. Alternatively, they are received as a pot of loose maggots, which then have to be held in the wound with dressings. The skin surrounding a wound is protected by an adherent dressing (usually a colloid) while the maggots are in the wound. They are held in by a light mesh that adheres to the colloid dressing. The mesh is covered with saline-soaked gauze swabs to prevent the larvae from drying out and the whole area is bandaged lightly with a *permeable* dressing (the maggots must not suffocate). They are left in place for a maximum of 3 days, when they are flushed out (or the 'bag' removed), and replaced with a new batch if necessary.

Research has shown that the maggots are able to eat all bacteria in a wound (including meticillin-resistant *Staphylococcus aureus*; Figure 4.10), and can resolve multiple-drug-resistant wound infections in 24–48 hours without recourse to antibiotics.

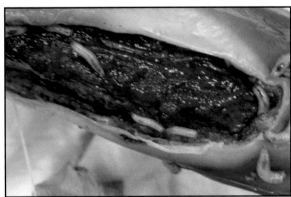

4.10 These larvae have been used to treat a wound infected with MRSA. Three days after application the wound is healthy and no longer infected. The skin surrounding the wound is protected by an adherent hydrocolloid and the maggots will be flushed out of the wound using sterile saline.

Silver

Silver and its salts have antiseptic and antibacterial properties. Traditionally, silver was available as a cream for the management of infected burn wounds (and is a human prescription-only medicine). In the presence of wound exudate, the silver in the dressing ionizes to release active silver ions into the wound. It is not entirely understood how the silver ions exert their antibacterial effect, but there is no selectivity or resistance. Nanocrystalline silver has been developed as a product that rapidly releases particularly high concentrations of silver into an infected wound. Dressings are available that can be left in the wound for up to 7 days, and there are other dressings, such as hydrocolloids, which are available impregnated with silver.

Primary (contact) layer wound dressings

Dressings perform the following functions:

* Debridement of necrotic or infected tissue
* Absorption of exudate
* Analgesia
* Protection of the wound from adherence of the secondary bandage layers
* Prevention of infection or strike-through of the bandage
* Promotion of wound healing.

Topical agents (see above) all have to be held in place in the wound and although larval preparations arrive with a pack of mesh and hydrocolloid, generally the veterinary surgeon needs to select a primary layer dressing to apply to the wound surface before the rest of the bandage is placed. The contact layer should be chosen based on the clinical assessment of the wound.

Optimal healing occurs under the following conditions:

* Moist (not too wet or macerated)
* No infection/necrosis
* No toxins/particles/loose fibres
* Optimum temperature (35–37°C – i.e. warmer than normal skin temperature)
* Undisturbed
* pH approximately 6 (inhibits bacterial proliferation).

Modern dressings achieve many of these goals and, in addition, some dressings can provide other roles in managing the wound, such as debridement, stimulation of granulation or control of exudate. The dressings are provided sterile and should be handled appropriately to prevent contamination of the surface on application. Dressings are usually fairly conformable so that they are in close contact with the wound surface, preventing the accumulation of fluid and debris in the space above the wound where it could be inflammatory or allow bacterial proliferation.

PRACTICAL TIP
It is good clinical practice always to wear gloves whenever a dressing is changed, to prevent nosocomial contamination.

Adherent contact layers

There are few indications for adherent dressings, and they are only used in the very early stages of wound management when the wound still requires debridement. They are very useful in the management of infection, as they rapidly remove necrotic material and bacteria/exudate, allowing the natural tissue defences to control bacterial numbers (Figure 4.11). Adherent dressings are applied dry or wet to a wound and allowed to absorb exudative material and then to dry in order to lift this material out of the wound on removal of the dressing. It is helpful to put a non-adherent dressing over the top of the adherent one, just to make it easier to remove the secondary bandage layer later. They are not suitable for leaving on a wound longer than 24 hours, and should not be allowed to dry into a hard crust.

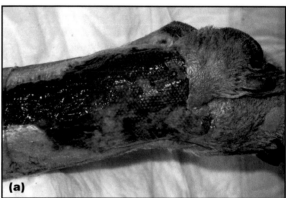
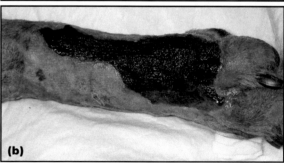

4.11 A chronic shearing injury was presented with a soaked bandage that had been in place for several days. The granulation tissue was foul-smelling and the foot was painful and very swollen. **(a)** An adherent dressing (dry-to-dry in this case as the wound was so wet) was applied and changed every 12 hours. **(b)** After 24 hours, the foot was no longer swollen and was much less painful. The infection had resolved and exudate levels were manageable.

Dry-to-dry dressings

These are used for wounds that are very exudative and have a signficant amount of necrotic, purulent or foreign material in them, or where surgical debridement is not immediately possible. Dry open-weave sterile gauze swabs are packed into the wound, which is then bandaged. The dressing is left in place long enough to allow the exudate to dry into the gauze swabs so that it is removed at the dressing change 12–24 hours later. Removal of these dressings can be extremely painful, as they tend to remove a layer of viable surface tissue from the wound at the same time, and they may need to be changed under anaesthesia.

Wet-to-dry dressings
Wounds with necrotic or foreign material that have less exudate or a more viscous exudate can be dressed with gauze swabs soaked in sterile saline or lactated Ringer's (Hartmann's) solution. The swabs are squeezed out so they are not too wet and are applied to the wound. The moisture in the swabs dilutes viscous exudate, enabling it to be drawn out of the wound, and also rehydrates necrotic tissue. The swabs are covered with a non-adherent dressing to separate them from the secondary layers, and the whole construct bandaged in place. This technique maintains a more physiological moist environment, but the principle remains that the exudate and necrotic material are loosened and dry into the swabs to be removed at the dressing change 12–24 hours later. It is important to change the dressing frequently so that the dressing does not become too wet and macerate normal tissue and so that strike-through does not occur to the outside of the bandage.

This technique is extremely useful for managing opportunistic infections with resistant organisms such as *Proteus* or pseudomonads. Such wounds should always be treated aggressively with wet-to-dry dressings before recourse to antibiotic therapy. Generally the signs of infection (odour, pain, swelling and inflammation of the surrounding skin) will resolve at the first or second dressing change.

Non-adherent contact layers
Most primary layer dressings in contact with the wound are designed to avoid adherent properties, as these damage tissue indiscriminately when they are removed. This is particularly important once granulation and epithelialization have started, although it is possible to apply different types of dressing to different parts of the wound, depending on the stage of healing. Once the wound is entering the granulation stage, it is important to absorb exudate and not to cause damage to the delicate cellular ingrowths in the wound. However, the wound should not be allowed to desiccate, and a moist environment needs to be maintained even if there is little exudate.

Petrolatum gauze
A wide-meshed bleached cotton gauze impregnated with petroleum or paraffin gel is hydrophobic and therefore does not adhere to the wound or the surrounding skin. It is very conformable and an easy solution. However, it can be occlusive, preventing oxygenation of the wound, and there is some evidence that it delays wound healing. There is no absorbent layer, so exudate must be absorbed into secondary layers, and the gauze can dry on to the wound surface. These dressings are cheap but may not be the best choice to promote wound healing.

Perforated films
These dressings are commonly used, particularly over sutured surgical wounds, to prevent adhesion to secondary bandage layers. The wound contact surface is a thin perforated polyurethane membrane with a light layer of absorbent backing. The films are fully permeable, so do not maintain a moist environment and in some circumstances they prove to be adherent when capillary loops and exudate get into the perforations.

Silicone and viscose mesh
Other non-adherent mesh dressings are available, made of silicone or viscose, which do not adhere to the skin or to the wet wound. They do not prevent drying and do not absorb, but they form an atraumatic surface over which other materials are applied. Some interesting data from human studies suggest that the silicone rehydrates scar tissue and reduces keloid or excessive scar formation.

Foams
Polyurethane foams are widely available in many shapes, sizes and formulations. They all have a high absorbent capacity, drawing fluid away from the wound surface and thereby removing inflammatory mediators. They usually have a semi-permeable membrane backing, which allows oxygen exchange and controlled evaporation, thus maintaining a moist but not wet environment at the wound surface.

> **WARNING**
> **Dry wounds do not benefit from foam dressings, as the foam does not provide any humidity on its own.**

The secondary layers can be applied directly over the top of the dressing, and foams are often used on top of other products (e.g. amorphous hydrogels) to hold them in place. Foam dressings are very comfortable and are often used to dress stoma sites, where the discharge can be absorbed and the skin is protected from the tube (e.g. cystostomy or gastrostomy tubes). The absorption of exudate can be seen from the outside of the dressing (Figure 4.12), which is removed when its absorption capacity has been reached.

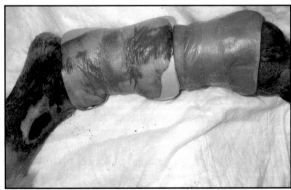

4.12 Foam dressing in place at presentation of the case shown in Figure 4.11. Prior to removal, heavy absorption of exudate by the foam is seen as a dark stain under the membrane outer surface.

Semi-permeable adhesive membranes

These are very thin conformable adhesive films that are applied stretched over the wound and adhere to the normal skin edges. There is no fluid absorption and they are therefore only suitable for shallow wounds with a low level of exudate. They allow oxygen exchange and controlled vapour loss and are particularly good for protection of abrasions. They are also used to protect skin, prevent pressure sores and as surgical incise-drapes.

Collagens

There are a number of collagen dressings available on the veterinary market. In principle, they aim to absorb fluid and form a moist gel on the surface of the wound. They may act to stimulate wound healing by providing growth factor presentation sites, thus increasing the responsiveness of the cells to endogenous growth factors.

Polymer dressings

Modern developments in wound management have resulted in the creation of dressings made up of various combinations of polymer composites. The molecules are able to donate water to the wound, thus liquefying thick exudate and rehydrating necrotic material. They can also trap water and thereby remove inflammatory exudate from the wound surface, reducing the level of inflammatory mediators at the wound surface.

Hydrogels: These are available as an amorphous gel or a sheet dressing (Figure 4.13) and consist of inert cross-linked polymers with a high water content. The gels can both donate and trap water, which means that they can absorb wound exudate as well as rehydrating and gently debriding necrotic material within the wound. The amorphous gel needs to be covered with a semi-permeable dressing so that it does not dry out and to hold it in the wound. The sheet hydrogels already have a semi-permeable backing attached and the secondary layers can be applied directly. Some amorphous hydrogels have been combined with antibiotics to debride deep abscesses and other wound-healing stimulants such as alginates. These hydrogels are an important substitute for adherent dressings to achieve wound debridement. They can be analgesic (especially if stored in the fridge) and do not damage areas of the wound that are healing. The high water absorbence will also reduce oedema and swelling in the surrounding tissues.

> **PRACTICAL TIP**
> Removal of the gel is painless, and the gel and trapped exudate and debris are lavaged out with sterile saline at each dressing change.

Hydrocolloids: Hydrocolloid dressings are made up of polymers suspended in an adhesive matrix. They are designed to adhere to the wound edges of the normal skin and are left *in situ* for a number of days, providing a moist controlled wound environment while absorbing exudate and preventing strike-through, as most are waterproof. The dressings actively stimulate wound healing and encourage debridement as they degrade on interaction with wound fluids. This has given them a bad reputation, as sometimes the wound appears to have enlarged at the first dressing change. The dressings swell and liquefy as they absorb exudate and have an unpleasant yellowish appearance after a few days, although this is normal. They are not used in the presence of active infection but are suitable for later stages of more subtle debridement combined with encouragement of granulation and epithelialization. The adherence to the wound edges may inhibit contraction of the wound by splinting it, although in veterinary patients adherence is often not complete.

> **PRACTICAL TIP**
> As with all dressing products, the wound should be lavaged at each dressing change to remove the degradation products.

Hydropolymers: These are another of the polymer matrix dressings that have been developed to control the environment of the wound by providing a huge absorbent capacity when the wound fluids are trapped in the dressing. Unlike the hydrocolloids, however, there is no degradation of the dressing itself and the material remains inert. They are more like the polyurethane foam dressings, but they have a greater capacity to trap fluids.

Alginates

Alginate dressings are derived from seaweed and consist of varying proportions of guluronic and mannuronic acids. The wound exudate interacts with

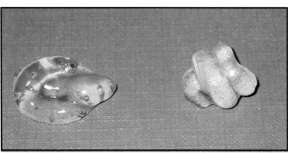

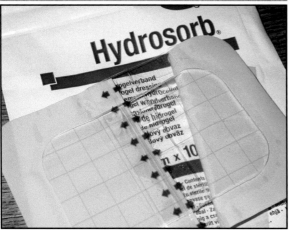

4.13 Hydrogel is available as an amorphous gel or a preformed sheet with a membrane backing.

the alginate to release cations that actively stimulate wound healing via the inflammatory cascade, allowing release of endogenous growth factors into the wound. The interaction with exudate transforms the alginate into a soft gel in the wound, which keeps the wound moist for a while. Dry wounds can be treated with alginates if they are pre-wetted with sterile saline and the skin edges protected from any dry fibres; thus, alginates can be used to stimulate wound healing or restart healing processes if there has been delayed activity.

Bandaging

Bandages should be constructed with care, using appropriate materials, and adequate *written* instructions on the care of a bandage should be given to the owner at the time of discharge from the hospital.

> **PRACTICAL TIP**
> If a bandage causes irritation or pain it should *always* be changed, as the risk of necrosis associated with leaving the bandage *in situ* is too high.

Early irritation from a bandage is likely to be due to numbness and tingling associated with superficial ischaemic injury in the skin, and this may be reversible if the bandage is removed promptly. However, damage related to deep ischaemia at a later stage may continue to develop due to the oedema that arises after bandage removal (reperfusion injury), and these injuries may threaten the limb or even result in the need for euthanasia.

Limbs should be prepared for bandaging carefully in order to minimize complications:

- Interdigital webs should be clean and dry
- Hair should either be clipped away or be clean, free of blood or exudate, and dry
- A small amount of padding is placed underneath the dew claw and gently separating each toe, with a twist of absorbent or non-adherent material in each interdigital web. This prevents the development of sores and keeps the glandular areas of skin clean and dry while confined in the bandage
- Grooming the fur during bandage changes, thereby stimulating the skin in the normal areas of the limb, is particularly important for injuries that are bandaged for a long period.

Secondary layers

The secondary layer is made of even turns of a light absorbent synthetic cotton material. The material is wrapped around the limb, overlapping on each turn by at least 50%. The number of layers depends on the degree of support the bandage is required to provide and also the quantity of exudate that will be absorbed. This absorbent material is then gently compacted using a stretch bandage (e.g. gauze) that is also applied in even turns around the limb with 50% overlap. This material is able to slide on itself as it is non-self-adherent, allowing slight movement in the bandage construction and slight expansion as the absorbent layers fill with exudate. Heavier bandages that are designed to splint the limb (such as Robert Jones; Figure 4.14) are often constructed with cotton wool roll, which is alternated with the stretch material that compacts it.

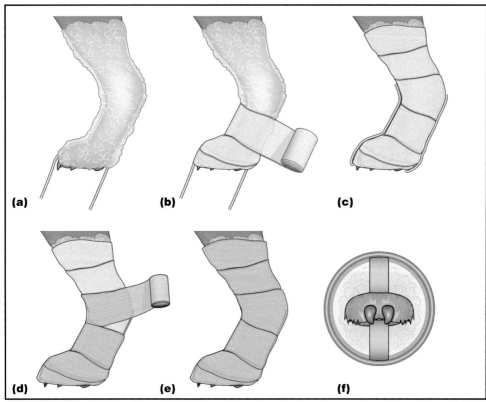

4.14

Modified Robert Jones bandage. **(a)** Cotton wool inner layer. **(b,c)** Conforming bandage is placed to compress the cotton wool as firmly and evenly as possible. **(d,e)** Cohesive dressing is placed over the bandage. **(f)** End-on-view showing bandage layers and the exposed middle toes.

PRACTICAL TIP
The pressure applied underneath a bandage is *inversely proportional* to the width of the bandage material and the circumference of the limb. Thus, a narrow part of the limb (such as just above the hock) is at risk of too high a pressure, as would be a compressing bandage applied using narrow bandage material. In order to prevent this effect, the secondary layers are applied in sufficient layers to even out the natural variations in circumference of the limb and therefore create a pressure gradient within the bandage that is lower at the top of the limb than at the bottom.

Tertiary layers

The tertiary layer is an adhesive or self-adherent layer that primarily provides some strength to the bandage construction and also protects the bandage from the environment and the animal. It is important to choose the material for this layer carefully, as it should allow some evaporation of vapour but be water-repellent. The elastic self-adherent materials can generate extremely high pressures underneath a bandage and should not be used where there is insufficient padding to control the pressure underneath. If a bandage is not required for direct application of pressure, it may be better to choose a conforming non-adherent gauze, which will slide on itself and allow some relaxation of the bandage and prevent the development of high pressure areas. The tertiary layer is applied in even turns around the limb, securing the final layer of secondary material. It should never adhere to the animal's skin or fur.

The bandage as a whole must be protected from becoming soiled or wet. Used intravenous fluid bags are useful to keep bandaged feet dry, but it is important that the bandage is not permanently kept in a plastic bag as this will cause maceration of the tissue and skin underneath.

Tie-over dressings

Some parts of the body are almost impossible to bandage. Wounds on the body may be dressed by applying a bandage over the whole body, although at the rear end of the animal this may involve placing an indwelling urinary catheter to protect the bandage from soiling, If this is not practical, dressings can be secured to the body using large loose sutures in the skin circumferentially around the wound, to anchor umbilical tape which is tied over the dressing and compresses it into place on the wound (Figure 4.15).

Pressure relief bandages

Pressure relief bandages have been described for the management of decubital ulcers or ischaemic injuries associated with bandages or casts. Rings of padding are used to surround a wound and allow a dressing to be applied without applying direct pressure on the wound. However, they are difficult to

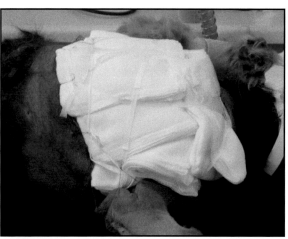

4.15 A tie-over dressing can be used to dress a wound in an area that is difficult to bandage. Tapes are secured to the skin surrounding the wound, using large loops of stay suture. The tie-over tapes can be undone to change the dressing and then looped together again when the fresh dressing is reapplied.

apply well and can cause an increased pressure on the surrounding skin, thereby delaying healing by reducing the blood supply.

Wound management strategy and planning

Wound management should be expected to be very expensive for the client. If done properly, it is not a quick process, but adequate wound management can achieve much better results and save them money in the long term.

All clinicians will have their own strategy for ongoing assessment and management of a wound, but it is helpful if all staff have a consistent system so that the clinical notes have some indication of consistency and simple rules applied to provide continuity of care.

WARNING
Wounds are most likely to become chronic and heal poorly in the face of inadequate clinical management and poor communication.

It is important to understand the normal process of healing and what the timeframe should be for normal tissue to achieve granulation, control of sepsis and epithelialization (see Chapter 1). One strategy that has been used to provide a system of assessment that ties into clinical decision-making is the TIME system (see also Chapter 2):

- **T**issue
- **I**nfection and Inflammation
- **M**oisture
- **E**pithelialization.

These parameters must be addressed and considered at every dressing change; management decisions are made based on the results (Figure

4.16). Many veterinary surgeons may run through these processes subconsciously as they look at a wound; recording the assessment and management decisions helps in being able to express and manage the expectations of clients and of the clinical staff who may need to deal with the wound when the primary clinician is unavailable.

1. Assess the patient:
   - How has the patient been feeling?
   - How painful is the wound?
   - What condition is the dressing in?
2. Lavage the wound at every dressing change:
   - Removes fragments of dressing material
   - Removes inflammatory fluids
   - Rehydrates the surface of the wound after exposure
   - May reduce the risks of contamination at the time of the dressing change.
3. Consider whether there is tissue that needs to be debrided from the wound:
   - Can this be done with dressings?
   - Does this need to be done surgically?
4. Assess and record the wound:
   - Size
   - Appearance of the wound – identify different areas
   - Appearance of the wound edges
   - Appearance of the skin surrounding the wound.
5. Make decisions:
   - What primary layer to apply
   - When you need to see the wound again
   - Whether or not tissue samples are necessary.
6. Re-dress the wound and make sure that the owner is informed about progress, deterioration, expectation and when to return.

4.16 Steps in continued wound management.

Wounds are frequently dressed regularly over a period of days to weeks and inevitably during this time there is some loss of continuity of care, with different people seeing the animal. Accurate records and a consistent method of recording data ensure that changes are identified early and can be responded to appropriately. A simple chart that is completed each time the animal is assessed helps provide historical information to the new clinician on the case and also reassurance to the owner that records are adequate and that discontinuity of care will not adversely affect the wound management (Figure 4.17). Photographs can help, particularly when different clinicians are involved at each dressing change. It is important to include a scale in the photograph; some dressings come with a sterile transparent template that can be used to trace the size of the wound at each change and placed in the clinical records.

Different wound dressings perform different tasks in the wound bed. If the TIME acronym is used, then dressings are used to treat specific problems that have been identified in the wound bed. For example, a wound that is considered to be 'too wet' may be dressed with a product that draws fluid through the wound and traps it off the surface, so that the wound maceration is controlled. Traditionally, dressings have been described in terms of categories of product, but often it is easier to describe them in terms of *what they do and when they should be applied;* this emphasizes their clinical action rather than the science (Figure 4.18).

Name: _____ Date: _____
Time since last visit: _____

General demeanour :   5   4   3   2   1
Lameness :   5   4   3   2   1
Condition of bandage: _____
Removal of bandage pain score :   5   4   3   2   1
Exudate level : _____
Exudate description : _____
Size of wound : _____
Description of edges : _____

TIME assessment : _____
T _____
Plan : _____
I _____
Plan : _____
M _____
Plan : _____
E _____
Plan: _____

Action :
Lavage ☐   Surgical debridement ☐   Biopsy ☐   Culture ☐
Dressing used : _____
Bandage placed: _____
Analgesic: _____

Next appointment: _____

Signed: _____

4.17 Example of a wound record sheet.

PRACTICAL TIPS

- **Expect to have to provide adequate pain relief at every dressing change and wound assessment.**
- **Expect to have to anaesthetize the patient sometimes to be able to manage the wound safely and without distress to the patient.**
- **Always wear gloves when changing a bandage, from the beginning to the end. Consider changing the gloves after you have lavaged the wound and prepare to re-dress it.**
- **Always protect the wound from the hospital environment and carry out the dressing change on a clean surface (such as a disposable incontinence pad).**
- **Protect the wound from cross-contamination from other ongoing cases by keeping all wound management materials completely separate from each case.**

Action required or wound characteristic	Examples	Comment
Control of exudate – prevention of maceration	Foams, hydropolymers, honey	Often very exudative wounds just need more frequent dressing changes – even twice daily if necessary. The inflammatory mediators in the fluid will perpetuate the problem unless it is removed
Necrotic, sloughy or contaminated requiring debridement	Adherent (wet-to-dry), hydrogels, larvae, honey or sugar pastes, hydrocolloids, enzymatic, acidic solutions	Consider surgical debridement if the wound is very necrotic
Rehydration of necrotic tissue or dry surfaces	Hydrogels, hydrocolloids (adherent wet-to-dry)	
Infection	Adherent (wet-to-dry), silver dressings, larvae	Debridement and frequent dressing changes should be the mainstay in managing wound infection
Stimulation of healing that appears to have slowed	Alginates, hydrocolloids, collagens	Identifying the cause of the slowed healing may be more important – e.g. healing may slow because the wound is too wet, or too dry or needs debriding
Maintenance of a humid environment or prevention of desiccation	Semi-permeable membranes, hydrogel sheets, hydrogel under foam	Semi-permeable membranes allow controlled evaporation of fluid and maintain a slightly humid environment. They also allow gaseous exchange. Sometimes it is necessary to provide a source of moisture to maintain the humidity

4.18 Clinical actions of wound dressings.

Further reading

Anderson DM and White RAS (2000) Ischaemic bandage injuries: a retrospective study in nine dogs and two cats. A review and discussion of the literature. *Veterinary Surgery* **29**, 488–498

Mathews KA and Dinnington AG (2002) Wound management using honey. *Compendium on Continuing Education for the Practicing Veterinarian* **24**, 53–60

Mathews KA and Dinnington AG (2002) Wound management using sugar. *Compendium on Continuing Education for the Practicing Veterinarian* **24**, 41–50

Morgan DA (2004) *Formulary of Wound Management Products.* Euromed Communications Ltd, Haslemere

Pavletic M (1993) *Atlas of Small Animal Reconstructive Surgery.* Lippincott, Philadelphia

Swaim S and Krahwinkel DJ (eds) (2006) Wound Management. *Veterinary Clinics of North America: Small Animal Practice* **36**(4)

CASE EXAMPLE 1:
Open wound management of a chronic shear injury prior to skin grafting

History
A 3-year-old male neutered DSH cat was presented 6 weeks after arthrodesis of the hock following severe injury in a road traffic accident. The wound had been dressed twice-weekly with a perforated film dressing but no consistent strategy.

Assessment and treatment
On presentation the wound was granulating but the tissue was smooth and macerated. There was excessive exudate and it was malodorous and painful. An adherent (wet-to-dry) dressing was put on and changed after 24 hours.

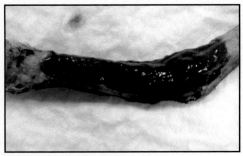
Wound on presentation.

The adherent wet-to-dry dressing was peeled off under general anaesthesia.

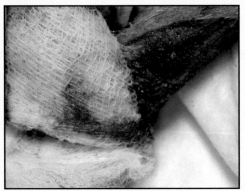
Removal of adherent dressing.

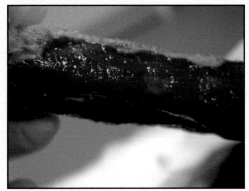
Exudate is already reduced, granulation tissue looks more normal (i.e. granular) and skin edges are smooth and dry.

The wound was dressed for a further 4 days using hydrocolloid dressings to maintain a moist environment and allow the healthy granulation tissue to establish. The hydrocolloid dressing was then removed.

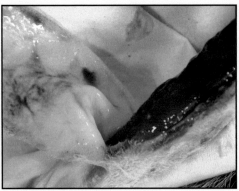
Removal of hydrocolloid dressing. There is characteristic yellowish liquefied colloid material where exudate has been absorbed. Skin edges are beginning to epithelialize.

Case Example 1 continues ▶

CASE EXAMPLE 1 continued:
Open wound management of a chronic shear injury prior to skin grafting

Prior to grafting, 7 days after initial presentation, there was healthy active granulation tissue. No antibiotics were used at any stage during preparation.

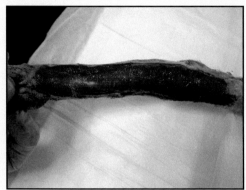

Healthy granulation tissue prior to grafting.

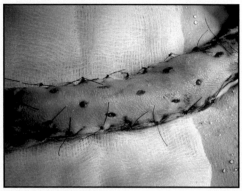

Free skin graft in place.

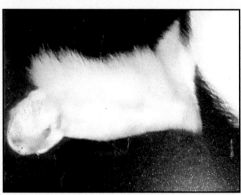

Foot with fur fully grown back 6 months later. Because the graft was harvested from the side of the body, the hair has grown back longer than the rest of the hair on the foot.

CASE EXAMPLE 2:
Management of an acute road traffic shear injury

History
A 2-year-old Border Collie was presented 20 minutes after being hit by a tractor in a muddy field. The dog was hyperventilating, very distressed, and had a large wound on the lateral aspect of the shoulder that was grossly contaminated with mud. He was tachycardic with pale mucous membranes and poor peripheral pulses.

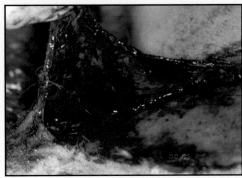
Wound on presentation.

Stabilization
Intravenous fluids were administered at 90 ml/kg/h and analgesia was provided (morphine 0.3 mg/kg i.m.). Broad-spectrum antibiotics were given (amoxicillin/clavulanate 20 mg/kg i.v.) and the dog was given oxygen via a mask. A lateral thoracic radiograph confirmed that the diaphragm was intact and there were no signs of pleural or pulmonary haemorrhage. Over the next half hour, the pulse rate and quality improved. The mucous membrane colour was pink and capillary refill time was rapid. The fluid rate was reduced and the dog was anaesthetized for wound assessment and treatment.

Wound assessment and treatment
The wound was lavaged with sterile isotonic fluids (lactated Ringer's (Hartmann's) solution). Once the wound was assessed, it was apparent that it might be possible to convert it to a clean wound.

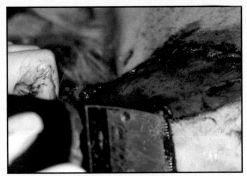
The wound was filled with sterile aqueous gel and the skin around the wound and along the thorax and neck was clipped.

After clipping, hair was removed from the wound through lavage of the gel. The skin surrounding the wound was then thoroughly cleaned with 1% povidone–iodine skin scrub until the area was considered clean enough for sterile surgery. The whole side was draped with sterile drapes and layered surgical debridement carried out.

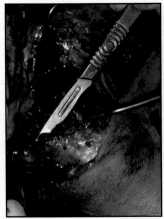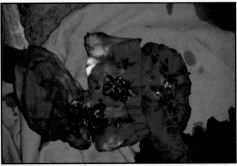
Using a scalpel blade and forceps, fascial layers were picked up and carefully cut away from the underlying fresh fascial planes.

Case Example 2 continues ▶

CASE EXAMPLE 2 continued:
Management of an acute road traffic shear injury

In some areas it was only necessary to remove the areolar tissue to expose clean tissue underneath. As each layer was exposed the instruments and surgeon's gloves were exchanged for clean ones (four times). At the final instrument change, the surgical drapes were also renewed.

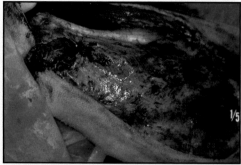

Wound following lavage and debridement.

Primary closure was achieved using advancement flaps from cranial and caudal to the wound and a suction drain was placed. The whole limb was bandaged for 24 hours to prevent postoperative swelling and seroma formation.

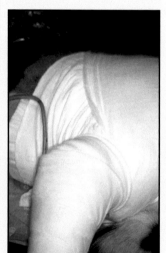

Bandaged wound.

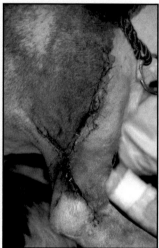

48 hours after surgery the bandage and drains were removed and the dog was discharged.

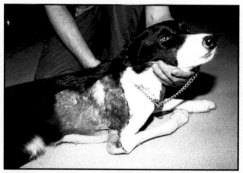

Wound appearance at 10 days when the dog returned for suture removal. The dog was sound.

5

Surgical drains in wound management and reconstructive surgery

Jane Ladlow

Introduction

A drain is a conduit placed in the wound to remove fluid and air. This usually refers to surgical implants, typically Penrose drains or closed suction drains; however, an autogenous drain, the omentum, can be used in selected cases. An alternative method of providing wound drainage is to leave part of the wound open. This technique is effective in open peritoneal drainage and can also work well with severely contaminated or necrotic skin wounds (see Chapter 4).

History of wound drainage

Hippocrates (c.460–377BC) first reported surgical drainage when he used hollow tubes for drainage of empyema. This was followed by Roman descriptions of ascitic abdominal drainage using hollow conical drains placed through the abdominal wall; intermittent drainage was achieved by removal of an adjustable plug. In the Middle Ages linen wicks were used to prevent premature wound closure and aid drainage.

Lorenz Heister developed capillary drainage in the early 1700s. The first American surgical textbook published in 1791 described leaving the dependent part of the wound open to aid drainage. Veterinary surgeons in the 1800s used a material called tow, which was coarse flax or hemp, to imbibe fluid and dilate canals. By the late 1800s rubber and glass tubes had been developed but high infection rates and failure rates were associated with wound drainage. Lister's advocation of antiseptics and wound drainage in the late 1800s increased wound drainage throughout Europe but veterinary surgeons continued to struggle with wound contamination. Charles Bingham Penrose designed the Penrose drain in 1897 by removing the end of a condom and placing gauze inside it. Rafe C. Chaffin produced the first commercial suction drain in 1932 and in 1954 Redon and Chaffe designed a portable closed suction drain that marked the beginning of the modern era of wound drainage.

Indications for drain usage

- Removal of fluid or air from a wound.
- Tissue apposition and obliteration of dead space.

> **WARNING**
> In the management of dirty wounds, such as bite injuries, it is important that appropriate wound debridement is combined with drain placement. Drain placement is not a substitute for good surgical technique (Figure 5.1). If a large amount of contamination is present or ongoing necrosis is anticipated, leaving the wound open for delayed primary closure or secondary intention healing may be preferable to closing over a drain.

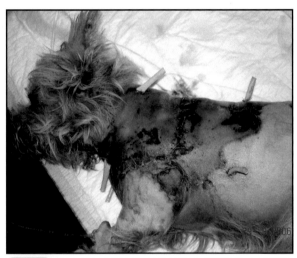

5.1 Inappropriate use of Penrose drains in a severe dogbite wound. Open management of this wound with wet-to-dry dressings would have been more appropriate.

The prophylactic use of drains to remove fluid that may occur after wound closure, thus avoiding seroma formation (Figure 5.2), is common practice, although there is very little evidence in the veterinary literature on the effectiveness of surgical drains used in this way. In human medical studies the use of closed suction drains following surgeries such as thyroidectomy, incisional hernia repair or orthopaedic procedures including joint replacements, cruciate ligament reconstruction or fracture fixation, is under debate. Recent studies have shown that surgical drainage in these cases has no benefit with respect to wound infection rates, pain scores, recovery times or wound dehiscence (Purushotham *et al.*, 2002; Lee *et al.*, 2006; Parker *et al.*, 2007).

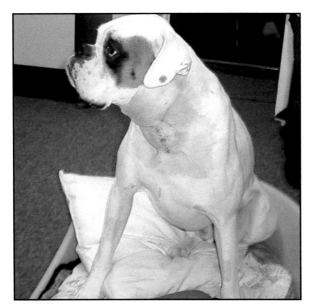

5.2 Seroma formation in a Boxer dog after resection of a thyroid carcinoma.

In veterinary medicine, however, there are wounds where anatomical closure of the dead space is not possible or, in the case of axial pattern flaps, undesirable as this may compromise the vascularity of the flap (Trevor *et al.,* 1992). Drain placement may also be beneficial for wounds in areas of high motion that may be more likely to develop seromas, for example the proximal limb, cervical area and tail base, particularly when the patient is not amenable to restricting movement.

Pressure dressings are an alternative method of reducing fluid build-up in a wound, but they are only effective at maintaining evenly dispersed topical pressure for a few hours. Pressure dressings are difficult to apply effectively to the cervical and head areas, axilla and tailbase. There are reports in the veterinary literature of tissue necrosis following Robert Jones dressings being applied to limbs (Anderson and White, 2000).

There are advantages to removing fluid that accumulates in a wound, such as decreasing the risk of wound infection and wound dehiscence. Wound fluid also increases susceptibility to infection due to the following mechanisms:

- The ability to opsonize bacteria for phagocytosis is lost
- The presence of fluid impedes the access of phagocytes into the wound
- Fluid provides a suitable substrate for bacterial growth
- Seroma formation may compromise the vascular supply to the wound.

WARNING
In oncological surgery, seroma formation may compromise future radiation fields if the seroma is aspirated through a clean tissue plane. Seroma formation in these patients also delays wound healing and hence the start of radiation therapy.

Although there are advantages to using drains in veterinary surgery, drains should not be used to compensate for poor haemostasis, inadequate wound debridement or lack of accurate tissue apposition.

Types of drain

There are a number of different drains available for use in wound management.
Drains are categorized as:

- active: a vacuum is attached to a closed circuit
- passive: a combination of capillary flow, overflow and gravity is used to remove fluid from the wound.

Materials
Drains were traditionally made of red rubber but this caused marked inflammatory reactions, so most tube drains are now produced from more inert materials such as silicone, polypropylene, polyvinylchloride and nylon. Penrose drains are produced from soft latex rubber. Ideally, drains should be soft and malleable to avoid wound trauma and should have a radiopaque marker so they can be visualized on radiography.

Passive drains
The advantages and disadvantages of passive drains are shown in Figure 5.3.

Advantages of passive drains
• Low cost, which enables multiple drains to be used if necessary
• Soft, malleable and less likely to cause tissue trauma when compared to the tube suction drains

Disadvantages and contraindications
• Not ideal for large wounds where extended drainage is likely to be required, as it is difficult to quantify fluid drained and difficult to manage dressings when fluid levels are high
• Of little use unless there is a gravitational flow of fluid from the wound and thus may not be suitable for some wounds on the head or dorsum
• Should be avoided in wounds of the thoracic wall that may communicate with the thoracic cavity, as they allow air into the wound and may therefore result in pneumothorax formation
• Should not be used to flush a wound, as the external part of the drain will be contaminated and flushing saline along the drain tract would be likely to flush bacteria and debris back to the wound

5.3 Advantages and disadvantages of passive drains.

Penrose drain
A Penrose drain consists of a tube or band of soft malleable radiopaque latex rubber (Figure 5.4). Wound fluid is drawn over or through the drain by capillary action (most of the flow is extraluminal) and then drains by gravitational flow from the drain as it exits the dependent part of the wound. Penrose drains can work well in small wounds where limited drainage is anticipated. Various widths of drain are available (6 mm to 5 cm), with 2–4 cm drains being suitable for most small animal wounds. The drainage obtained depends upon the surface area of the drain placed, with wider drains being more effective.

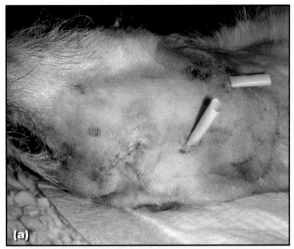

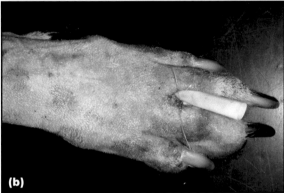

5.4 Penrose drains in place **(a)** after debridement of a dog bite wound; and **(b)** after resection of an interdigital foreign body. (a, © Alison L. Moores)

A Penrose drain can be modified to a cigarette drain by placing gauze through the lumen. This technique increases fluid flow by capillary action but increases the inflammatory reaction produced by the drain and is therefore rarely used.

Sump drain
Sump drains are double- or triple-lumen tube drains that act on the principle that more lumina result in more efficient drainage of the wound. The smaller-bore tube allows air to enter the wound and fluid drains via the larger tube(s). Sump drains are commercially available, or a Foley catheter – with the bulb and syringe adaptor removed and fenestrations placed – can be used as a sump drain.

Sump–Penrose drain
A sump drain can be placed within a Penrose drain to increase the surface area of the drain and thus increase efficiency.

If continuous negative pressure is applied to the outer tubing using a suction unit, sump drains and sump–Penrose drains can be used as active drains and are particularly useful in wounds with high fluid production. This method is cumbersome, however, compared with closed suction drains and results in drawing air through the wound, increasing the risk of infection. A bacterial filter placed in the drain will decrease contamination of the wound. This type of drain is rarely used in veterinary medicine.

Others
Other types of passive drains include corrugated drains, Yeates drains, dental dams, and tube drains.

Other uses of passive drains
A small-gauge tube drain (6–8 F) or catheter (18–20 gauge epidural catheter) with multiple fenestrations and sealed at one end can be placed in a wound bed at the end of surgery as a means of dispersing local anaesthetic agent on the wound. This technique is very useful for lateral thoracotomy, median sternotomy, total ear canal ablation, amputation, and after some major tumour resections. If a drain is also required for fluid removal in these procedures a second, wider-bore drain should be used. In these cases the wound drain should be occluded for 20 minutes after the administration of local anaesthetic through the wound drain.

Active drains: closed suction drains
Closed suction drain systems rely on a vacuum, which draws fluid through a rigid drain placed in the wound. The drain tubing exits the skin into a collection chamber.

Alternatively, rigid tube drains can be used, with intermittent suction applied with a syringe at least every 6 hours (Figure 5.5). This type of intermittent suction is more likely to become occluded than low-level continuous suction but it offers a cheaper alternative to a continuous drainage system.

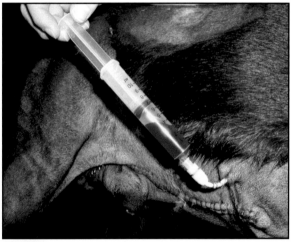

5.5 A tube drain with suction being applied with a syringe. Suction is applied to the drain at least every 6 hours. The tube is sealed when it is not being actively drained. (© P Neath)

There are a number of different active drains available: most rely on a collapsible collection chamber that has an inherent tendency to reinflate and therefore apply a vacuum; an alternative rigid collection chamber that has an internal spring mechanism and pre-applied vacuum is available. A one-way valve is present in some collapsible collection chambers, which prevents reflux into the wound if the patient lies on the chamber and compresses it. A separate spout allows emptying of the chamber when required.

The advantages and disadvantages of closed suction drains are shown in Figure 5.6.

Advantages of closed suction drains

- More effective at removing fluid than passive drains
- Closed system reduces the risk of nosocomial bacteria entering the wound
- System is easily portable
- Wounds do not require substantial dressings, which, in an exudative wound, can compensate for the extra cost of the drain
- Fluid can be collected and recorded, allowing a trend in fluid production to be observed. Many drains have a measuring facility on the collection chamber
- The constant low level of suction applied to the wound decreases the rate at which the drain is occluded

Disadvantages and problems

- Losing the vacuum, due to air entering the chamber, may occur if wound closure is not airtight. Placement of additional sutures or staples should resolve this problem. If the animal is awake, placing an impermeable dressing over the wound allows a vacuum to be placed. Alternatively, if the wound is left for 4–6 hours postoperatively a fibrin seal will form, making the wound airtight and allowing negative pressure to be applied
- Occlusion of the drain by clots: the use of continuous suction helps prevent occlusion. The Jackson–Pratt drain is less likely to become occluded due to the large number of fenestrations present. If the drain tubing does become occluded it is sometimes possible to aspirate the clot using a needle and syringe placed in the end of the drain, drawing the clot into the needle and then wrapping the clot around a cotton bud or gauze
- Premature removal of the drain: unless the drain is under a dressing the animal should wear an Elizabethan collar when the drain is in place

5.6 Advantages and disadvantages of closed suction drains.

Jackson–Pratt drain

This is a silicone drain available in different lengths, with a large flat end that contains multiple fenestrations (Figures 5.7). The flat end narrows to form a tube that exits the skin via a stab incision and attaches to a collapsible grenade-shaped collection chamber. The drain is malleable and easy to place. The large number of fenestrations means that it is less likely to become occluded by blood clots or tissue debris.

Redon/Red-O-Pack

These systems consist of a single piece of drain tubing, one end of which is fenestrated and is placed in the wound. The other end is attached to a needle, which is used to exit the drain through the skin. The needle is cut off the tubing and the tube is attached to the corrugated collection chamber (Figure 5.8).

Redovac

This system is similar to the Redon drain, with a tube drain that attaches to a collection system. The collection system is rigid, with a spring-loaded vacuum mechanism. There is a vacuum indicator on the collection chamber. When this is at the MIN setting the chamber should be emptied. Suction can be reapplied to these units using a suction unit or syringe after emptying the drain of fluid. It may be preferable to switch collection chambers when full if fluid volumes are anticipated to be low.

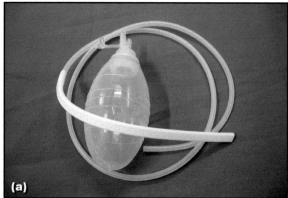
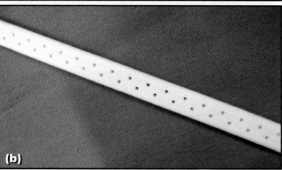
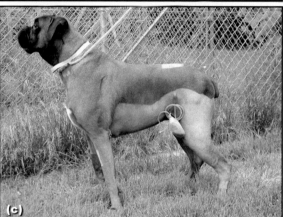

5.7 Jackson–Pratt drain. **(a)** Drain and collection chamber. **(b)** Flat end with fenestrations. **(c)** A Boxer dog with a Jackson–Pratt drain in place. The collection system is sutured to the flank, making the drain system portable. (c, © P Neath)

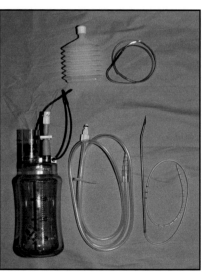

5.8

Redon drains with corrugated (top) and rigid (bottom) collection chambers. (© Alison L. Moores)

Vacuum syringe drain

A simple and inexpensive closed suction drain can be constructed using an 18-gauge needle, a 20, 30 or 60 ml syringe and a 19-gauge butterfly giving set (Figure 5.9). After removal of the catheter section of the butterfly giving set, multiple fenestrations can be placed in the tubing with a scalpel blade. Each fenestration should not exceed 30% of the tube diameter to avoid the tube kinking or breaking on removal. The tubing is placed via a stab incision through adjacent skin into the wound and the syringe is connected to the hub of the tubing. After drawing approximately 5 ml of air into the syringe the plunger is drawn back to create a vacuum and a hypodermic needle is placed across the syringe to secure it in place. The tip of the needle should be removed after passing the needle through the syringe.

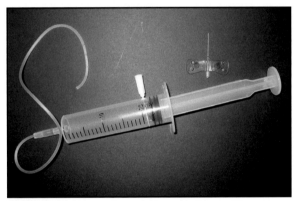

5.9 Vacuum syringe drain made from a 19-gauge butterfly catheter and a 20 ml syringe.

The suction on the drain can be tested intermittently by drawing back the syringe and observing the plunger collapse back. The drain should be emptied as necessary; a three-way tap placed between the syringe and the tubing facilitates emptying without contamination of the tubing. The lack of a one-way valve in the vacuum syringe system means that contamination of the wound is possible, so careful handling is required when emptying the drain.

This drain is suitable for small wounds where a relatively moderate drainage rate is anticipated (5–10 ml per 4 hours). Attaching the needle of a butterfly catheter into a vacutainer can produce a similar type of drain, though this is only suitable for small wounds where a very limited amount of fluid drainage is anticipated, such as an aural haematoma.

Drain placement

Principles of drain insertion are listed in Figure 5.10.

Penrose drain

Placement of a Penrose drain is described and illustrated in Operative Technique 5.1. The proximal part of the drain is secured in the wound by a single suture that passes through the skin and the drain, and the distal part of the drain exits through a stab incision in the dependent part of the wound, creating a single-exit drain.

- Before placement of a drain, the hair should be clipped from a large area surrounding the drain and the site surgically prepared.
- The drain should be placed using aseptic technique.
- The drain should exit through a stab incision adjacent to the wound rather than through the wound incision, to allow primary closure and healing of the wound.
- With passive drains the exit hole should be of a size that allows adequate drainage but prevents herniation of tissue. With active suction drains the exit hole is ideally the same size as the largest part of the drain to allow easy removal, but if this hole is larger than the drain tubing, as can occur with the Jackson–Pratt drain, a purse-string suture can be used to reduce the size of the exit hole.
- Passive drains should exit the dependent or ventral part of the wound.
- The length of the drain should be recorded at insertion to determine whether any part of the drain is left in the wound if removed accidentally or prematurely.
- If the animal is to have further treatment, such as radiotherapy, this should be considered before drain placement and the drain exit site should not be placed at a great distance from the wound. The drain exit site should be noted for the oncologist to include it in the radiation field.

5.10 Principles of drain insertion.

Traditionally Penrose drains were placed across a wound with the proximal and distal part of the drain exposed. This technique only aids drainage when pressure is placed on the wound site and is more likely to result in nosocomial infection than a single-exit drain. In certain areas, such as the axilla or inguinal area, the placement of a drain exiting proximally and distally from the wound may prevent air being sucked into the wound when the animal moves, although the author has not found this to be a problem with a single-exit drain in these areas.

> **WARNING**
> **Placing multiple holes in Penrose drains makes them less effective, as they decrease the efficiency of the capillary flow and reduce the drain surface area. They also make the drain more likely to tear when the skin suture is cut and the drain is removed.**

Closed suction drains

Placement of a closed suction drain is described and illustrated in Operative Technique 5.2. The drains leave the wound through a small stab incision, or by passing the needle attachment (if present) to the drain through the skin adjacent to the suture line. The drain tubing should be well secured to the skin, for example with a Chinese finger-trap suture (Figure 5.11). Any redundant external tubing can be cut off after placing the drain and before attaching the tubing to the collection system. The collection chamber can be attached to the patient by placement of a suture or a bandage to make the system easily portable. If the drain system has a single-use collection system where the vacuum cannot easily be recreated (e.g. Redovac drain), the drain is not opened to the collection system until a fibrin seal has formed over the wound i.e. after 4–6 hours.

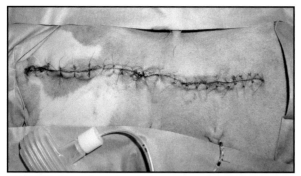

5.11 Closed suction drain exiting adjacent to a primary wound. The drain tubing is secured to the skin with a Chinese finger-trap suture.

If the drain is placed after wound closure to drain a seroma or haematoma, a small stab incision is made adjacent to the wound and a long pair of forceps, such as Rochester Carmalt or Doyen forceps, are used to tunnel the drain through the subcutaneous tissue and into the fluid pocket. A purse-string suture placed around the drain tubing aids vacuum placement.

Applying a vacuum to a closed suction drain

The amount of vacuum that should be placed on the drain should be sufficient to obliterate dead space but not so high that it results in tissue damage. A vacuum of −80 mmHg has traditionally been recommended. High-vacuum suction (−700 to −800 mmHg) evacuates more fluid initially but may cause more damage to tissues. Human studies have found little difference between high- and low-vacuum drainage in volume and duration of seroma formation or wound complications. The different closed suction drains used in veterinary medicine vary markedly in the negative pressures applied to the wound, with rigid containers having a significantly greater initial negative pressure. With manually compressible drains, two-hand compression results in significantly greater negative pressure compared to one-hand compression (Halfacree *et al.*, 2006). The suction applied by the drain decreases as the reservoir fills with fluid, with suction pressures of between 13 and 20% of initial pressure when the collection chamber is half full.

> **PRACTICAL TIP**
> It is difficult to know what negative pressure is being applied to a wound. It is therefore advisable to empty containers and reapply the vacuum once collection chambers approach half full.

A low continuous rate of fluid production indicates that an effective pressure is being used.

Postoperative and drain care

With all types of drain, an Elizabethan collar is strongly advisable to avoid premature removal of the drain, particularly in animals in which the drain is uncovered. The drain is likely to cause some irritation and pain in the wound and analgesic drugs should be given whilst it is in place.

Passive drains

After placement of a Penrose drain, a sterile dressing should be placed over the drain to decrease the risk of nosocomial infection; this should be changed as often as necessary to avoid fluid strike-through (often twice daily). In areas that are difficult to dress effectively, such as the cervical, submandibular and inguinal areas, a sterile adhesive dressing is beneficial. The drain exit site should be cleaned when the dressing is changed, using saline or dilute chlorhexidine.

In the rare cases where a dressing cannot be placed, petroleum jelly (Vaseline) or a topical antibiotic ointment can be placed around the drain exit site to protect the skin.

Closed suction drains

The chamber should be emptied of fluid or air as necessary to maintain suction on the wound, i.e. when it is 50% full. The drain should be handled with gloves when emptying the chamber or reapplying the vacuum. With rigid collection chambers, checking the collapsible button on the chamber can assess the vacuum. If the vacuum has been released, the chamber should be replaced or emptied and the vacuum reapplied. Practically, once the chamber is over half full the vacuum has usually gone. The Redovac collection chambers have a vacuum indicator; when this reaches MIN the bottle should be changed or the vacuum reapplied using dosage tipped 60 ml syringes.

> **PRACTICAL TIP**
> To decrease the risk of nosocomial infection, the drain should be handled with gloves when emptying the chamber or reapplying the vacuum.

Drain removal

Active drains are removed when fluid production decreases, usually after 2–5 days, although with some large oncological resections fluid production may continue for up to 3 weeks. There is little information in the veterinary literature about fluid production by drains. In human surgery the majority of wound fluid is drained by 48 hours after surgery but seroma formation occurs in 10–50% of patients following drain removal (Tadych and Donegan, 1987).

> **PRACTICAL TIP**
> Accepted practice is to remove active suction drains when fluid production is <2–4ml/kg/24h, as this amount may be expected to occur from the inflammatory reaction elicited by the presence of the drain in the wound. If the volume of fluid draining from a wound stays constant for more than 5 days, then removal of the drain is sensible on the basis that the presence of the drain may be contributing to persistent wound drainage.

The optimal time to remove a passive drain is more difficult to assess, but the amount and appearance of the discharge on the dressing can be used as a rough guide. Once fluid production has markedly decreased, the drain should be removed.

> **PRACTICAL TIP**
> If the drain is exposed at both the proximal and distal aspects of the wound, the exposed proximal part should be cut off before withdrawing the rest of the drain from the distal exit point, so that exposed drain is not drawn through the wound.

Cytological analysis of fluid draining from a bite wound will aid in assessing whether the wound is still contaminated. It may also help to assess whether a previously clean wound has become contaminated or infected, as prolonged drainage times increase the risk of postoperative infection.

If the drain has been in place for more than 7–10 days or if the wound was initially contaminated, culture of the tip of the drain is advisable following removal. However, unless the wound appears clinically infected, antibiotic treatment is not warranted in most cases, even if a positive culture result is obtained.

Once the drain has been removed, the exit hole is left to seal by second-intention healing.

If seroma formation occurs after drain removal and leads to wound dehiscence or respiratory problems, or becomes markedly increased in size, it may be necessary to place another drain (see Chapter 12).

Complications

Possible complications associated with the use of drains are:

- Increased risk of infection
- Decreased rate of healing
- Premature removal
- Increased duration of hospitalization.

Risk of infection
The presence of drains in wounds has been shown to increase infection rates in human studies. An experimental study on rabbits demonstrated that retrograde migration of *Streptococcus* spp. along a drain tract from the skin to the peritoneum was significantly less using closed suction drainage (incidence 20%) compared to simple conduit drainage (incidence 90%) (Raves *et al.*, 1984). Similar results were obtained in dogs that had Penrose drains placed experimentally into the peritoneal cavity: after 7 days a positive culture of the same organism that had been placed on the external tip of the drain was obtained from the peritoneum of 90% of the dogs (Nora *et al.*, 1972). The use of closed suction drains is associated with lower infection rates in human surgical wards than are passive drains; however, bacteria can still migrate along the interior of suction tubing and the closed system is compromised when the collection chamber is emptied. Closed collection systems may theoretically reduce the risk of infection.

Decreased rate of healing
The presence of latex drains adjacent to oesophageal and colonic anastomoses has been shown to increase leakage from the anastomosis site in rats (Smith *et al.*, 1982; Cui and Urschel, 2000). Silastic, polyvinyl-chloride and Teflon drains have no effect on healing. The possible detrimental effects of drain placement should be considered alongside the delayed healing that can occur from seroma or haematoma formation if a drain is not used.

Premature removal
Premature removal of drains should be avoided by the use of Elizabethan collars and dressings where appropriate. If the animal traumatizes the drain and there is any suspicion that drain material may be left in the wound, a radiograph should be used to exclude this possibility. Any drain fragments that are left in wounds should be surgically removed to avoid the possibility of persistent wound drainage and fistula formation.

Drains in specific surgeries

Skin grafts
Skin graft survival is dependent upon maintaining close contact between the graft and the recipient bed, so that initial nourishment can occur by imbibition, followed by revascularization of the graft (see Chapter 8). Haematoma or seroma formation is detrimental to graft take. Pope and Swaim (1986a,b) performed a study of the effect of four different drainage techniques (continuous low level suction, piecrust incisions, non-expanded mesh graft and a control group (sheet graft, no drainage)) on graft take. They demonstrated that the continuous suction drain yielded the most fluid from under the graft, followed by the non-expanded mesh graft. Drainage from the continuous suction drain decreased after day 4, at which time the graft was adhered to the wound bed. Survival rates for all grafts were 90%, and cosmetic appearance was similar for all grafts. The authors therefore recommended mesh incisions for drainage of full-thickness skin grafts (Figure 5.12).

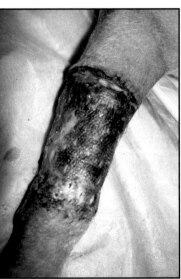

5.12

Meshed skin graft to allow drainage from under a full-thickness skin graft.

Total ear canal ablation and lateral bulla osteotomy

A retrospective study comparing primary closure *versus* the placement of drains after total ear canal ablation and lateral bulla osteotomy demonstrated no difference in short- or long-term complication rates (Devitt *et al.,* 1997). The authors recommended meticulous haemostasis, debridement of devitalized tissue and accurate apposition of tissue planes instead of drain placement.

Aural haematoma

Closed suction silicone drains have been used successfully to treat aural haematomas in dogs (Kagan, 1983; Swaim and Bradley, 1996). This technique, which involves drain placement for 7–28 days after stab incision into the haematoma, resulted in healing with no deformation of the pinna. Compressive dressings were not required.

References and further reading

Anderson DA and White RA (2000) Ischemic bandage injuries: a case series and review of the literature. *Veterinary Surgery* **29**, 488–498

Bonnema J, van Geel AN, Ligtenstein D A *et al.* (1997) Prospective randomized trial of high versus low vacuum drainage after axillary dissection for breast cancer. *American Journal of Surgery* **173**, 76–79

Cui Y and Urschel JD (2000) Latex rubber (Penrose drain) is detrimental to esophagogastric anastomotic healing in rats. *Journal of Cardiovascular Surgery* **41**, 479–481

Devitt CM, Seim HB, Willer R *et al.* (1997) Passive drainage versus primary closure after total ear canal ablation-lateral bulla osteotomy in dogs: 59 dogs (1985–1995). *Veterinary Surgery* **26**, 210–216

Donner GS and Ellison G (1986) The use and misuse of abdominal drains in small animal surgery. *Compendium on Continuing Education* **8**, 705–712

Halfacree ZJ, Wilson A and Baines SJ (2006) In vitro performance of active suction drains. *American College of Veterinary Surgeons Symposium* **35**, E9–E10 [abstract]

Kagan KG (1983) Treatment of canine aural hematoma with an indwelling drain. *Journal of the American Veterinary Medical Association* **183**, 972–974

Lee AH, Swaim SF and Henderson RA (1986) Surgical drainage. *Compendium on Continuing Education* **8**, 94–103

Lee SW, Choi EC, Lee YM *et al.* (2006) Is lack of placement of drains after thyroidectomy with central neck dissection safe? A prospective, randomized study. *Laryngoscope* **116**, 1632–1635

Nora PF, Vanecko RM and Bransfield JJ (1972) Prophylactic abdominal drains. *Archives of Surgery* **105**, 173–176

Parker M, Livingstone V, Clifton R *et al.* (2007) Closed suction surgical drainage after orthopaedic surgery. *Cochrane Database System Review* July 18(3), CD001825

Pope ER and Swaim SF (1986a) Wound drainage from under full-thickness skin grafts in dogs. Part I. Quantitative evaluation of four techniques. *Veterinary Surgery* **15**, 65–71

Pope ER and Swaim SF (1986b) Wound drainage from under full-thickness skin grafts in dogs. Part II. Effect on cosmetic appearance. *Veterinary Surgery* **15**, 72–78

Purushotham AD, McLatchie E, Young D *et al.* (2002) Randomized clinical trial of no wound drains and early discharge in the treatment of women with breast cancer. *British Journal of Surgery* **89**, 286–292

Raves JJ, Slifkin M and Diamond DL (1984) A bacteriologic study comparing closed suction and simple conduit drainage. *American Journal of Surgery* **148**, 618–620

Smith SR, Connolly JC, Crane PW *et al.* (1982) The effect of surgical drainage materials on colonic healing. *British Journal of Surgery* **69**, 153–155

Swaim SF and Bradley DM (1996) Evaluation of closed-suction drainage for treating auricular hematomas. *Journal of the American Animal Hospital Association* **32**, 36–43

Tadych K and Donegan WL (1987) Postmastectomy seromas and wound drainage. *Surgery of Gynecology and Obstetrics* **165**, 483–487

Tokunaga Y, Nakayama N, Nishitai R *et al.* (1998) Effects of closed-system drain in surgery: focus on methicillin-resistant *Staphylococcus aureus*. *Digestive Surgery* **15**, 352–356

Trevor PB, Smith MM, Waldron D *et al.* (1992) Clinical evaluation of axial pattern skin flaps in dogs and cats: 19 cases (1981–1990). *Journal of the American Veterinary Medical Association* **201**, 608–612

Williams J, McHugh D and White R (1992) Use of drains in small animal surgery. *In Practice* **3**, 73–81

CASE EXAMPLE 1:
Drainage of a flank abscess

History
A 6-year-old male neutered 14 kg Springer Spaniel was presented with a 2-week history of reluctance to walk, lumbar pain, inappetence and lethargy.

Assessment and investigation
Clinical examination revealed focal pain along the right flank, in an area where the muscle felt 'doughy'. Haematology profile revealed a mature neutrophilia; biochemical profile was within normal limits. On ultrasound examination the retroperitoneum was of mixed echogenicity. Magnetic resonance imaging of the abdomen revealed fluid pockets in the right flank muscles compatible with abscess formation. Abnormal tissue was also seen in the midline, ventral to lumbar vertebrae 1–2.

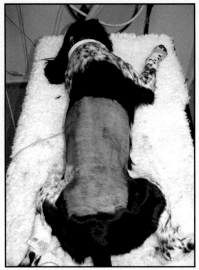

Right flank swelling.

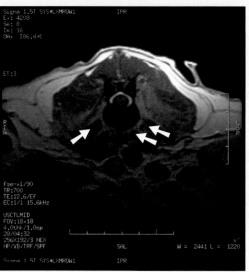

MRI showing changes in the epaxial muscles ventral to L2 (arrowed).

Treatment
A coeliotomy was used to retrieve a grass seed foreign body, which was located in the epaxial muscles adjacent to the second lumbar vertebra. The flank abscess was opened; the purulent discharge was drained and cultured, and the abscess lavaged. A closed suction Jackson–Pratt drain was placed in the wound before closure.

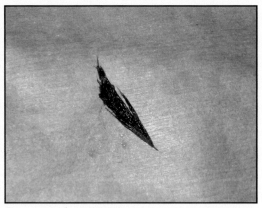

Grass seed foreign body.

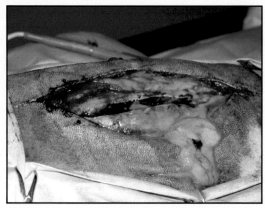

Abscess drainage and lavage.

Case Example 1 continues ▶

CASE EXAMPLE 1 continued:
Drainage of a flank abscess

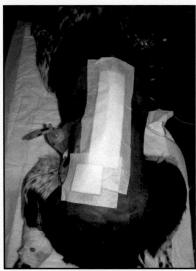

Jackson–Pratt drain in place.

The drain was left in place for 5 days, at which stage <30 ml of serosanguineous discharge was being produced over 24 hours (2 ml/kg/24h). Culture results from the abscess yielded a mixed growth, including *Bacteroides, Peptostreptococcus* and *Actinomyces.* Culture of the tip of the drain at removal was not performed, as the dog was being treated with antibiotics (amoxicillin/clavulanate), which were continued for 3 weeks postoperatively. Recovery postoperatively was uneventful.

CASE EXAMPLE 2:
Surgical management and drainage of a chronic mucocele

History
A 3-year-old female neutered 23 kg Labrador Retriever was presented with a chronic (2-year) swelling ventral to the right mandible. The fluid-filled mass had previously been diagnosed as a salivary mucocele but no treatment had been given. Although the owner did not feel it was bothering the dog, the mass appeared to be increasing in size.

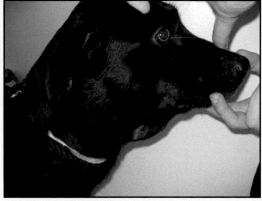

Submandibular swelling.

Assessment and management options
The swelling was compatible with a chronic mucocele originating from the right mandibular and sublingual glands. No oral ranula was evident. The right mandibular salivary gland was palpably enlarged and uneven in texture. The diagnosis was confirmed by aspiration of some fluid and cytological analysis, including periodic acid–Schiff staining, which confirmed the fluid contained mucin. Surgical excision of the right mandibular and sublingual salivary glands was advised, with drainage of the mucocele.

Treatment
The right mandibular and sublingual glands were surgically excised and the damaged area of the sublingual duct was identified. The mucocele was drained via a surgical incision, and a closed suction drain was placed. The drain was in place for 7 days, at which stage <40 ml/24h (1.7 ml/kg/24h) of serosanguineous fluid was being aspirated. Culture of the mucocele and of the drain tip when removed yielded no bacterial growth.

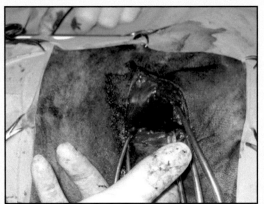

Opening of the mucocele after surgical excision of the mandibular and sublingual salivary glands.

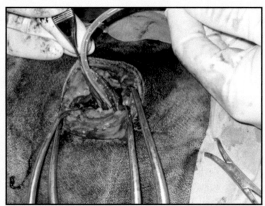

Placement of a closed suction tube drain into the capsule of the mucocele.

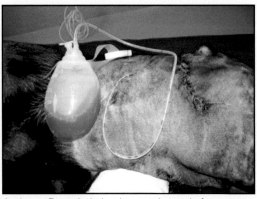

Jackson–Pratt drain in place at the end of surgery.

OPERATIVE TECHNIQUE 5.1:
Placement of a Penrose drain

Positioning
Depends on individual case.

Assistant
Not necessary.

Equipment extras
Penrose drain; haemostat forceps.

Surgical technique
Prior to inserting the drain it should be measured so that in case of premature removal the surgeon will know if any part of the drain has been left in the wound.

1. Place the drain into the wound, avoiding neurovascular bundles.

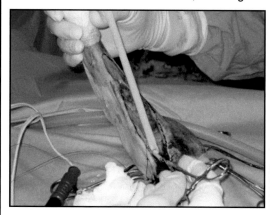

The Penrose drain is placed into the wound and secured proximally by a skin suture that incorporates the drain.

2. Use the haemostat forceps to tunnel from the ventral aspect of the wound to the skin ventral to the wound.
3. Push the haemostats to pull the skin taut and make an incision with a scalpel blade over the top of the haemostat forceps. The exit hole should be 1½ to 2 times larger than the width of the drain to allow easy fluid drainage.

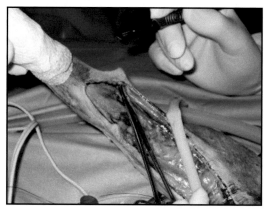

Haemostats are used to make the skin taut so that a scalpel stab incision can be made.

OPERATIVE TECHNIQUE 5.1 continued:
Placement of a Penrose drain

4. Push the forceps back through the skin into the wound. Grasp the tip of the Penrose drain and pull it so it exits the wound. The drain should be exited from the wound adjacent to the primary suture line rather than through the suture line.

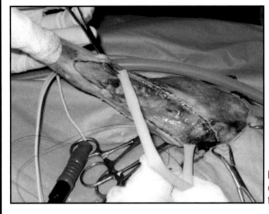

Forceps pull the end of the drain through the exit hole.

5. Fix the drain in place proximally by encircling it with a skin suture placed adjacent to the primary suture line. A second skin suture may be placed at the exit hole, penetrating the drain. Contact between the primary suture line and the drain is avoided by suturing subcutaneous tissue over the drain or directing the drain to the side of the wound.
6. Close the wound.

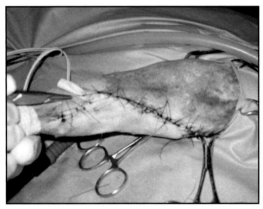

The wound is closed, with the drain exiting ventral to the wound and secured at the exit hole.

If a Penrose drain is placed in a wound that is already closed (such as an abscess), a stab incision is made ventral to the wound and a long pair of forceps, such as Rochester Carmalt or Doyen forceps are used to tunnel the drain through the subcutaneous tissue and into the fluid pocket. The tip of the forceps can be felt through the skin and a skin suture can be placed to encircle the drain in the proximal part of the wound. The drain is also sutured at the exit point, as described above.

Postoperative care
The wound and drain are covered with a dressing, which is changed as soon as strike-through is noticed. Cutting the skin sutures will allow removal of the drain.

OPERATIVE TECHNIQUE 5.2:
Placement of an active suction drain

Positioning
Depends on individual case.

Assistant
Not necessary.

Equipment extras
Active suction drain; haemostat forceps.

Surgical technique
Prior to inserting the drain it should be measured so that in case of premature removal the surgeon will know if any part of the drain has been left in the wound.

1. Place the drain in the wound, ensuring that any holes in the drain will not exit the skin. Avoid neurovascular bundles and, if possible, do not place the drain directly below the skin suture line.

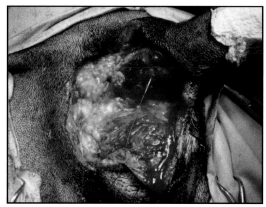

A wound next to the anus, caused by resection of a mast cell tumour. The site is considered contaminated.

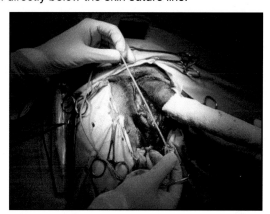

A closed suction drain is selected and measured.

2. If the drain system has a needle attached to the end of the drain tubing, push this through the subcutaneous tissue and skin. Remove the needle and secure the drain tubing in place with a Chinese finger-trap suture of non-absorbable suture material around the drain near the exit hole.

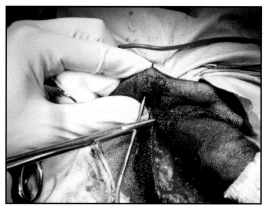

The needle attachment to the drain is exited from the wound.

OPERATIVE TECHNIQUE 5.2 continued:
Placement of an active suction drain

3. If the drain is not attached to a needle, use a pair of small haemostat forceps to tunnel from the wound though the subcutaneous tissue to the skin. Push the forceps to tent the skin, and make an incision over them. Pass the forceps through the skin into the wound; place the drain between the teeth of the forceps and pull it out of the wound. Secure the drain in place with a Chinese finger-trap suture.
4. Close the primary wound.
5. Connect the drain to the collection chamber and apply negative pressure. If the drain system has a single-use collection system, where the vacuum cannot be re-created (e.g. Redovac drain), the drain tubing is kept closed until a fibrin seal has formed over the wound, i.e. after 4–6 hours.

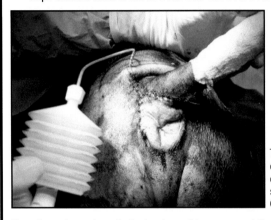

The wound is closed and the drain connected to the collection chamber after being secured to the skin with a Chinese finger-trap suture.

If a closed suction drain is placed in a wound that is already closed (such as an abscess), a stab incision is made adjacent to the wound and a long pair of forceps, such as Rochester Carmalt or Doyen forceps, are used to tunnel the drain through the subcutaneous tissue and into the fluid pocket. The drain is secured with a Chinese finger-trap suture, as described above.

Postoperative care
When possible the drain exit should be covered by a sterile adhesive dressing. A stockinette dressing around the abdomen may be used to secure the collection chamber. Cutting the Chinese finger-trap suture will allow drain removal.

6

Tension-relieving techniques and local skin flaps

Philipp Mayhew

Introduction

Most skin defects seen in small animal patients are created either by traumatic injury or by surgical resection of a diseased area of tissue. In cats and dogs the elasticity of skin, along with the frequent presence of adjacent loose skin in many areas of the body, allows the primary closure of many wounds. However, techniques to reduce tension or to harvest skin from adjacent areas can help, in some cases, to produce a tension-free closure that is less likely to result in wound-healing complications. A working knowledge of such techniques is essential, as their required use cannot always be predicted preoperatively. In situations where primary closure was anticipated but cannot be achieved due to unforeseen circumstances, these techniques can become invaluable. Many of the techniques described in this chapter are very simple and will often be used in combination during wound reconstruction.

Blood supply to the skin

The blood supply to the skin is similar in dogs and cats. It is based on a series of well documented direct cutaneous arteries that supply blood to the subdermal plexus (Figure 6.1), which provides blood supply to the dermis and epidermis. The subdermal plexus is located both superficial and deep to the cutaneous trunci muscle, which is present over the head, neck, thorax and abdomen, being absent only over the distal aspect of the limbs; in those areas the subdermal plexus lies within the deep areolar tissue. When undermining skin, dissection below the subdermal plexus is essential to maintain blood supply and avoid necrosis. In the distal limb this is achieved by dissecting in the plane between the subcutaneous fat and the deep fascia covering skeletal muscle below.

Skin tension

Intrinsic factors

- Different dog breeds possess very different skin characteristics that will profoundly affect the way wound reconstruction is approached: sighthounds have less mobile and less elastic skin than many other breeds; Basset Hounds and Shar-peis have large rolls of skin that will often facilitate primary closure of large wounds.
- Cats have highly elastic skin that can be easily mobilized to cover surprisingly large defects.
- The location of a wound profoundly affects tension. Wounds on the distal limbs are difficult to

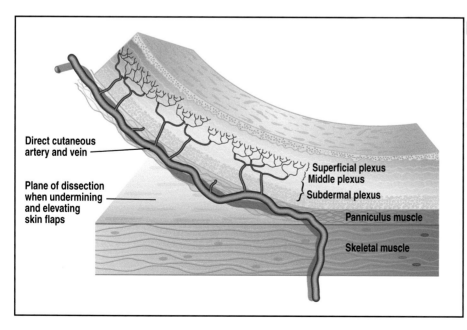

6.1 Vascular supply to canine and feline skin is through direct cutaneous vessels that emerge from the underlying skeletal muscle to supply the subdermal plexus located at the level of the panniculus muscle.

Direct cutaneous artery and vein

Plane of dissection when undermining and elevating skin flaps

Superficial plexus
Middle plexus
Subdermal plexus

Panniculus muscle

Skeletal muscle

close due to the relative dearth of skin that can easily be recruited to these areas. Wounds located over joints will experience significant motion, and tension may vary considerably as the joint moves through its range of motion.
* Other factors such as wound geometry can affect tension. Wounds of identical geometry can be closed in a number of different ways, with each technique potentially resulting in a different amount of tension.

Tension lines of the skin have been well described (Figure 6.2). When a choice exists as to which direction a wound is closed, the long axis of the wound is aligned parallel to the line of tension in that area. Thus, for the thoracic and abdominal wall the long axis of the closure will be directed dorsal-to-ventral rather than cranial-to-caudal. On the limbs the tension lines are less well described; the veterinary surgeon is advised to manipulate the skin gently in opposite directions and then conclude which direction of closure is most likely to result in the least amount of tension.

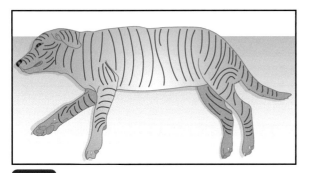

6.2 Tension lines of the skin.

Adverse effects
Excessive tension can lead to dehiscence, either from tearing of sutures through the tissues or through the compromising effect of tension on the cutaneous microcirculation. In highly mobile areas, such as over joints, the effect of tension is likely to be magnified by excessive motion. Excessive scar tissue formation and increased postoperative pain are other detrimental effects of high-tension wound closure. Over the distal limb it is possible to create a tourniquet effect that, within a very short period of time, can result in loss of blood supply to the distal limb and possibly tissue necrosis (Figure 6.3).

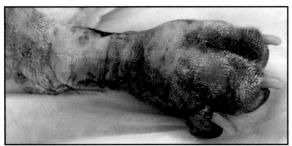

6.3 Excessive tension during closure of a lateral defect on the distal limb has created a tourniquet effect that must be alleviated immediately to avoid foot necrosis.

> **WARNING**
> The rapid development of distal limb oedema and coolness after surgery should prompt: immediate removal of sutures to re-establish blood flow to the foot; and consideration of alternative methods of wound closure.

Techniques to overcome skin tension

Patient positioning
When patients are positioned on a surgical table it is possible to change the degree of tension on a wound dramatically purely by altering patient positioning. For example, a large wound over the back will exhibit greater tension during closure if the animal is positioned in sternal recumbency with the pelvic limbs drawn forward beneath the animal compared to when the limbs are pulled out caudally. The use of positioning aids, such as sandbags under the thoracic or pelvic limb girdles may maximize local skin available for closure of wounds on the trunk and neck. Considering the optimal patient position in this way can greatly facilitate wound closure. Conversely, it is also possible to position the patient on the operating table in such a way as to decrease tension artificially in a way that is not reflected in the animal's awake or weightbearing position. This may lead to a dramatic increase in tension postoperatively, with subsequent complications.

Undermining
A combination of blunt and sharp dissection below the cutaneous trunci muscle on either side of a wound constitutes undermining. It is one of the simplest and most effective ways of harnessing the elasticity of skin and allows a significant reduction in tension at the wound margin (Figure 6.4). Undermining alone can often obviate the need for more complex reconstruction and should always be considered ahead of more complex techniques.

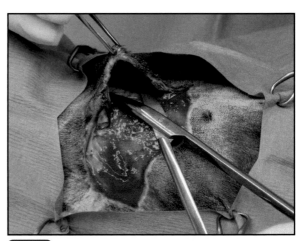

6.4 Undermining below the subdermal plexus.

Manipulating wound geometry

Closure of certain shaped wounds in different ways can have an effect on the amount of tension placed on the wound margin and can affect cosmesis. When circular, square or rectangular defects are closed by simple apposition they will inevitably result in the formation of large 'dog ears'. Conversion of such wounds into an ellipse will require removal of a greater amount of skin, so may only be possible where there is plenty of loose skin available for wound closure, but will usually result in a much improved cosmetic appearance (Figure 6.5a). Circular and square wounds can also be closed by creation of a triangulating or star-shaped closure made up of small flaps that form as skin is advanced inward from the sides of the circle (Figure 6.5b) or square (Figure 6.5c). This may result in less tension at the wound margin, although the point in the centre where these flaps meet has a tendency to dehisce. This may be due to compromised vascular supply at the tip of the flaps or remaining excessive tension.

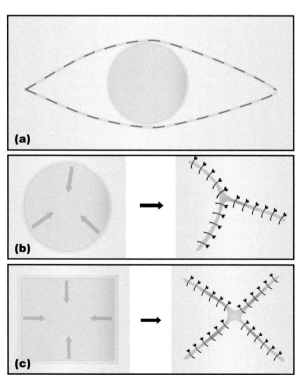

6.5 Manipulation of wound geometry.
(a) Conversion of circular, square or rectangular defects into an ovoid configuration can facilitate closure and improve cosmesis. **(b)** Circular defects can be closed by bringing together three triangular flaps. **(c)** Square defects can be closed in an X-configuration.

Walking sutures

The placement of walking sutures allows undermined skin to be pulled towards the centre of the wound, as well as reducing tension where the skin margins meet. Monofilament absorbable suture material is usually used. Initially, a 'bite' of the wound bed beneath the undermined skin is taken. Subsequently, a 'bite' of the underside of the undermined skin through the cutaneous trunci muscle is taken in a position 1–2 cm further from the centre of the defect than the first bite in the wound bed (see Operative Technique 6.1). As the suture is tightened the undermined skin is pulled towards the centre of the wound. Multiple walking sutures are usually placed in one or more rows that progressively advance skin towards the centre of the wound.

Suture patterns

To achieve uneventful healing of skin it is essential to relieve tension at the skin margin by placement of sutures in the subcutaneous tissues such that the dermis and epidermis are in tension-free apposition.

Interrupted tension-relieving suture patterns are generally used for the subcutaneous tissues and include 'bites' taken through the cutaneous trunci muscle as it has good suture-holding ability. In the limbs where the cutaneous trunci muscle is absent, tension-relieving sutures can be placed in the deep fascia (if it has been incised) or in the deep areolar tissue above the fascia.

If needed, further tension relief can be achieved by placement of a continuous line of intradermal sutures in the deep dermis. Skin sutures or staples can be placed for added security but are not always necessary if good apposition has been achieved simply with the use of the intradermal pattern.

In situations where moderate tension at the skin margin still exists despite placement of sutures in the deeper tissues, tension suture patterns can be used. Vertical mattress, horizontal mattress, 'far-near-near-far' and 'far-far-near-near' patterns (see Chapter 3) can all be used to reduce tension at the skin margin if necessary. Sutures can also be buttressed by passage of the suture through a stent at the skin margin that acts to distribute tension over a greater surface area and minimizes the risk of the sutures cutting through the skin.

Multiple relaxing incisions

The creation of multiple small incisions on one or both sides of a wound can aid in closure of a primary defect. This technique can be especially useful on the distal limbs, where local flaps are not easily created (Figure 6.6). The small incisions are oriented in a plane parallel to the primary defect and the skin between them and the defect is undermined. Separation of the relaxing incisions allows the skin to be stretched into the primary defect. If multiple rows are created, they should be staggered to reduce compromise to the blood supply.

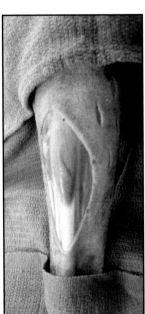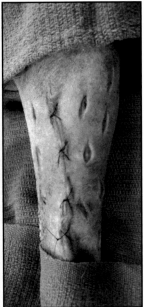

6.6 Multiple relaxing incisions can be created to allow tension relief at the closure of a primary defect over the limb. Illustrated on a cadaver specimen.

This is a very simple technique but does have some disadvantages: vascular compromise can lead to necrosis; and healing of the small incisions with extensive scar tissue formation may mean the cosmetic outcome is not as good as with a local flap.

Skin stretching

When a tensile force is placed across intact skin, an expansion in effective skin area occurs over time. This phenomenon is termed 'mechanical creep' and arises due to the stretching of dermal collagen fibres in line with the direction of the tensile force. This occurs in combination with a phenomenon termed 'stress relaxation', where the fibres no longer require as much force to stay in this alignment. Recognition of these physiological events has given rise to the concept of skin stretching.

Skin stretching (see Operative Technique 6.2) is a non-invasive technique that requires basic and inexpensive equipment and is simple to execute. It can be used preoperatively to harness greater elasticity in the skin, so that when surgery is performed it becomes much easier to close the defect. It can also be used postoperatively to reduce tension on a wound closure, which can then be exposed to progressively greater tension over the course of healing. In general, skin stretching is easiest over the thorax and abdomen where it is easy to retain tension when the animal is weightbearing or moving around.

Tissue expanders

Tissue expanders are inflatable vessels, available in many different shapes and sizes, which are surgically placed adjacent to the defect that is to be closed. They are progressively inflated over time and result in stretching of the overlying skin in a manner similar to that which occurs when skin stretchers are applied. Once they are fully inflated they are removed and the loose skin created is elevated and moved into position. They are usually used in the distal limbs where few other reconstruction methods are available. Their major disadvantages, and the reasons they are no longer used frequently, are manifold: they require a two-step procedure for placement and then reconstruction; necrosis of skin overlying the vessel can occur if there is excessive pressure compressing the subdermal plexus; the vessel is a large foreign body and is prone to infection.

Incisional 'plasty' techniques

Several plasty techniques exist that are designed to provide a moderate degree of tension relief for situations where primary wound closure is not possible due to excessive tension but raising a local flap is not deemed necessary. Their aim is to reduce or redistribute tension in such a way that either the tension at the primary wound margin is reduced, or its magnitude or direction is altered so that it does not have a detrimental effect on function.

should be evaluated preoperatively by palpation of the area. If excessive scar tissue exists and the skin is not movable the desired effect may not occur or will be diminished.

V–Y plasty

V–Y plasty is a very simple technique used to obtain a modest reduction in tension at the primary wound margin. It has been described for management of cicatricial ectropion of the eyelid, where the tension relief provided can aid in reducing corneal exposure.

A V-shaped incision is made adjacent to the primary wound margin with the tip of the V pointing away from the wound (see Operative Technique 6.3). The skin between the V and the wound is undermined, after which the primary wound is closed. In doing so the V incision will assume a Y-shaped configuration and tension relief will be realized at the primary closure site. Closure of the now Y-shaped incision completes the plasty.

PRACTICAL TIP
A V–Y plasty will cause only a modest reduction in tension at the wound margin and is usually used in small peripheral defects. If more significant wound tension exists it may be necessary to use flap or graft techniques instead.

Z-plasty

A chronic non-healing wound over the lateral stifle (Figure 6.7) is a good indication for Z-plasty closure.

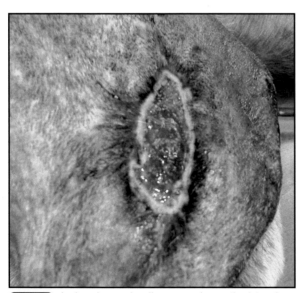

6.7 A chronic non-healing wound over the lateral stifle is a good indication for Z-plasty.

In a Z-plasty (see Operative Technique 6.4) two adjacent equilateral triangular flaps are created, whose alignment is altered to increase the magnitude of their long axis length and reduce tension at the primary wound site. This plasty is designed to provide a moderate reduction in tension at the primary wound site, although multiple Z-plasties can be aligned in series to increase the amount of tension relief.

The increase in length obtained by Z-plasty, and the subsequent degree of tension reduction obtained, can theoretically be calculated based on the size and number of Z incisions and the angles between the arms of the Z. However, in a clinical situation it actually depends upon several factors that are difficult to control, such as the region of the body and the amount of laxity in the skin between the Z-plasty and the primary wound site. In general, as the dimensions of the Z are increased, the magnitude of tension relief becomes greater but the ability to move the flaps becomes harder.

WARNING
This technique is only beneficial if the skin around the Z can be undermined easily and is loose. In areas of extensive scar tissue formation where skin is immobile, tension may not be alleviated.

PRACTICAL TIP
If local anatomy precludes the formation of one large Z, multiple smaller Z-plasties can be created in series, the resulting tension relief from each Z-plasty being additive, though smaller than one large Z (Figure 6.8).

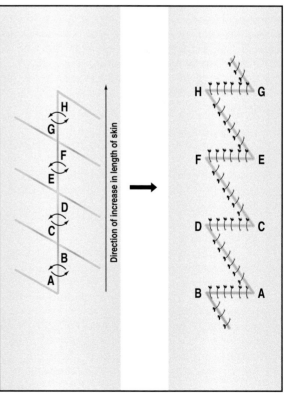

6.8 Multiple Z-plasties can be aligned in series, oriented perpendicular to the long axis of a wound. The cumulative magnitude of tension relief will be additive. The tip of each triangle for each Z (A, B, C, etc.) is transposed into its opposing wound bed and sutured.

Local subdermal plexus flaps

- Pedicle grafts denote all techniques that involve elevation of an area of skin that in some way remains attached to its vascular bed.
- Axial pattern flaps (see Chapter 7) incorporate a direct cutaneous artery and vein and have very reliable and well described vascular angiosomes capable of providing blood supply to large areas of skin.
- Local subdermal plexus flaps are, by definition, flaps that have a vascular supply provided by the subdermal plexus from the flap base, without the known inclusion of a direct cutaneous artery and vein.

Local subdermal plexus flaps are mostly harvested from skin adjacent to the primary defect. They cannot be made into an 'island' flap (i.e. the base cannot be severed) and they are generally capable of supporting smaller areas of skin than axial pattern flaps. They are, however, one of the most frequently used flap types in general practice, due to their simplicity and versatility. Certain guidelines need to be followed to ensure optimal results.

Blood supply

Local flaps possess a less reliable blood supply than axial pattern flaps, as they are dependent upon the subdermal plexus alone. The dimensions of a flap are critical in determining flap survival and depend to a large extent on vascular supply, although factors such as tension, motion and trauma also play significant roles. No linear relation exists between flap dimensions and flap survival. Therefore, it is difficult to give accurate guidelines that surgeons can use when elevating flaps. In general the following points should be observed:

- Create flaps that are only just large enough to cover the primary defect and avoid flaps that are very long
- Maximize the width of the base of the flap as much as possible. A 2:1 flap length:base width ratio is a good guideline

PRACTICAL TIPS
- In general, a greater base width to flap length ratio will not guarantee flap survival if the flap is too long but it will maximize the chances of inadvertently including larger cutaneous vessels.
- When large defects are to be covered, the surgeon should consider the use of axial pattern flaps, multiple local flaps or a combination of reconstruction techniques.

Flap elevation

With any defect there is always a choice of harvest sites for local flap creation. Selection of flap type is based on several factors but in all cases the simplest flap type that is likely to be successful should be chosen. Flaps can be created by advancing skin in a straight direction (advancement flap) or a rotational pattern (rotation flap), or skin can be transposed into position by pivoting it 30 to 120 degrees from its base (transposition flap). When flaps are created there remains a donor bed that is usually closed primarily. The defect created must not expose vital structures. It must not be in a high motion area and ideally it should not be difficult to close. There must be adequate elasticity and motion of the flap or movement into the primary defect will not be possible. Areas with extensive scarring are not good potential flap beds.

The elevation of local flaps can be done in several ways. The preferred technique is to incise skin sharply with a scalpel blade. Use of a carbon dioxide laser has been described; it results in improved haemostasis but may be associated with delayed healing and possibly a higher incidence of flap dehiscence. Once the skin has been incised, elevation of the flap proceeds by undermining deep to the subdermal plexus.

Once the flap has been elevated, careful handling is essential. Gentle tissue handling includes the use of fine-gauge stay sutures or the use of fine tissue forceps, such as Adson toothed thumb forceps or Adson–Brown thumb forceps, and is helpful in minimizing trauma, especially to the tip of the flap, which has the most tenuous blood supply.

PRACTICAL TIP
Towel clamps can be used to hold the flap in position temporarily during the planning stages of wound closure, but they should be used judiciously as they will cause some tissue trauma.

Single pedicle advancement flap
This is a very simple flap to elevate (see Operative Technique 6.5) and does not create a 'donor' bed defect, as skin is simply advanced in a straight direction into the defect, but the technique does have some disadvantages. The amount of skin coverage that can be achieved depends heavily on how much loose skin is available adjacent to the wound, which will vary with region, and with species and breed of the animal.

WARNING
Advancement of too great an area of skin will result in significant wound tension through the 'elastic recoil' that tends to occur with this flap; this may promote dehiscence.

Care must be taken that resulting tension does not alter the function of essential structures close to the wound margin; for example, when the flap is used to close the eyelid margin it is possible for the lid margin to be distorted. The technique is very useful for closure of defects on top of the head (Figure 6.9), where the abundant skin on the dorsum of the neck (in most breeds) can be utilized.

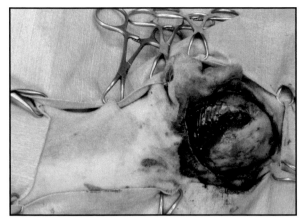

6.9 Defects on the head are especially amenable to single pedicle advancement flap development.

If a large defect is present and loose skin is available on either side of the defect, opposing single pedicle advancement flaps can be raised, such that an H-plasty is created (Figure 6.10). This is often a better option than one large single pedicle flap.

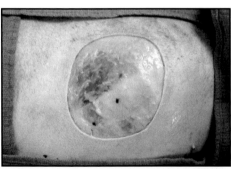

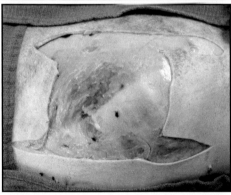

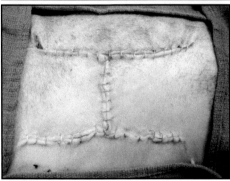

6.10 H-plasty. When a single pedicle advancement flap provides inadequate tension relief, two opposing flaps can be created and sutured in place in an H configuration. Illustrated on a cadaver specimen.

With most single pedicle advancement flaps and H-plasties some 'dog ear' formation will occur at the base of the flap. If small, these can be ignored and they will remodel over time. If they are substantial, they can be excised by resection of the so-called Burow's triangles – triangular pieces of skin that form the 'dog ears'. They are easily excised but care must be taken to remove them in such a manner that flap base width remains uncompromised (Figure 6.11).

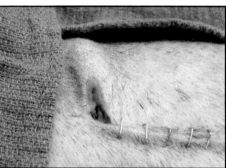

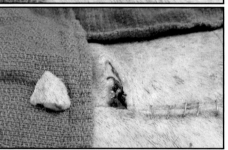

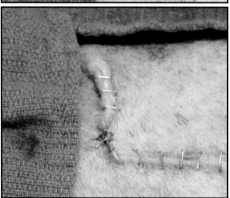

6.11 Large 'dog ears' can be excised but their excision should not narrow the base of axial pattern or subdermal plexus flaps. Illustrated on a cadaver specimen.

Bipedicle advancement flap
This simple flap has two vascular pedicles that remain intact at either end (see Operative Technique 6.6), thus assuring a more reliable blood supply than a single pedicle advancement flap when similar flap dimensions are compared.

> **WARNING**
> **Vascular compromise can arise if the flap is too narrow.**

This flap is essentially synonymous with a large releasing incision. Its disadvantage is that a second wound is created that has to heal by secondary intention (Figure 6.12) or needs to be closed with a second reconstructive procedure. The flap is planned in such a way that the secondary defect is a fresh wound with intact deep fascia and muscle and a good blood supply, representing a good healing environment. Bipedicle advancement flaps are frequently used on the extremities where few other options exist for closure of large wounds and may be useful to close wounds over orthopaedic implants.

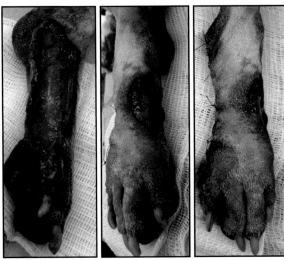

6.12 Defects on the lateral or medial metatarsal region are good candidates for bipedicle advancement flaps as few other reconstructive procedures are possible in these areas. The releasing incision was left open to heal by secondary intention after closure of the primary defect.

Rotation flap

Rotation flaps (see Operative Technique 6.7) are classically used to close triangular defects by creating a semicircular incision from the base of the triangle and extending the incision until there is enough laxity to the flap to allow tension-free closure of the defect. The semicircular incision is continued until enough skin has been advanced to close the defect, which typically occurs with an incision approximately four times the length of the defect margin. Rotational flaps can be used to close incisions of many configurations, not just triangular ones (Figure 6.13).

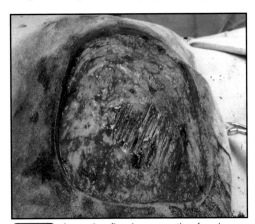

6.13 A rotation flap is one option for closure of a large ovoid shaped defect created by resection of a tumour over the lateral thigh (see Operative Technique 6.7).

Transposition flap

This is a very versatile local flap that can be created from most areas of the body apart from the distal extremities, where closure of the 'donor' bed is usually challenging. Transposition flaps (see Operative Technique 6.8) are created by selecting a rectangular area of loose elastic skin, one of whose borders forms one border of the defect. Once the skin to be transposed has been selected, the flap is elevated and transposed into the defect by pivoting on the point of the flap base that is farthest from the defect. Transposition flaps are usually pivoted through 45–90 degrees. While they can be pivoted to a greater degree, this will result in significant shortening of the flap.

A similar pivoting flap where there is no contact between the flap and the defect is termed an interpolation flap but is not frequently used. Axial pattern flaps are transposition or interpolation flaps that contain a direct cutaneous artery and vein rather than relying upon the subdermal plexus for a blood supply (see Chapter 7).

Axillary and inguinal fold flaps

These subdermal plexus flaps are capable of closing comparatively large defects over many different areas of the trunk, ventral thorax and abdomen, as well as the medial and lateral aspects of the proximal limbs. Their size and reliability is mainly attributed to the abundance of loose skin that exists in the axillary and inguinal folds and the fact that once the flap is elevated its lateral and medial surfaces, when combined, create a flap that is in effect twice the surface area that it initially appears. Depending upon the way they are used, some fold flaps could also be termed rotation or transposition flaps. In each case the fold flaps have four attachments to the body: a proximal and distal attachment to the trunk; and a medial and lateral attachment to the proximal limb. Any three of these four attachments are incised to create a flap whose base is continuous with the trunk or proximal limb. The techniques are illustrated in Operative Techniques 6.9 and 6.10.

Distant direct flaps

A distant direct flap can be either single pedicled (hinge) or bipedicled (pouch) and is used to reconstruct distal limb deficits by moving the affected limb to the flank, where the flap is created.

> **PRACTICAL TIP**
> Prior to creating a distant direct flap it is advisable to bandage the patient's limb to the flank for 24–48 hours to ensure that it will tolerate the limb being held in that position for an extended period of time.

The flap is raised over the flank, the exact position depending upon which limb is affected and the precise location of the wound. The width of the flap should be slightly wider than that of the defect (to allow for contraction), with the length of the flap being based on the size of the defect. In general, smaller wounds are managed by use of a single pedicle flap whilst a bipedicled flap is ideally suited for circumferential defects. In the author's experience it is usually preferable to create a bipedicled flap, as there seems to be less tension on the flap compared with using a single pedicle flap. It may not be possible to use a bipedicled flap in distal thoracic limb wounds in some dogs, however, as it is not always possible to rotate the limb into the flap; in such cases a single pedicle flap must be used.

- In creating the flap, as with all flaps in the dog and cat, it is essential to incise and undermine deep to the cutaneous trunci muscle (Figure 6.14).
- The flap edges are then sutured to the wound using a suitable gauge monofilament nylon or polypropylene.
- Either a suction drain or a Penrose drain is placed to prevent fluid accumulation in the ventral part of a bipedicled flap or a ventrally based hinge flap.
- The limb is then secured in place with a 'body bandage' for 14 days. The bandage is changed every 2–3 days.

- After this the flap is severed as a staged procedure to ensure that the risk of flap ischaemia is kept to a minimum. It is recommended to section each flap attachment over 2 days, i.e. the base of a hinge flap is incised halfway across on day 14 and the incision sutured, and the second half is sectioned on day 15. On day 15 the sutures placed on day 14 are removed and the 'free end' of the flap is sutured to the wound defect on the limb. With a bipedicled flap the procedure is repeated on the second base on days 16 and 17 before releasing the flap to cover the wound.

This is a time-consuming and often expensive technique, due to the number of dressing changes required and the fact that patients often require sedation to carry them out. It is now less popular due to the use of simpler, less intensive techniques (e.g. free skin grafting or axial pattern flaps) but should still be considered for difficult distal extremity wounds where the patient will tolerate it.

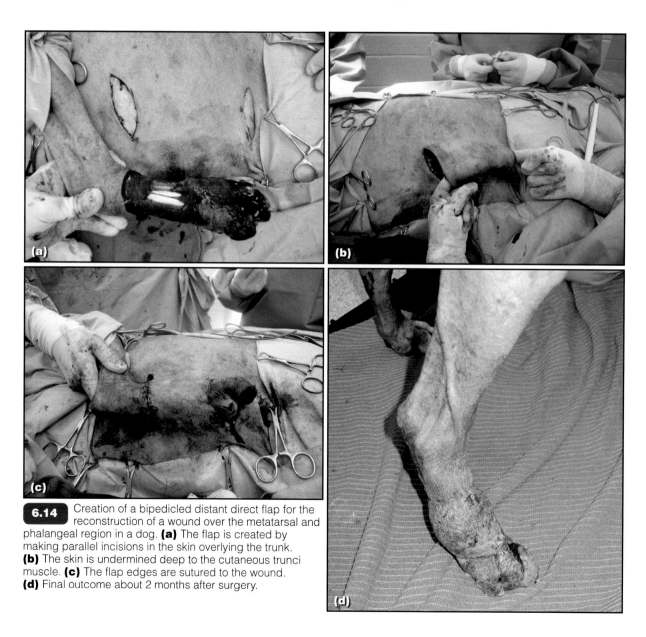

6.14 Creation of a bipedicled distant direct flap for the reconstruction of a wound over the metatarsal and phalangeal region in a dog. **(a)** The flap is created by making parallel incisions in the skin overlying the trunk. **(b)** The skin is undermined deep to the cutaneous trunci muscle. **(c)** The flap edges are sutured to the wound. **(d)** Final outcome about 2 months after surgery.

Complications of skin flaps

Most complications of local skin flaps result from technical errors but may also be caused by self-trauma.

Seroma formation (see Chapter 12) occurs, especially with reconstruction of larger wounds. When significant dead space is present, the placement of a closed suction drain, such as a Jackson–Pratt drain, is helpful in avoiding seroma formation as it pulls serous fluid from the dead space and, in so doing, promotes adhesion of the underside of the flap to the wound bed (see Operative Technique 6.7). Reconstruction of large wounds that involve the thigh or inguinal areas are especially prone to seroma formation. Prevention is better than cure but when small seromas do arise they will usually self-resolve, although bandaging may hasten their resolution. Very large seromas can be opened and a drain placed to minimize recurrence.

WARNING
Drains should be used with caution in large oncological resections, as their exit at a location distant from the primary surgery site may dramatically increase the size of any subsequent resections (if incomplete resection or tumour recurrence occurs) or radiation therapy treatments.

Flap dehiscence is usually the result of excessive tension. All attempts should be made to remove tension from the skin margin by placement of sufficient sutures in the subcutaneous tissues. Sufficient undermining of local flaps is essential to allow tension-free movement of the flap into place. If excessive tension is deemed to exist postoperatively, bandaging to reduce motion, or postoperative skin stretcher placement to reduce tension for the first few days after surgery, can be considered.

Distal flap necrosis is usually the result of technical error or trauma to the flap blood supply (see Case Example 1). It usually becomes obvious 2–5 days postoperatively. Care must be taken when planning flap margins to maximize the width of the flap base in relation to the flap length. Gentle tissue handling is essential to minimize trauma to the distal flap blood supply. Attempts at minimizing flap tip necrosis have been used, such as hyperbaric oxygen or thrombolytic agents, but are not very practical in most clinical situations.

Further reading

Hunt GB, Tisdall P, Liptak JM *et al.* (2001) Skin-fold advancement flaps for closing large proximal limb and trunk defects in dogs and cats. *Veterinary Surgery* **30**, 440–448
Mison MB, Steficek B, Lavagnino M *et al.* (2003) Comparison of the effects of the CO_2 surgical laser and conventional surgical techniques on healing and wound tensile strength of skin flaps in dogs. *Veterinary Surgery* **32**, 153–160
Pavletic MM (1999) *Atlas of Small Animal Reconstructive Surgery, 3rd edn.* WB Saunders, Philadelphia

CASE EXAMPLE 1:
Hemimaxillectomy and transposition flap for a maxillary mass

History

A 5-year-old Hungarian Vizsla was presented with a mass over the right maxillary area that had been progressively enlarging over the previous month. An incisional biopsy led to a diagnosis of fibrosarcoma.

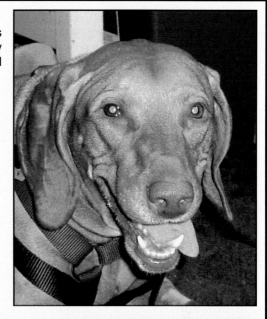

Treatment

A right-sided hemimaxillectomy was performed to remove the tumour. This left a large defect extending from just cranial to the medial canthus of the right eye almost to the margin of the nasal planum. A small margin of skin was deliberately left intact so that skin transposed into the defect did not have to be sutured to the nasal cartilages.

This defect was challenging for many reasons: it was in an area without a large amount of loose skin available, that was difficult to immobilize and protect from self-trauma, and very visible to the owner, making an acceptable cosmetic result even more desirable.

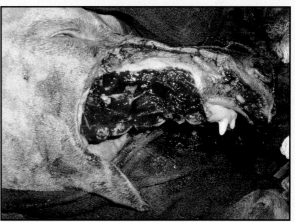

Several options could be considered. The simplest techniques for closure of smaller lip and maxillary defects involve taking advantage of the loose and abundant amounts of skin in the lips of many breeds of dog; this allows labial advancement or buccal rotation flaps to be created. The superficial temporal axial pattern flap could also be considered, although this is usually brought down between the eyes to cover more midline defects and probably would not have extended far enough ventrally to allow coverage of this aspect of the wound. A transposition flap was used in this case and rotated approximately 120 degrees into position to close the defect.

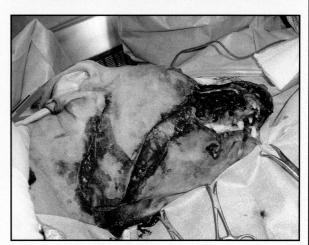

Case Example 1 continues ▶

CASE EXAMPLE 1 continued:
Hemimaxillectomy and transposition flap for a maxillary mass

Initially the flap incorporated the superficial temporal artery and vein, but these were severed as they were acting to tether the flap and prevent it reaching the cranial margin of the defect, likely resulting in significant loss of vascular supply. The flap was rotated into position and its borders were sutured with a layer of interrupted horizontal mattress sutures in the subcutaneous tissues, followed by interrupted cruciate skin sutures. A section of lower lip margin that was not resected was advanced as a labial advancement flap to try and maintain as much normal mucocutaneous junction as possible on the upper lip.

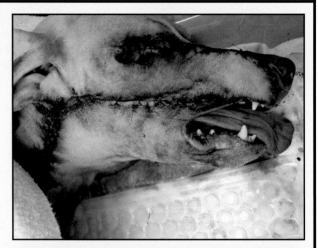

Complications
Four days after the initial surgery necrosis of the distal tip of the flap was evident.

This area was debrided and the remainder of the flap pulled more cranially to cover as much of the remaining defect as possible. This case highlights the inability of the subdermal plexus alone to ensure a sufficient blood supply to large or long flaps. Unfortunately it is difficult to predict distal flap necrosis as there is extensive regional variation in vascular density.

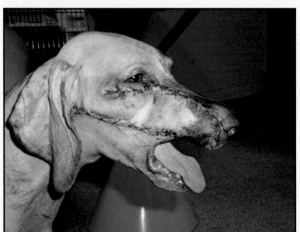

Outcome
After debridement the flap healed uneventfully. A small area at the cranial margin was left to heal by secondary intention, resulting in a suboptimal cosmetic outcome but one the owners were satisfied with.

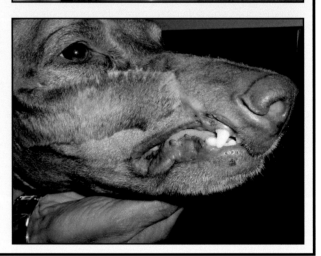

CASE EXAMPLE 2:
Axillary fold flaps after excision of a thoracic mass

History
A 9-year-old Cairn Terrier presented with a 3-month history of a progressively enlarging mass over the ventral thorax. The owners reported that the mass had been growing rapidly. Cytological evaluation of fine needle aspirates revealed a mast cell tumour. The dog was otherwise healthy.

Treatment
Management options
Mast cell tumours have traditionally been treated with wide surgical excision, incorporating a 3 cm margin of grossly normal tissue lateral to all grossly visible tumour margins, and resection of at least one fascial plane deep to the tumour. Recent evidence has suggested that a 2 cm margin may be adequate for achieving a 'clean margin' of resection in grade I and II tumours (Fulcher *et al.*, 2006). Unfortunately the grade of the tumour cannot be obtained from cytology and so is rarely available prior to resection. In cases such as this where wound closure may be difficult, taking a 2 cm margin can significantly reduce the size of the defect, facilitating closure by reducing tension and minimizing the chance of dehiscence. However, in areas where there is adequate skin it is still recommended that a 3 cm margin of resection be taken.

In this case primary closure would have been impossible due to excessive tension. Bilateral single pedicle advancement flaps elevated from the ventral neck and caudal abdomen could be considered, although excessive tension would remain a concern. Delayed free skin graft application following confirmation of a 'clean' surgical resection on biopsy would be possible, although this is an area that is difficult to immobilize and one that receives significant direct pressure when the dog lays on the area. Elevating thoracodorsal axial pattern flaps would be an option, although positioning during surgery is challenging due to the need for access to the dorsum of the dog as well as its ventral thorax.

Bilateral axillary fold flaps were used in this case. The axillary fold provides a surprisingly large area of easily mobilized skin adjacent to the wound.

Surgical technique
A marker pen was used to delineate the grossly palpable tumour tissue and a 2 cm margin of normal tissue was resected around the tumour.

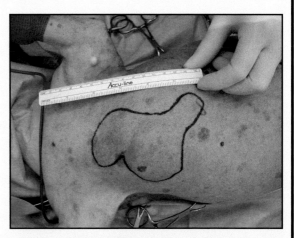

A skin incision was made along this margin. To achieve a deep margin the superficial and deep pectoral muscles that lay directly beneath the tumour were resected, rather than just peeling the fascia from these muscles. The less aggressive approach can be used in some cases but this tumour was not well circumscribed and was relatively well fixed to the pectoral muscles beneath. It was therefore felt that removing these muscles *en bloc* with the tumour would increase the likelihood of achieving a 'clean' deep margin.

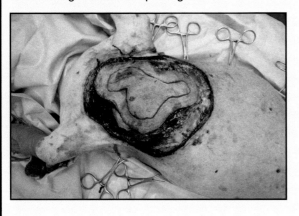

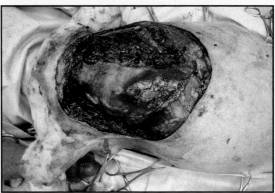

Case Example 2 continues ▶

CASE EXAMPLE 2 continued:
Axillary fold flaps after excision of a thoracic mass

Once the tumour had been removed, the axillary fold flaps were mobilized by incising their medial, lateral and distal attachments and rotating them 90 degrees on to the ventral thorax. To aid with surgical planning they were held in place using towel clamps; care was taken not to cause too much tissue trauma, especially to the tips of the flaps. Using stay sutures may be a less traumatic alternative.

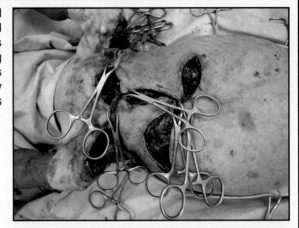

Once in place, all flaps were sutured using interrupted horizontal mattress sutures of 2 metric (3/0 USP) polydioxanone in the subcutaneous tissue incorporating the cutaneous trunci muscle. Interrupted cruciate skin sutures were then placed using 2 metric nylon.

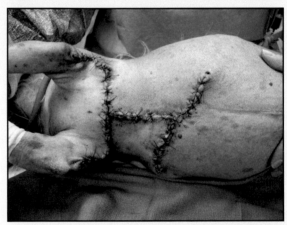

Postoperative management and outcome
After surgery, non-adherent dressings were placed over the wound and incorporated into a bandage around the chest for 5 days. Dressings were changed daily to absorb any wound discharge and provide some degree of immobilization. The owner was advised to give the dog strict rest and keep it in a well padded area to minimize direct pressure when it was lying down. Biopsy results revealed the mass to be a grade III mast cell tumour with no neoplastic cells seen at the margins of the resected specimen. Appropriate postoperative analgesia is imperative in these cases, as the site remains very painful for several days after surgery. This dog healed well and made a good recovery.

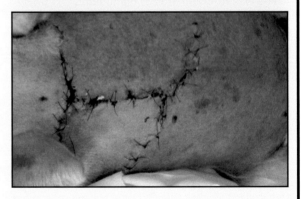

Reference
Fulcher RP, Ludwig LL, Bergman PJ *et al.* (2006) Evaluation of a two-centimeter lateral surgical margin for excision of grade I and grade II cutaneous mast cell tumors in dogs. *Journal of the American Veterinary Medical Association* **228**, 210–215

OPERATIVE TECHNIQUE 6.1:
Walking sutures

Patient positioning
Depends on location of the wound.

Assistant
Helpful to elevate skin margin during suture placement.

Equipment extras
None.

Surgical technique
1. Undermine the skin deep to the subdermal plexus to free up the skin to be advanced in order to close the wound.
2. Take a 'bite' of the undermined dermis with 1.5 to 2 metric (4/0 to 3/0 USP) monofilament absorbable suture material.
3. Take a 'bite' through the deep muscle fascia in the wound bed, in a location 1–2 cm closer to the defect margin. Alternatively, the suture can be placed first in the wound bed followed by the undermined dermis.

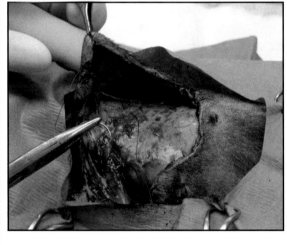

Placement of a walking suture in the wound bed is demonstrated. A bite of the underlying wound bed is taken, followed by a bite of the deep dermis 1–2 cm more distant from the wound margin.

4. Tighten the suture; this advances the undermined skin towards the defect, resulting in a decrease in tension at the wound margin.
5. One or multiple staggered lines of walking sutures can be placed on each side of the wound in order to create an equal decrease in tension across the entire length of the wound closure.

WARNING
Walking sutures are sometimes unknowingly placed around vessels in the subdermal plexus, resulting in vascular compromise. For this reason the minimal number judged necessary should be used and they must not be placed close together.

Postoperative care
Standard postoperative wound care for any wound includes minimizing motion by enforcement of strict rest. Observation for evidence of developing wound dehiscence or infection is important.

OPERATIVE TECHNIQUE 6.2:
Skin stretching

Positioning
Depends on location of the defect.

Assistant
Not required.

Equipment extras
A skin-stretching kit.

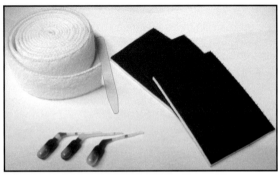

Skin-stretching kit: self-adherent
Velcro-covered skin patches;
elastic connecting tape; and
tissue glue (cyanoacrylate).
These can be purchased from
department stores.

Surgical technique
If skin stretchers are to be applied over an open wound, standard bandaging should be applied first and the skin stretchers placed over the wound dressing. The skin must be clean and dry prior to skin stretcher placement.

1. Clip the hair closely over an area at least 10 cm wide around the wound. Wash the area thoroughly with a surgical scrub; then apply an alcohol preparation. Allow the skin to dry completely.
2. Apply cyanoacrylate glue to the underside of the self-adherent patches prior to their application to the skin.
3. Place the patches on to the skin 5–10 cm away from the wound margin. Patches are placed on all sides of the wound to allow multidirectional skin stretching.

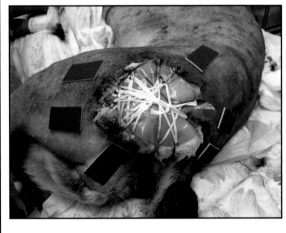

The wound has been packed
with dressing and a tie-over
bandage applied. Adhesive
patches have been applied
to the clean and dry skin
around the wound.

OPERATIVE TECHNIQUE 6.2 continued:
Skin stretching

4. Once patches are in place and the glue has dried, place the elastic connecting tapes on to the Velcro patches, exerting mild tension across the defect.

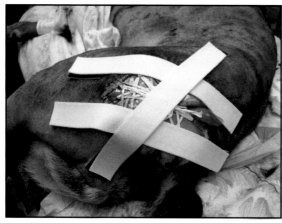

Stretching tapes in place.

5. Increase the tension in the elastic tapes by a small amount every 6 hours for 24–96 hours.

WARNING
Applying extreme tension as soon as the stretchers are placed will usually lead to the patches peeling off prematurely.

Postoperative care
Strict rest should be enforced to minimize motion at the wound site. An Elizabethan collar should be placed to prevent self-trauma. Once skin stretching is complete, the pads can be gently peeled off the skin. If the glue is difficult to remove, application of nail polish remover will facilitate this.

PRACTICAL TIP
Skin stretchers can also be used postoperatively for 3–5 days to reduce tension at suture lines and decrease the chance of dehiscence.

OPERATIVE TECHNIQUE 6.3:
V–Y plasty

Positioning
Depends on location of the wound.

Assistant
Not required.

Equipment extras
None.

Surgical technique

1. Make a V-shaped incision no less than 3 cm from the margin of the defect to be closed, with the tip of the V directed *away from* and *perpendicular to* the long axis of the defect.

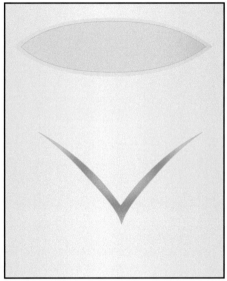

V-shaped incision.

2. Undermine the skin around the V incision and the defect as much as is necessary.
3. Close the original defect. The skin on the inside of the V will be pulled towards the incision, thereby reducing tension at the defect closure.

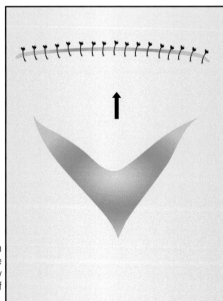

The skin has been undermined and the defect closed. The arrow shows the direction of movement of the skin.

OPERATIVE TECHNIQUE 6.3 continued:
V–Y plasty

4. The incision will then assume a more Y-shaped configuration and can be sutured closed following this pattern.

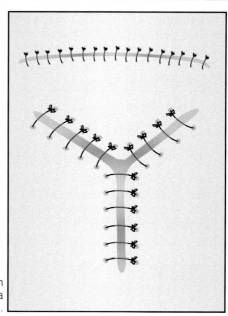

The incision is closed in a Y shape.

Postoperative care
Standard postoperative wound care for any wound includes minimizing motion by enforcement of strict rest. Observation for evidence of developing wound dehiscence or infection is important.

OPERATIVE TECHNIQUE 6.4:
Z-plasty

Positioning
Depends on location of the wound.

Assistant
Not required.

Equipment extras
None.

Surgical technique

1. Make a Z-shaped incision, starting 3–5 cm from the primary wound margin, with the central limb *perpendicular* to the long axis of the primary wound. The arms of the Z are usually placed at 60 degrees to its central limb. The length of the arms of the Z will depend on location and availability of free skin in the area, but is typically 3–8 cm.

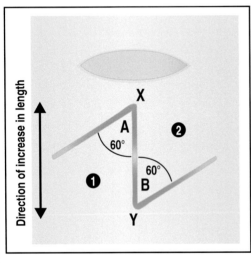

Planning a Z-plasty. The arms are of equal length and at 60-degree angles to the central limb, which is perpendicular to the wound. The tip of triangle 1 (A) will be moved to opposite position Y, and the tip of triangle 2 (B) will be moved to opposite position X. This will allow stretching of the skin in the direction of the X–Y axis.

2. Undermine the skin of the two triangular flaps and the skin between the Z and the defect. The central limb of the Z will be seen to lengthen as tension at the primary defect is redirected.
3. Transpose the two triangular flaps from their original wound beds into their respective opposite wound beds and suture them into place.

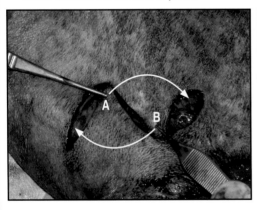
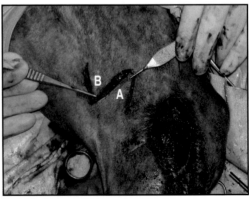

Z-plasty used to close a defect over the lateral stifle (see Figure 6.7). Triangular skin flaps are transposed into their opposing wound beds.

OPERATIVE TECHNIQUE 6.4 continued:
Z-plasty

4. The primary defect can now be closed with reduced tension.

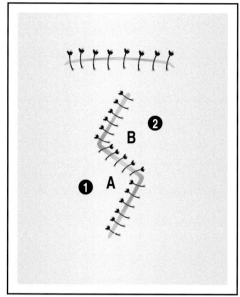

The tips of triangles 1 and 2 are shown in their new positions. After primary wound closure the Z is seen to elongate.

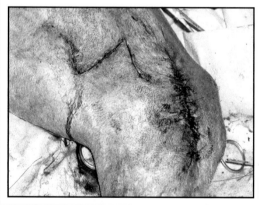

The Z and the primary defect have been closed.

Postoperative management
Standard postoperative wound care for any wound includes minimizing motion by enforcement of strict rest. Observation for evidence of developing wound dehiscence or infection is important. Avoid self-trauma to the incisions by bandaging extremities, using Elizabethan collars.

OPERATIVE TECHNIQUE 6.5:
Single pedicle advancement flap

Positioning
Depends on location of the wound.

Assistant
Not required.

Equipment extras
None.

Surgical technique

1. Palpate the skin in the proposed donor site to ensure that sufficient elasticity exists for advancement.
2. The leading edge of the flap will form one border of the defect; thus, the width of the flap is equal to the width of the defect. Make two, slightly diverging, skin incisions to create the flap length. This ensures a base to the flap that is slightly wider than the tip, minimizing compromise to the vascular supply. Flap length generally equals the length of the defect.
3. Undermine the skin deep to the subdermal plexus and gradually pull the skin flap forward with the help of stay sutures or careful forceps handling.

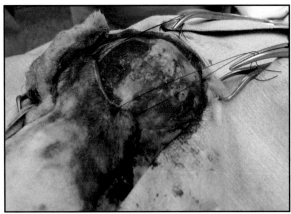 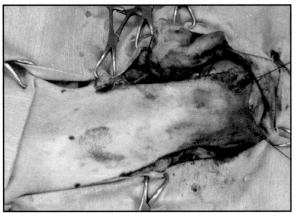

The flap is gradually advanced over the defect by progressive lengthening and undermining. Tension can be judged by exerting traction on stay sutures placed in the flap tip.

4. Once the flap is judged to stretch far enough to cover the defect without excessive tension it can be sutured into place. The flap can be lengthened as necessary to close the defect, as long as a flap of excessive length is not created.

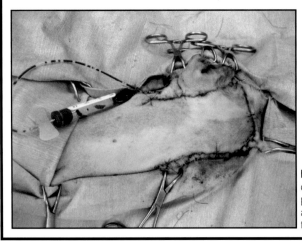

Flap sutured in place. A small closed suction drain has been placed to drain dead space and promote flap adhesion to the wound bed.

OPERATIVE TECHNIQUE 6.5 continued:
Single pedicle advancement flap

91

5. Any 'dog ears' that form at the base of the flap can either be left alone or excised if they are large. Any excision must be done in such a way that the width of the flap base is not compromised.

Postoperative care
Standard postoperative wound care for any wound that is closed with some tension includes minimizing motion by enforcement of strict rest. Observation for evidence of developing wound dehiscence or infection is important.

OPERATIVE TECHNIQUE 6.6:
Bipedicle advancement flap (releasing incision)

Positioning
Depends on location of the wound.

Assistant
Not required.

Equipment extras
None.

Surgical technique

1. Make an incision parallel to the long axis of the primary defect at least 2–10 cm from the wound margin, depending upon the size of the animal. This ensures that blood supply to the flap is preserved. It can be curved slightly with the concave side facing the defect.

   WARNING
   Do not make the distance between the primary wound and the releasing incision too small, as this may compromise the subdermal plexus blood supply from the dual pedicles.

   PRACTICAL TIP
   A bipedicle advancement flap can be created on either side of the defect to further minimize tension when the defect is closed.

2. Undermine the skin between the primary defect and the releasing incision deep to the subdermal plexus to allow tension relief when the primary defect is closed.
3. The defect created by closure of the primary incision can be left to heal by secondary intention or another reconstructive technique can be used to close it. Apply a non-adherent wound dressing to the surface of the open wound if the defect created is not primarily reconstructed.

Postoperative care
If the releasing incisions are left open to granulate it will be necessary to bandage the area to avoid contamination at least until a bed of granulation tissue has formed, which usually occurs within 3–5 days. Bandage changes should be performed as required during this time. The patient should be strictly rested for 2 weeks and the area inspected regularly for evidence of wound infection or signs of dehiscence.

OPERATIVE TECHNIQUE 6.7:
Rotation flap

Positioning
Depends on location of the defect.

Assistant
Not required.

Equipment extras
None.

Surgical technique

1. Make a semicircular incision, extending from one side of the defect. The extent of the semicircular incision is dependent on the amount of tension that remains when the flap is advanced into position. A full 180 degrees semicircle only needs to be completed if deemed necessary to relieve tension at the leading edge of the flap.

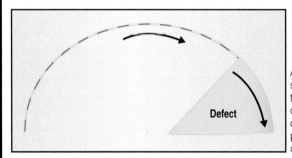

A semicircular incision starting from one tip of a triangular or square defect creates a flap that can be rotated over a primary wound in the direction of the arrows.

2. Undermine the flap deep to the subdermal plexus. Rotate the free point of tissue thus created at the tip of the flap to close the defect, and suture it into position.

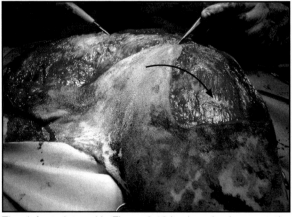
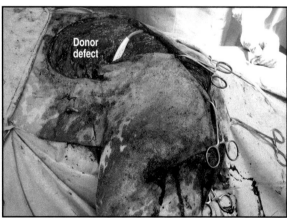

The defect pictured in Figure 6.13 is closed using a rotation flap. The donor defect will be closed primarily.

PRACTICAL TIP
Two rotational flaps located on opposite sides of a defect can be used to close a large or rectangular defect.

OPERATIVE TECHNIQUE 6.7 continued:
Rotation flap

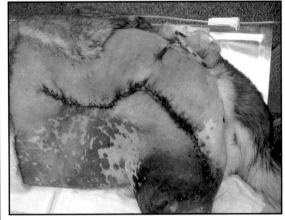

The flap has been sutured in position over a closed suction Jackson–Pratt drain.

Postoperative care
Standard postoperative wound care for any wound includes minimizing motion by enforcement of strict rest. Observation for evidence of developing wound dehiscence or infection is important. Avoid self-trauma to the incisions by bandaging extremities and using Elizabethan collars.

OPERATIVE TECHNIQUE 6.8:
Transposition flap
(see also Chapter 7 for Axial pattern flaps)

Positioning
Depends on location of the defect.

Assistant
Not required.

Equipment extras
None.

Surgical technique

1. Create a rectangular flap with one side of the flap forming part of the defect. The width of the flap is the same as the width of the defect. The length of the flap is equal to the distance from the pivot point of the flap (located at the base of the flap on the side farthest from the defect margin) to the tip of the defect.

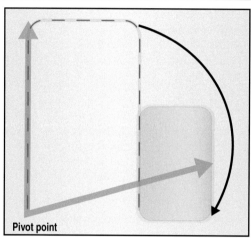

90 degrees transposition flap. The red arrows show that the length of the flap is equal to the length from the pivot point to the distal margin of the defect. The black arrow shows the direction of rotation of the flap to cover the defect.

Pivot point

2. Undermine the flap deep to the subdermal plexus.
3. Rotate the flap into position to close the defect. The angle of transposition is usually 45 to 90 degrees.

> **WARNING**
> **Greater rotation of the flap is possible but will create greater tension at the closure site and can lead to significant kinking of the base, which can result in vascular compromise.**

4. After the flap has been sutured into the defect, the skin around the donor site can usually be closed primarily.

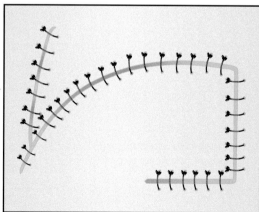

Once the transposition is complete the flap is sutured into place and the donor site is sutured. There will be some kinking of the skin at the flap base, which increases with the degree of rotation.

Postoperative care
Standard postoperative wound care for any wound includes minimizing motion by enforcement of strict rest. Observation for evidence of developing wound dehiscence or infection is important. Avoid self-trauma to the incisions by bandaging extremities, using Elizabethan collars.

OPERATIVE TECHNIQUE 6.9:
Axillary fold flap

Positioning
Dorsal recumbency for defects located on the ventral thorax/sternal area or medial aspect of the humerus. Lateral recumbency for lateral thoracic wall or shoulder defects.

Assistant
Not required.

Equipment extras
None.

Surgical technique
There are four attachments of the axillary skin fold to the body: medial and lateral attachments to the thoracic limb; and proximal and distal attachments to the trunk. Any three of these four attachments can be incised, depending upon the location of the defect to be closed.

1. Harvest the axillary fold flap, undermine the skin below the subdermal plexus and rotate it into position.

Defect on the ventral thorax/sternum: Incise the lateral and medial attachments of the fold, followed by the distal attachment to the trunk proximal to the elbow. Do not extend into the thickened skin over the elbow that cushions the olecranon as pressure necrosis can result. Rotate the flap 90 to 180 degrees into position over the defect.

> **PRACTICAL TIP**
> **Bilateral axillary fold flaps can be used to close very large ventral wounds (see Case Example 2).**

Defect over the lateral shoulder/lateral thorax: Leave the distal attachment to the body wall intact. Rotate the flap dorsally and either cranially or caudally, depending on the location of the lesion.

Defects on the proximal limb: Incise the proximal and distal attachments to the trunk. Maintain either the medial or lateral attachment to the limb in order to close defects on either aspect of the proximal limb.

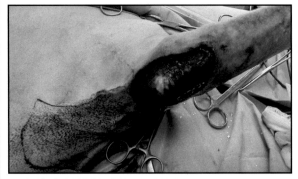
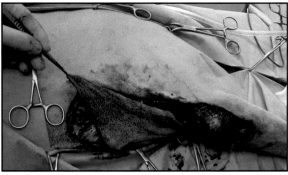

For closure of this wound over the elbow joint an axillary fold flap was created by incising the proximal, distal and lateral sides of the axillary fold. The flap's base was its medial attachment to the thoracic limb.

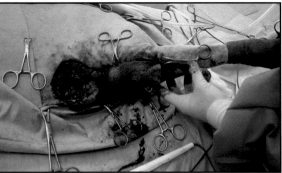

OPERATIVE TECHNIQUE 6.9 continued:
Axillary fold flap

2. Suture the flap into the recipient bed. Placement of an active or passive surgical drain should be considered when a large defect or defect with significant dead space is present.

Postoperative care
Care should be taken to avoid direct pressure on the flap, especially when older sedentary dogs lie in sternal recumbency. Placing a padded bandage over the wound for the first few days, followed by the placement of a T-shirt and providing confinement to a modestly sized crate or pen area that is well bedded is important.

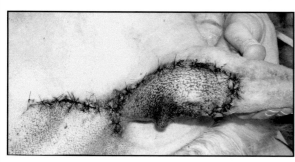

Flap sutured into position. This flap will need protection from pressure necrosis over the point of the elbow. Deep bedding and strict rest, possibly in combination with spica splinting of the limb, should be considered.

OPERATIVE TECHNIQUE 6.10:
Inguinal fold flap

Positioning
Dorsal recumbency for defects located on the ventral abdomen and groin areas. Lateral recumbency for defects of the lateral body wall and thigh.

> **PRACTICAL TIP**
> **Do not tie the animal to the surgical table such that the limb cannot be manipulated, as tension on the closure of ventral abdominal wounds is significantly affected by limb position.**

Assistant
Not required.

Equipment extras
None.

Surgical technique
There are four attachments of the inguinal fold to the body: medial and lateral attachments to the pelvic limb; and proximal and distal attachments to the trunk. Any three of these can be cut to allow flap rotation into the defect.

1. Harvest the inguinal fold flap, undermine the skin below the subdermal plexus and rotate it into position.

Defects of the proximolateral thigh: incise the proximal and distal attachments to the trunk and leave the flap base medially. Elevate the flap and rotate it into position.

Defects of the lateral abdominal wall: The medial, lateral and distal attachments can be incised and the flap based on its proximal attachment to the proximal thigh or body wall depending on the exact location of the defect.

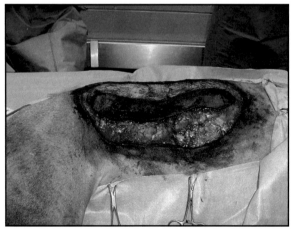 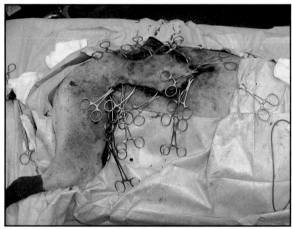

A large defect was present over the lateral abdomen, from the excision of a tumour that was not cleanly resected at the first attempt. An inguinal fold flap was created by incision of its medial, lateral and distal attachments and was rotated dorsally into the defect.

Defects of the ventral abdomen/groin: incise the proximal and distal attachments to the limb, leaving a laterally based flap to be rotated into the groin or ventral abdominal area. Bilateral inguinal fold flaps can be used to cover large ventral abdominal defects.

OPERATIVE TECHNIQUE 6.10 continued:
Inguinal fold flap

2. Suture the flap into the recipient bed.

PRACTICAL TIP
In most ventral abdominal wound closures a significant amount of dead space is present, which can lead to seroma formation. Use of a closed suction drain is often helpful for the first 2–4 days to prevent fluid accumulation at this site.

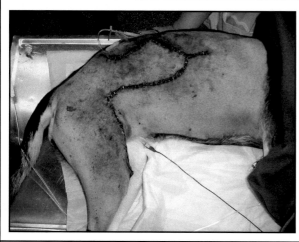

Flap sutured into place over a closed suction drain.

Postoperative care
Strict rest is important to minimize motion on the suture lines. Good drain management is necessary if a drain is placed, including secure fastening of the drain to the body with sutures or a bandage and regular emptying of closed suction drain collection devices to prevent ascending infection.

7

Axial pattern flaps

Alison Moores

Introduction

Reconstruction of large skin defects following trauma or radical excision of neoplastic masses can be problematical, particularly when wounds occur on the extremities where there is not enough skin for primary closure. Options for management include: axial pattern flaps; local subdermal plexus flaps; skin grafts; and second intention healing. There may, however, be insufficient skin adjacent to the wound to allow second intention healing or the use of local subdermal plexus flaps. Second intention healing may also result in formation of fragile epithelium or wound contracture.

Axial pattern flaps are used for the one-stage reconstruction of wounds. Flaps are usually raised from the trunk, neck or proximal limbs, where there is sufficient loose skin to allow closure of the donor site with minimal morbidity. They provide durable full-thickness skin with a predictable vascular supply, resulting in normal to near-normal hair growth and minimal visible scar tissue, although hair growth is in the opposite direction and may be of different length and texture to the hair in the local area. Functional results after successful axial pattern flap use are good, although some owners are dissatisfied with cosmetic results.

The advantage of axial pattern flaps over subdermal plexus flaps is the larger size of flap that can be raised: axial pattern flaps have a 50% greater survival area than subdermal plexus flaps of the same size (Pavletic, 1981). Whereas survival of subdermal plexus flaps is not related to flap width, increasing the axial pattern flap width increases the chances of incorporating the direct cutaneous vessels in the flap.

Advantages of axial pattern flaps over free skin grafts include: the ability to place the flap over poorly vascularized tissue, e.g. bones, nerves and previously irradiated tissue, as the flap is not reliant upon the wound bed for vascularization; and the greater tolerance to movement, so that immobilization of the surgical site postoperatively is not required.

Secondary axial pattern flaps are those in which skin is transferred over a direct cutaneous artery and allowed to establish a blood supply, then raised as an axial pattern flap as a later procedure. Their use is rarely necessary.

Traumatic wounds should undergo a period of wound management prior to surgery (see Chapter 4).

Blood supply and axial pattern flaps

In dogs and cats the main blood supply to the skin is from direct cutaneous arteries that branch to form the deep or subdermal plexus and, in turn, the middle and superficial plexuses (see Chapter 6). Direct cutaneous arteries and veins travel parallel to the skin between the subcutaneous fat and cutaneous musculature where present, and provide a vascular supply to skin of a large area. Direct cutaneous vessels are not present in the distal limb.

Skin flaps are classified according to their blood supply:

* *Subdermal plexus flaps* are based on the terminal cutaneous branches of direct cutaneous arteries and veins (the subdermal plexus). Flap length and width are limited by the attenuation of these vessels (see Chapter 6)
* *Axial pattern flaps* are based on direct cutaneous arteries and veins. The area of flap that can be raised depends upon the vascular territory (primary angiosome) of the direct cutaneous artery. An *angiosome* is the three-dimensional composite 'block' of tissue served by a named source artery.

Direct cutaneous vessels and angiosomes vary in size between locations. Some direct cutaneous arteries, including the thoracodorsal and caudal superficial epigastric arteries (Figure 7.1a), have angiosomes of large areas and long lengths.

There may also be variations in branching of direct cutaneous vessels between individual animals that may affect the size of the angiosome. The mean length and width of flaps used in clinical cases in dogs and cats in one study was 19 cm and 6.5 cm, respectively (Trevor *et al.*, 1992).

PRACTICAL TIP
Direct cutaneous vessels that have been described in small animals have predictable locations relative to local palpable anatomical landmarks. Thus, flaps can be raised without direct visualization of the vessels.

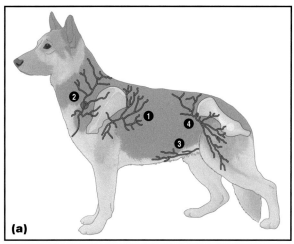

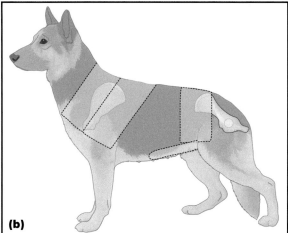

7.1 **(a)** The thoracodorsal (1), superficial cervical (2), caudal superficial epigastric (3) and deep circumflex iliac (4) direct cutaneous arteries are the largest direct cutaneous arteries supplying the skin of the dog. These axial pattern flaps **(b)** are therefore the most robust and have the most predictable survival.

> **WARNING**
> **Care should be taken when planning flap size based on data from experimental studies, as the area of flap survival in clinical cases may not be as great. Conversely, in some flaps it may be possible to harvest longer flaps than those described in the literature.**

To minimize distal flap necrosis, some authors do not recommend the routine use of long flaps, in particular those that extend beyond the primary angiosome (Kostolich and Pavletic, 1987; Aper and Smeak, 2003). Others recommend maximizing flap length and treating tip necrosis if it occurs, in order to guarantee coverage of the skin defect (Trevor *et al.*, 1992).

> **PRACTICAL TIP**
> **If a long flap is raised, e.g. a thoracodorsal flap that extends beyond the dorsal midline, owners should be warned of the risk of distal flap necrosis and the need for subsequent surgical procedures to manage remaining skin deficits.**

To prevent necrosis, flap vasculature comprising the direct cutaneous vessels and the subdermal plexus must be preserved. The four major direct cutaneous arteries and veins (thoracodorsal, caudal superficial epigastric, superficial cervical and deep circumflex iliac) (see Figure 7.1) are relatively large; thus, flap survival is relatively predictable. Other vessels, e.g. the superficial brachial artery and the genicular branch(es) of the saphenous artery, are relatively small and are at greater risk of surgical trauma that may result in complete flap necrosis. To protect the subdermal plexus the flap must be undermined beneath the cutaneous musculature; this is absent on the limbs, so dissection is performed deep to the dermis. Extra protection can be obtained by dissecting deep to fascia.

Terminal branches of direct cutaneous vessels may anastomose with each other; the vascular territory supplied by these vessels is termed the *secondary angiosome*. Blood flow from the primary angiosome through 'choke' vessels into the secondary angiosome may allow longer flaps to be raised. Examples include: anastomosis of thoracodorsal or superficial cervical vessels with the contralateral vessel on the dorsal midline; and anastomosis of the caudal auricular vessels with the superficial cervical vessels. Flow through vessels in the secondary angiosomes is reversed, and viability of the distal flap is less predictable, possibly due to spasm of choke vessels, particularly if the animal becomes dehydrated, hypovolaemic or hypothermic during or after surgery. It may therefore be prudent to harvest longer flaps only when greater experience with harvesting axial pattern flaps has been obtained.

> **WARNING**
> **Many direct cutaneous arteries have been mapped in dogs, but to date only thoraco-dorsal, caudal superficial epigastric, reverse saphenous conduit, superficial temporal and caudal auricular flaps have been described for cats. Care should be taken when using canine data for raising flaps in cats, particularly as there are differences in the amount of skin that can be raised and in skin coverage of defects by flaps.**

Classification of axial pattern flaps

Most axial pattern flaps are harvested in a *peninsular* or standard configuration, i.e. a rectangular shape (Figure 7.2a,b).

L-shaped (or 'hockey stick') flaps have two arms, usually joining each other at 90 degrees on the dorsal midline (Figure 7.2c). The resultant flap is shorter and wider than a peninsular flap; suturing the inner arms at the distal end of the flap can create even wider flaps (Pavletic, 1981). L-shaped flaps are useful for wide or irregular wounds close to the donor site, or if additional wounds or areas of excess tension preclude raising a peninsular flap.

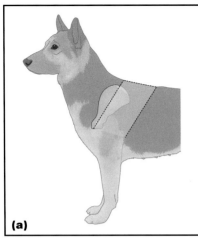
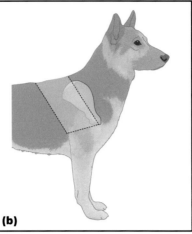
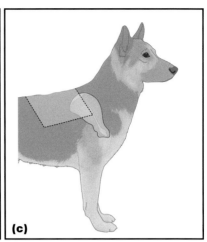

(a) **(b)** **(c)**

7.2 Flaps can be created in a peninsular (rectangular) or L shape. **(a)** Left peninsular thoracodorsal flap extending to the dorsal midline. **(b)** Left peninsular thoracodorsal flap that has crossed the dorsal midline to include the secondary angiosome of the right thoracodorsal vessels. **(c)** Left thoracodorsal flap that has crossed the dorsal midline and is continued at right angles to give an L-shaped flap.

Island flaps are raised in a similar way to peninsular flaps, but the skin at the base is incised so that the flap is tethered to the underlying tissue only by the direct cutaneous vessels (Figure 7.3). Island flaps are also created when the wound or defect lies adjacent to the base of the flap. These flaps are more mobile than peninsular or L-shaped flaps and can easily be rotated through 180 degrees into defects. There is no evidence that flap survival is greater in peninsular than in island flaps, but there is a risk of vessel damage when creating island flaps if meticulous surgical technique is not used.

Raising an axial pattern flap

Flap selection
The decision to close a wound using an axial pattern flap is based on several factors, including wound location and size. Where more than one axial pattern flap could be used to close a defect, preference may be given to flaps supplied by medium to large arteries, including the thoracodorsal, caudal superficial epigastric, superficial cervical and deep circumflex iliac arteries (see Figure 7.1), as these flaps are larger and have more predictable survival. If these flaps have already been raised or if the direct cutaneous vessels have been damaged, flaps supplied by smaller arteries that can reach the same position can be raised, such as the lateral thoracic and superficial brachial flaps instead of a thoracodorsal flap (Figure 7.4).

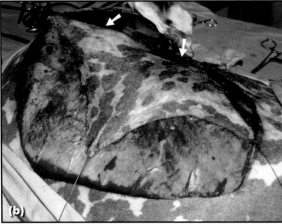

Dorsal

Caudal

(a)

(b)

7.3 **(a)** Thoracodorsal flap raised as a peninsular flap. **(b)** The pedicle is incised to create an island flap (arrows). (Courtesy of John M Williams)

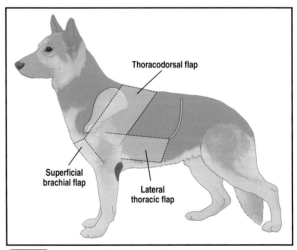

Thoracodorsal flap

Superficial brachial flap

Lateral thoracic flap

7.4 A defect of the caudal elbow can be closed using a thoracodorsal, lateral thoracic or superficial brachial flap. The thoracodorsal flap is preferred, if intact, as it has more predictable survival.

Patency of arteries should be established prior to surgery in cases where wounds or previous surgical procedures may have damaged them. Ultrasonography can be used to identify thoracodorsal, deep circumflex iliac and caudal superficial epigastric arteries with a high level of success (Reetz *et al.*, 2006). It is harder to identify superficial cervical arteries and it is likely that arteries supplying smaller flaps would be difficult to identify without angiography.

Preoperative planning

> **PRACTICAL TIP**
> As part of surgical planning, it is useful to make a list of which axial pattern flaps are available to close individual defects.

Careful preoperative planning is required to ensure that a flap of sufficient size to reach and fill the defect is raised. Ability of flaps to reach defects may be affected by species, skin elasticity and body conformation, e.g. trunk to limb length. Flap width is limited by ability to close the donor site, although other reconstructive techniques can be used to achieve this. Skin elasticity means that flaps may be stretched to fill defects that are wider than the donor site in some animals.

Planning the size of the flap

It is useful to draw the planned surgical procedure on paper before the animal is anaesthetized, including anatomical landmarks and actual measurements from the animal. The surgical planning diagram should include:

- The defect – location and maximum length and width. If the defect shares a common border with the pedicle of the flap an island flap will be created
- The anatomical landmarks for planning the flap
- The origin and direction of the direct cutaneous vessels
- The outline of the flap based on anatomical

landmarks – initially the drawing shows the maximum size the flap can be raised to. The distal tip of the flap can be rounded or rectangular depending upon the shape of the defect. The shape does not affect the incidence of tip necrosis
- The flap pivot point – this is located at the pedicle of the flap furthest away from the defect. During rotation of the flap into a defect the flap moves away from the pivot point (see Figures 7.5 to 7.8).
- The distance between the pivot point and the furthest point of the defect. This is equivalent to the length of the flap that will be raised (see Figures 7.5 to 7.8). Extra length is required to accommodate the effective shortening that occurs during rotation of the flap into the defect, especially if flaps are rotated through 180 degrees. The length required may be shorter than the flap outline based on anatomical landmarks. If the length required is longer than the flap outline based on anatomical landmarks, a different flap or surgical procedure should be considered.
- The width of the flap, based on anatomical landmarks. This must be equivalent to or wider than the width of the defect (see Figures 7.5 to 7.8). If the defect is too wide, an L-shaped flap should be considered
- The flap rotated into the defect and the resultant defect of the donor site
- The planned closure of the donor site – usually primary closure but in rare cases a local subdermal plexus flap may be required to close the donor site defect.

If the defect is adjacent to one arm of the flap, the flap is planned as for a transposition flap (see Chapter 6) (Figure 7.5).

If the defect is not adjacent to the flap, the distance between the pivot point and the furthest point of the defect includes the skin between the defect and the flap (Figures 7.6 and 7.7).

If the pedicle of the flap is adjacent to the defect an island flap is created (Figure 7.8).

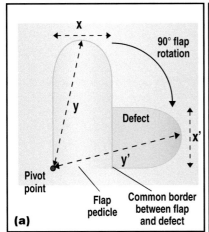
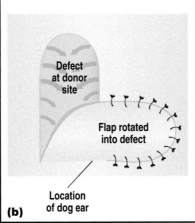
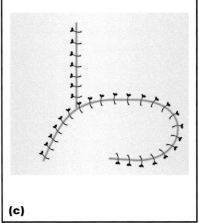

7.5 **(a)** Creation of an axial pattern flap where one border of the flap is adjacent to the defect and the flap is rotated through 90 degrees. The width of the flap (x) equals the width of the defect (x'). The distance from the pivot point to the furthest point of the defect (y') is equal to the length of the flap from the pivot point to the flap tip (y). The distal tip of the flap is transposed into the defect. **(b)** Flap rotated and sutured into the defect. Arrows show the direction of closure at the donor site. A 'dog ear' is often created in the base of the flap furthest from the pivot point, but this is not excised in case there is inadvertent damage to the direct cutaneous vessels. **(c)** Donor site closed.

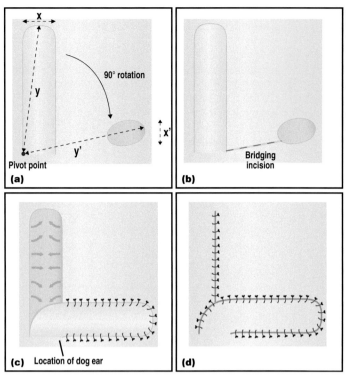

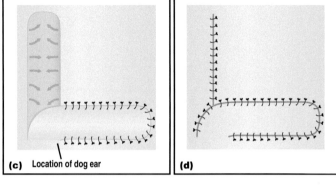

7.6 **(a)** Creation of an axial pattern flap where the flap is not adjacent to the defect and the flap is rotated through 90 degrees. The dimensions of the flap are planned as in Figure 7.5, but the distance from the pivot point to the furthest point of the defect (y') includes the defect *plus* the tissue between the flap and the defect. **(b)** Bridging incision between the base of the flap and the defect. **(c)** Flap rotated and sutured into the defect. **(d)** Donor site closed.

7.7 **(a)** Creation of an axial pattern flap where the flap is not adjacent to the defect and the flap is rotated through 180 degrees. The dimensions of the flap are planned as in Figure 7.6. **(b)** Bridging incision between the base of the flap and the defect. **(c)** Flap rotated and sutured into the defect. **(d)** Donor site closed.

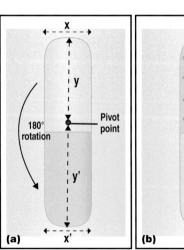

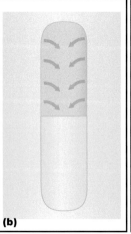

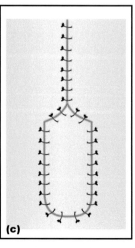

7.8 **(a)** Creation of an island axial pattern flap where the flap pedicle shares a common border with the defect (creating an island flap) and the flap is rotated through 180 degrees. The flap is tethered to the underlying tissue by the direct cutaneous vessels alone. **(b)** The flap is rotated and sutured into the defect. **(c)** The defect at the donor site is closed.

Surgical procedure

Details of raising and rotating an axial pattern flap are given in Operative Technique 7.1. Rotation through 180 degrees is usually tolerated in more durable flaps but limiting rotation to 90 degrees has been suggested to limit flap failure in flaps with small vessels, e.g. superficial temporal flaps (Fahie and Smith, 1999). The only sutures placed are those in the subcuticular tissues and skin between the edges of the flap and the defect (and bridging incision where present).

Using axial pattern flaps

Specific flaps are chosen based on the anatomical location of the defect (Figures 7.9 and 7.10).

Location of defect	Axial pattern flaps available
Oral cavity/palate	Superficial cervical (modified) Angularis oris
Orbit/forehead	Superficial temporal Caudal auricular
Maxillofacial region	Superficial cervical Superficial temporal
Ear	Superficial cervical Caudal auricular
Neck	Thoracodorsal Superficial cervical
Axilla	Thoracodorsal Superficial cervical
Shoulder	Thoracodorsal Superficial cervical
Proximal thoracic limb	Thoracodorsal Lateral thoracic
Elbow	Thoracodorsal Lateral thoracic Superficial brachial
Antebrachium	Thoracodorsal Superficial brachial
Carpus	Thoracodorsal (cats only)
Trunk	Thoracodorsal
Ventral thorax/sternum	Thoracodorsal Cranial superficial epigastric

Location of defect	Axial pattern flaps available
Lateral thorax	Deep circumflex iliac (dorsal branch) (caudal thorax only)
Lateral abdomen	Cranial superficial epigastric Caudal superficial epigastric Deep circumflex iliac (ventral branch) Deep circumflex iliac (dorsal branch)
Gluteal region	Lateral caudal Deep circumflex iliac (dorsal branch)
Sacrum/dorsal pelvis/ tailbase	Deep circumflex iliac (ventral branch) Caudal superficial epigastric Deep circumflex iliac (dorsal branch) Lateral caudal
Perineum	Caudal superficial epigastric Lateral caudal
Prepuce	Caudal superficial epigastric
Inguinal region	Caudal superficial epigastric
Proximal pelvic limb	Caudal superficial epigastric Deep circumflex iliac (dorsal branch)
Stifle	Caudal superficial epigastric
Crus	Caudal superficial epigastric Genicular
Hock	Caudal superficial epigastric (depends upon breed) Genicular (depends upon breed)
Metatarsal region	Caudal superficial epigastric (cats only) Reverse saphenous conduit

7.9 Axial pattern flaps that can be used to close defects, based on anatomical location.

Flap	Potential uses	Operative Technique
Angularis oris	Palate	
Caudal auricular	Maxillofacial region, orbit, ear	7.13
Caudal superficial epigastric	Flank, inguinal region, perineum, prepuce, medial and lateral thigh, stifle, crus, hock (depends on conformation in dogs), metatarsus/phalanges (cats only)	7.4
Cranial superficial epigastric	Lateral abdomen, ventral thorax/sternum	7.8
Deep circumflex iliac (dorsal branch)	Caudal thorax, lateral abdomen, flank, lateral lumbar region, pelvic region, lateral and medial thigh, greater trochanter	7.7
Deep circumflex iliac (ventral branch)	Lateral abdomen, pelvic region (island flap), sacrum (island flap)	7.6
Genicular	Lateral and medial tibia, hock (depends on conformation in dogs)	7.10
Lateral caudal	Perineum, dorsal pelvic region	7.14
Lateral thoracic	Caudal humerus, elbow	7.5
Reverse saphenous conduit	Dorsal, medial and plantar metatarsus	7.11
Superficial brachial	Elbow, antebrachium	7.9
Superficial cervical (omocervical)	Maxillofacial area, orbit, pinna, neck, shoulder, axilla, oesophagus	7.3
Superficial temporal	Maxillofacial region, orbit	7.12
Thoracodorsal	Neck, thorax, axilla, shoulder, proximal thoracic limb/brachium, elbow, antebrachium, carpus (cats only), flank	7.2

7.10 Uses of axial pattern flaps.

Flap	No. of cases	Flap length (cm)	Flap width (cm)	Mean flap survival	Range of flap survival
Caudal auricular	3	9–12	4.5–7	100%	100%
Caudal superficial epigastric	8	20–23	6–8	100%	100%
Reverse saphenous conduit	18	8	4	100%	100%
Superficial temporal	5	6.5–7	2	98% of length	92–100% of length
Thoracodorsal	8	9–12	9–9.5	98% of area	96–100% of area

7.11 Flap size and survival in experimental studies in cats.

Flap	No. of cases	Flap length (cm)	Flap width (cm)	Mean flap survival	Range of flap survival
Caudal auricular	12	15–23	5–8	85% of length	70–100% of length
Caudal superficial epigastric	8 [a]	17.8–30.5	3.8–8	100% of length	100% of length
Cranial superficial epigastric	6	N/R	N/R	N/R	47–100% of area [b]
Deep circumflex iliac (dorsal branch)	10	25–30	10–15	N/R	90–100% area
Genicular	8	18–20	6–9	89% of length	67–100% of length
Lateral caudal	5	Most of tail used		78% of length; 78% of area	N/R
Lateral thoracic	1	20	7	100%	100%
Reverse saphenous conduit	15	12–20	4–6	100%	100%
Superficial brachial	5	12–15	5.5	98% of length	92–100% of length
Superficial cervical (omocervical)	10	25–45	10–15	N/R	80–100% area
Superficial temporal	9	10	3.6	92% of length; 93% of area	N/R
Thoracodorsal	10	25–40	10–15	N/R	90–100% area [c]
	10 [a]	15–20	6–15	87% area	47–98% area

7.12 Flap size and survival in experimental and clinical studies in dogs. [a] Clinical case series; [b] if normal vasculature 87–100%; [c] 99% in 8/10 cases; N/R = not recorded.

The survival of a range of flaps in experimental studies in cats and in experimental and clinical studies in dogs are shown in Figures 7.11 and 7.12.

Flaps raised from the trunk

Thoracodorsal axial pattern flap

Thoracodorsal axial pattern flaps are the most versatile and robust flaps available for closing defects in the cranial part of the body. They can extend to the thorax, flank, neck, axilla, shoulder, brachium, elbow and mid-antebrachium in dogs. In cats, flaps can also extend to the carpus.

The cutaneous branches of the thoracodorsal artery and vein are medium-sized and arise at the caudal shoulder depression adjacent to the dorsal point of the acromion (see Figure 7.1a). The vessels are bordered by the latissimus dorsi muscle caudally, the long head of the triceps muscle ventrally and the spinous head of the deltoideus muscle cranially. The angiosome lies caudal to the scapular spine and ventral to the dorsal midline.

Peninsular or L-shaped flaps are raised, depending upon the length and width of the defect. Extending the flap over the dorsal midline can capture the secondary angiosome of the contralateral thoracodorsal artery to create a larger flap (see Figure 7.2).

Key points of thoracodorsal axial pattern flaps, plus planning and performing a procedure are illustrated in Operative Technique 7.2.

- In experimental cats, flaps of 9–12 cm x 9–9.5 cm were raised with mean survival of 98% (range 96–100%) (Remedios *et al.*, 1989).
- In medium-sized experimental dogs, flaps of 25–40 cm x 10–15 cm were raised with 90–100% area survival (99–100% survival in 8/10 flaps) (Pavletic, 1981).
- In canine clinical cases where the flap was rotated to the axilla or thoracic limb (Aper and Smeak, 2003) flap length was 15–20 cm and flap width 6–15cm. Flap necrosis at the distal end of the flap or overlying the olecranon occurred in 7/10 dogs, and 6 required a second surgical

procedure to achieve complete skin coverage of the defect. Overall mean flap survival area was 87%. Greater flap necrosis in clinical cases may be related to greater rotation of the flap, movement of the flap during joint flexion or pressure necrosis, all of which may compromise vasculature.

Superficial cervical (omocervical) axial pattern flap
Superficial cervical axial pattern flaps (see Operative Technique 7.3) can be used to close skin defects of the shoulder, axilla, neck, maxillofacial area, ear and oral cavity. Wounds in these areas can also be closed by thoracodorsal, caudal auricular and superficial temporal axial pattern flaps.

The cervical cutaneous branch of the superficial cervical artery (previously called the omocervical artery) originates from the subclavian artery and emerges between the trapezius and omotransversarius muscles adjacent to the prescapular lymph node. The angiosome is an area of cervical skin cranial to the scapula.

As with thoracodorsal flaps, superficial cervical axial pattern flaps can extend beyond the dorsal midline, and the flap may be raised in a peninsular or L-shaped configuration. In experimental dogs, flaps of 25–45 cm long and 10–15 cm wide had a survival area of 80-100%, suggesting that smaller flaps should be used for clinical cases (Pavletic, 1981). Thoracodorsal flaps tend to have greater survival than superficial cervical flaps of the same size.

Caudal superficial epigastric axial pattern flap
Caudal superficial epigastric axial pattern flaps (see Operative Technique 7.4) are the most versatile flaps for closing defects in the caudal part of the body. They have been used to reconstruct defects of the flank, inguinal region, perineum, prepuce, medial and lateral thigh, stifle, crus and hock (the latter depends upon breed conformation). Comparatively longer flaps can be created in short-legged breeds, whereas flaps may only reach the stifle in long-legged breeds. In cats, flaps can extend as far distally as the metatarsal or phalangeal regions. Use of bilateral caudal superficial epigastric axial pattern flaps has been described but results in an extensive defect at the donor site (Mayhew and Holt, 2003).

The caudal superficial epigastric artery and vein arise from the external pudendal artery and vein at the inguinal ring and supply the caudal three mammary glands (mammary glands 3–5 in dogs and 2–4 in cats) and overlying skin. Vascular anastomoses with cranial superficial epigastric vessels allow longer flaps to be raised.

- In canine clinical cases where the flap was rotated to the inguinal region or pelvic limb, flap length was 18–30 cm and flap width 4–8 cm and there was almost 100% flap survival (Aper and Smeak, 2005). The cranial border of the flap was between mammary glands 1 and 3 in individual dogs.

- In another study in dogs and cats, mean survival area was 91% (Trevor et al., 1992).
- In experimental cats, flaps of 20–23 cm long and 6–8 cm wide were raised with no flap necrosis, suggesting that it may be possible to raise even longer flaps (Remedios et al., 1989).

> **WARNING**
> **The flap includes intact mammary tissue, which may be more prominent in intact older females. Lactation and development of neoplasia may still occur in mammary tissue in a heterotopic location, so ovariohysterectomy should be considered in females.**

Lateral thoracic axial pattern flap
The lateral thoracic axial pattern flap (see Operative Technique 7.5) can be used for the closure of wounds overlying the caudal humerus and elbow, and a flap of 20 cm long and 7 cm wide has been described (Anderson et al., 2004). The artery arises from the axillary artery adjacent to the first rib and cranioventral to the thoracodorsal artery. The angiosome is a small area of skin caudal to the axillary fold. There may be variations in vasculature in individual dogs and the artery may not supply an angiosome at all, particularly in dogs with poorly developed axillary skin folds.

Deep circumflex iliac axial pattern flap (dorsal and ventral branches)
The deep circumflex iliac artery (see Figure 7.1a) arises from the aorta and exits the abdomen cranioventral to the wing of the ilium. The large ventral branch supports a flap (see Operative Technique 7.6) that can extend to the lateral abdomen and, if used as an island flap, may extend to defects over the pelvis and sacrum. An inguinal fold flap incorporates part of the ventral branch. A smaller flap based on the small dorsal branch (see Operative Technique 7.7) is more versatile and can be used to reconstruct defects of the caudal thorax, lateral abdomen, flank, lateral lumbar region, medial and lateral thigh, pelvic region and over the greater trochanter.

Flaps based on the dorsal branch of the vessels of 25–30 cm long and 10–15 cm wide, raised in experimental dogs, had 90–100% survival area of the flap (Pavletic, 1981). In three clinical cases in dogs and cats there was complete flap survival. Flaps can be extended over the dorsal midline and can be raised in a peninsular or L-shaped configuration. Smaller flaps may be necessary to avoid problems of donor site closure.

Cranial superficial epigastric axial pattern flap
Flaps based on the cranial superficial epigastric artery and vein (see Operative Technique 7.8) can be used to reconstruct defects over the sternum.

The cranial superficial epigastric artery arises from the cranial epigastric artery and supplies the skin and third mammary gland in dogs. Aberrant vasculature has been described, including perforating branches of the cranial epigastric artery and vein located several centimetres caudal to the origin of the cranial superficial epigastric vessels. The cranial superficial epigastric vessels are small in diameter in these dogs. The perforating vessels should be preserved if present as they may provide a significant contribution to the vascular supply of the skin. Area of flap survival varied from 87 to 100% in experimental dogs with normal vasculature (Sardinas *et al.*, 1995). Due to necrosis commonly occurring at the distal end of the flap, and difficulty in closing the donor site when it is adjacent to the prepuce, flap length is limited to the cranial aspect of the prepuce.

Flaps raised from the limbs

Superficial brachial axial pattern flap

Flaps based on the superficial brachial vessels (see Operative Technique 7.9) can be used to reconstruct defects of the elbow and antebrachium. Wounds in this area may also be reconstructed using thoracodorsal or lateral thoracic flaps.

The superficial brachial artery branches from the brachial artery 3 cm proximal to the elbow on the medial aspect. The primary angiosome overlies the craniomedial aspect of the distal humerus. In medium-sized experimental dogs, flaps of 12–15 cm in length and 5.5 cm in width were raised with a mean survival length of 98% (Henney and Pavletic, 1988), suggesting that it may be possible to harvest larger flaps that will extend to the carpus. The superficial brachial artery lies medial to the cephalic vein, which is preserved during dissection, but the artery is small and often hard to identify. Meticulous surgical technique is required to raise this flap and unnecessary dissection around the pedicle of the flap is avoided. Closure of the donor site creates a T-shaped incision adjacent to the flap that may result in a small area of dehiscence, which is usually treated conservatively and allowed to heal by second intention.

Given the potential risk of damage to vessels and subsequent flap failure, consideration should be given to raising a thoracodorsal flap in preference to a superficial brachial flap. Advantages of the superficial brachial flap include: smaller donor site; easier access to both the donor site and the defect; and the potential for the flap to reach the carpus in dogs.

Genicular axial pattern flap

Flaps based on the genicular vessels (see Operative Technique 7.10) can be used to reconstruct defects of the lateral and medial tibia and can extend to the tibiotarsal joints in some dogs, depending upon body conformation. Wounds in these areas may also be reconstructed using caudal superficial epigastric flaps.

The genicular artery is a short branch of the saphenous artery on the medial aspect of the stifle, which may be single or paired. The genicular vein drains into the medial saphenous vein. The primary angiosome is on the proximolateral aspect of the thigh. The vessels are small, so meticulous surgical technique is required in raising the flap.

In medium-sized experimental dogs, flaps of 18–20 cm in length and 6–9 cm wide were raised with mean survival length of 89% (range 67–100%)

(Kostolich and Pavletic, 1987). Differences in flap viability may be related to different vascular patterns in individual dogs. Donor site dehiscence was described in 25% of dogs.

Reverse saphenous conduit axial pattern flap

Flaps based on the cranial and caudal branches of the saphenous artery and medial saphenous vein can be used to reconstruct defects overlying the dorsal, medial and plantar metatarsus (see Operative Technique 7.11).

There are no major direct cutaneous vessels in the distal pelvic limb. The saphenous artery supplies a number of small direct cutaneous arteries to the skin, thereby acting as a conduit. The saphenous artery and medial saphenous vein arise from the femoral artery and vein and divide into cranial and caudal branches distal to the stifle. Ligation and division of the saphenous vessels close to the femoral artery and vein is possible due to vascular connections between:

- The cranial branch of the saphenous artery and the superficial branch of the cranial tibial artery
- The caudal branch of the saphenous artery and the perforating metatarsal artery via medial and lateral plantar arteries
- The cranial branch of the medial saphenous vein and the cranial branch of the lateral saphenous vein
- The cranial and caudal branches of the medial saphenous veins distal to the tibiotarsal joint.

These vascular connections allow blood flow to and from the distal limb in a reverse direction through arteries and veins, despite the presence of valves in veins.

- Flaps of 12–20 cm in length and 4–6 cm wide were raised in medium-sized experimental dogs with 100% survival (Pavletic *et al.*, 1983).
- In experimental cats, flaps of 8 cm long and 4 cm wide were raised with complete survival (Cornell *et al.*, 1995).

WARNINGS
- **Care must be taken when using this flap in traumatic wounds of the distal limb that the vessels supplying the flap and the rest of the distal limb are intact, and that the vascular supply to the distal limb is not reliant upon the saphenous vessels. Angiography is recommended in such cases.**
- **If the flap is tubed, care must be taken to ensure that the flap is not under tension during hock extension.**

Flaps raised from the head, neck and tail

Superficial temporal axial pattern flap

Superficial temporal axial pattern flaps (see Operative Technique 7.12) can be used to reconstruct defects of the rostral maxillofacial area, including the orbit, cheek, lips and nose.

- Mean flap length and width in experimental dogs was 10 cm and 3.6 cm, with 92% and 93% of the length and area of the flap surviving. Longer flaps were associated with skin necrosis (Fahie and Smith, 1999).
- Cats had comparatively longer mean survival length than dogs, with flaps of 6.5–7cm long and 2 cm wide achieving a mean survival area of 98% (range 92–100%) (Fahie and Smith, 1997).

Caudal auricular axial pattern flap
Flaps based on the caudal auricular vessels (see Operative Technique 7.13) can reconstruct defects overlying the orbit, face, forehead and ear.

Two sternocleidomastoideus branches of the auricular artery and vein arise caudal to the base of the pinna in a palpable depression between the lateral aspect of the wing of the atlas and the vertical ear canal. The primary angiosome lies in the middle third of the lateral aspect of the neck. Flaps can be raised to the level of the scapular spine due to anastomotic connections between caudal auricular and superficial cervical vessels with reversed blood flow occurring in the latter. Flap width depends upon the ability to close the donor site and is comparatively greater in cats than dogs.

- In experimental medium-sized dogs, flaps of 15–23 cm in length and 5–8 cm in width were raised with mean survival length of 85% (range 70–100%) (Smith *et al.*, 1991).
- In feline clinical cases, flaps of 9–12 cm long and 4.5–7 cm wide were raised with complete survival (Spodnick *et al.*, 1996).
- In five clinical cases in dogs and cats mean survival was 99% (Trevor *et al.*, 1992).

Lateral caudal axial pattern flap
Lateral caudal axial pattern flaps (see Operative Technique 7.14) can be used to close defects of the perineum or the dorsal pelvic region, depending upon the location of the flap pedicle.

The lateral caudal arteries arise from the caudal gluteal arteries and lie ventral to the transverse processes of the coccygeal vertebrae. Studies in experimental dogs show that the length of this flap should be limited to 75% of tail length to minimize distal flap necrosis (Saifzadeh *et al.*, 2005). Mean survival in two clinical cases was 93%. Amputation of the tail means the cosmetic change associated with the use of this flap is more noticeable than with other flaps.

Complications and flap failure

Technical errors may result in: failing to raise a flap of sufficient size to close the defect, or inability to close the donor site by raising too wide a flap. Technical errors can be excluded by careful pre-operative planning.

Dehiscence
The most common complication of axial pattern flap use in clinical practice is dehiscence, seen in one third of cases. It occurs most commonly along the flap–defect interface but usually only along a small portion of the suture line (Figure 7.13). Causes include excessive wound tension, irregular wound interfaces and movement. Dehiscence of the donor site may also occur but can be minimized by careful pre-operative planning to ensure it can be closed without tension. Dehiscence can be minimized by using tension-reducing suture patterns and restricting exercise postoperatively. In most cases wounds will heal by second intention if managed conservatively.

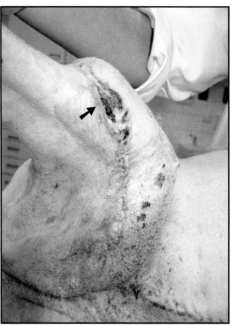

7.13 Partial wound breakdown at the edge of a caudal superficial epigastric flap rotated into a stifle wound. There is also discharge within the wound and on the skin (arrowed). (© Alison L Moores)

Discharge
Wound discharge may be associated with wound dehiscence (see Figure 7.13). Mild to moderate serosanguineous to purulent discharge may also be seen from surgical drains for up to a week.

Seroma
Failure to place surgical drains commonly results in seroma formation (see Chapter 12). Options for treatment include: conservative therapy with warm compresses and local hydrotherapy; removing sutures from the dependent portion of the flap to allow drainage; placement of a surgical drain if one is not present; or aspiration and bandaging via the skin around the flap to avoid vessel damage.

Flap necrosis
Bruising and oedema are commonly noted in the flap in the first few days postoperatively. In some cases this may be an indicator of pending flap necrosis, which may be partial or complete (Figures 7.14 and 7.15). In three studies of clinical cases in dogs and cats, the mean area of flap survival was 91–100%, depending on flap type (Trevor *et al.*, 1992; Aper and Smeak, 2003, 2005). The greatest area of flap necrosis recorded was 53%.

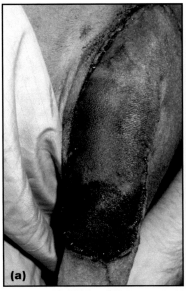
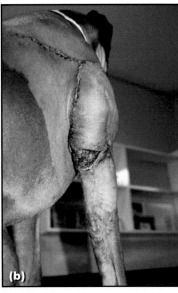

7.14 **(a)** Partial (distal) flap necrosis of a thoracodorsal flap used to close a defect of the elbow. **(b)** The necrotic tissue has been debrided and the wound has been left to heal by second intention. (© Alison L Moores)

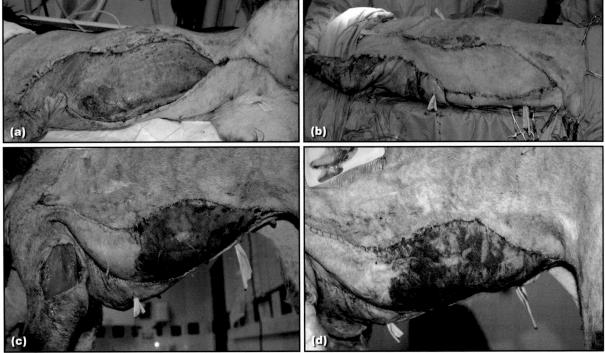

7.15 **(a)** Large skin defect, including the left mammary chain and skin of the left thoracic/abdominal wall, secondary to sloughing of a large subcutaneous abscess of unknown origin. **(b)** A thoracodorsal flap has been raised and rotated 90 degrees caudally into the defect. The distal end of the flap is over the dorsal midline at the contralateral scapulohumeral joint and therefore includes the secondary angiosome. The defect is adjacent to and shares a common border with the caudal aspect of the flap. Penrose drains have been placed in dependent positions under the flap and the donor site. A small amount of postoperative haemorrhage noted from the drains is within normal limits. **(c)** Appearance 2 days postoperatively. There is marked bruising of the distal half of the flap, with a clear line of demarcation between normal and bruised skin. This represents the area of vascular communication between the primary and secondary angiosomes on the dorsal midline. There is serosanguineous discharge from the drains. **(d)** Appearance 4 days postoperatively. The distal half of the flap is necrotic, there is dehiscence of the flap in the caudal aspect of the wound and purulent discharge from the drains. The distal portion of the flap was removed along the line of demarcation with normal skin. (© Alison L Moores)

Initial indicators of necrosis are noted within 24 hours of surgery and include red to purple skin discoloration and decreased surface temperature. Full-thickness skin necrosis will then occur within 2–6 days of surgery in most cases.

Necrotic tissue should be debrided and the resulting wound can often be left to heal by second intention with good cosmetic results. In cases with more extensive necrosis, or if the wound is in a high motion area, further surgical intervention may be required, e.g. advancement of the remaining part of the flap into the defect. If complete flap necrosis occurs, other attempts at wound closure are required.

PRACTICAL TIPS

The risk of complete flap necrosis can be minimized by avoiding damage to the direct cutaneous vessels and subdermal plexus. This is achieved by careful surgical technique to avoid vessel damage and arteriolar vaso-constriction, undermining deep to the cutaneous musculature and not placing sutures in the flap. Care must be taken not to damage the vessels in the postoperative period by careful application of bandages (where used) and by not incising or aspirating through the flap.

Harvesting long flaps that include a secondary angiosome, use of flaps with small direct cutaneous vessels and individual variation in vessel size may increase the risk of partial or total flap failure. Using thoracodorsal or caudal superficial epigastric axial pattern flaps in preference to flaps based on smaller vessels may improve flap survival.

Infection

Infection occurs in 15–30% of clinical cases but does not affect flap viability or survival. Infection should be managed with antibiotics and local wound care. Use of prophylactic antibiotics does not affect infection rates (Trevor *et al.*, 1992).

References and further reading

Anderson DM, Charlesworth TC and White RAS (2004) A novel axial pattern flap based on the lateral thoracic artery in the dog. *Veterinary and Comparative Orthopaedics and Traumatology* **17**, 73–77

Aper R and Smeak D (2003) Complications and outcome after thoracodorsal axial pattern flap reconstruction of forelimb skin defects in 10 dogs, 1989–2001. *Veterinary Surgery* **32**, 378–384

Aper RL and Smeak DD (2005) Clinical evaluation of caudal superficial epigastric axial pattern flap reconstruction of skin defects in 10 dogs

(1989–2001). *Journal of the American Animal Hospital Association* **41**, 185–192

Cornell K, Salisbury K, Jakovljevic S *et al.* (1995) Reverse saphenous conduit flap in cats: an anatomic study. *Veterinary Surgery* **24**, 202–206

Fahie MA and Smith MM (1997) Axial pattern flap based on the superficial temporal artery in cats: an experimental study. *Veterinary Surgery* **26**, 86–89

Fahie MA and Smith MM (1999) Axial pattern flap based on the cutaneous branch of the superficial temporal artery in dogs: an experimental study and case report. *Veterinary Surgery* **28**, 141–147

Henney LH and Pavletic MM (1988) Axial pattern flap based on the superficial brachial artery in the dog. *Veterinary Surgery* **17**, 311–317

Kostolich M and Pavletic MM (1987) Axial pattern flap based on the genicular branch of the saphenous artery in the dog. *Veterinary Surgery* **16**, 217–222

Mayhew PD and Holt DE (2003) Simultaneous use of bilateral caudal superficial epigastric axial pattern flaps for wound closure in a dog. *Journal of Small Animal Practice* **44**, 534–538

Pavletic MM (1980a) Vascular supply to the skin of the dog: a review. *Veterinary Surgery* **9**, 77–80

Pavletic MM (1980b) Caudal superficial epigastric arterial pedicle in the dog. *Veterinary Surgery* **9**, 103–107

Pavletic MM (1981) Canine axial pattern flaps, using the omocervical, thoracodorsal, and deep circumflex iliac direct cutaneous arteries. *American Journal of Veterinary Research* **42**, 391–406

Pavletic MM, Watters J, Henry RW *et al.* (1983) Reverse saphenous conduit flap in the dog. *Journal of the American Veterinary Medical Association* **182**, 380–389

Reetz JA, Seiler G, Mayhew PD *et al.* (2006) Ultrasonographic and color-flow Doppler ultrasonographic assessment of direct cutaneous arteries used for axial pattern skin flaps in dogs. *Journal of the American Veterinary Medical Association* **228**, 1361–1365

Remedios AM, Bauer MS and Bowen CV (1989) Thoracodorsal and caudal superficial epigastric axial pattern skin flaps in cats. *Veterinary Surgery* **18**, 380–385

Saifzadeh S, Hobbenaghi R and Noorabadi M (2005) Axial pattern flap based on the lateral caudal arteries of the tail in the dog: an experimental study. *Veterinary Surgery* **34**, 509–513

Sardinas JC, Pavletic MM, Ross JT *et al.* (1995) Comparative viability of peninsular and island axial pattern flaps incorporating the cranial superficial epigastric artery in dogs. *Journal of the American Veterinary Medical Association* **207**, 452–454

Smith MM, Payne JT, Moon ML *et al.* (1991) Axial pattern flap based on the caudal auricular artery in dogs. *American Journal of Veterinary Research* **52**, 922–925.

Spodnick GJ, Hudson LC, Clark GN *et al.* (1996) Use of a caudal auricular axial pattern flap in cats. *Journal of the American Veterinary Medical Association* **208**, 1679–1682

Trevor PB, Smith MM, Waldron DR *et al.* (1992) Clinical evaluation of axial pattern skin flaps in dogs and cats: 19 cases (1981–1990). *Journal of the American Veterinary Medical Association* **201**, 608–612

CASE EXAMPLE 1:
Superficial cervical axial pattern flap for a face wound in a cat

History
A 2-year-old DSH cat was presented with a wound to the right side of the face.

Assessment
The wound consisted of an area of dark, dry, hard skin that was cool to the touch, non-pliable and hairless. This area of ischaemic skin extended across a large part of the right side of the face, rostrally as far as the lateral half of the lower eyelid and the lateral quarter of the upper eyelid, and was approximately 5 cm x 6 cm. Two small puncture wounds were evident within the centre of the area of dead tissue.

Second intention healing and primary closure were not selected, as they would have compromised eyelid function. Options for reconstruction included: superficial cervical and caudal auricular axial pattern flaps; and local subdermal plexus flaps, such as a transposition flap.

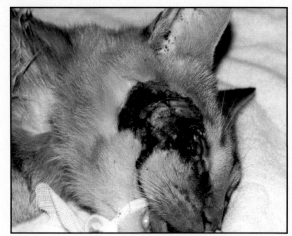
The wound on presentation.

Treatment
A superficial cervical axial pattern flap was performed. The landmarks have not yet been described in the cat, so those described for the dog were used. Although this flap can be successfully extended beyond the dorsal midline in the dog, there is no evidence that this can be done in cats, so anticipation of complications such as distal tip necrosis should be considered.

The cat was given intravenous antibiotics, due to a presumed cat bite abscess. The ischaemic tissue was excised and the underlying tissue lavaged.

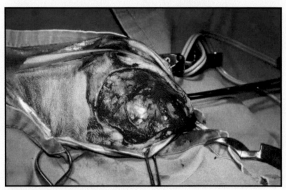
Wound after debridement and lavage.

The anatomical landmarks and flap margins were drawn on to the skin. The flap was harvested to a point between the dorsal midline and the contralateral scapulohumeral joint. A bridging incision was made along the length of the neck, from the base of the flap to the base of the recipient site. The flap was rotated to lie within the space created by the bridging incision and to cover the recipient site. The Luer lock was removed from two 19-gauge butterfly catheters. These were partially fenestrated and placed underneath the flap, exiting through a separate stab incision dorsal to the flap, and secured with Chinese finger-trap sutures. The flap was sutured to the skin margins of the bridging incision and the wound, using subcutaneous sutures and skin staples, and the donor site was closed.

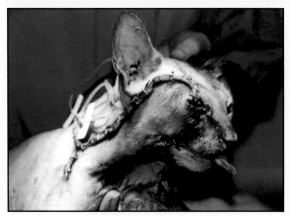
Flap in place and wounds closed.

Case Example 1 continues ▶

CASE EXAMPLE 1 continued:
Superficial cervical axial pattern flap for a face wound in a cat

The lower and upper eyelids of the right eye were closed together with a horizontal mattress suture to prevent corneal irritation by the ends of the suture material. The butterfly catheters were attached to 10 ml vacutainers to create active suction drains. The vacutainers were bandaged to the dorsum via a well padded chest dressing.

The closed drainage system was maintained for 7 days postoperatively. On the seventh day the mattress suture apposing the eyelids on the right side was removed. Eyelid function was good and there was no irritation of the cornea. Sutures and staples were removed 15 days postoperatively.

Outcome
Four weeks postoperatively the cat was well and eyelid function was good, with only slight lower lid ectropion.

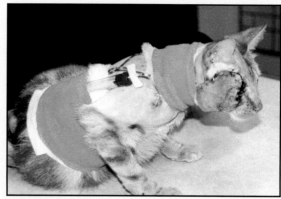

Active suction drain in place.

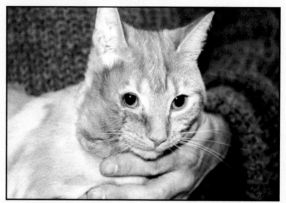

The cat 4 weeks after the flap procedure.

CASE EXAMPLE 2:
Thoracodorsal axial pattern flap for an elbow wound in a dog

History
A 1-year-old male neutered Rhodesian Ridgeback was presented with a 3 cm wound overlying the right elbow. The wound had been created by the resection of an infected hygroma; attempted closure techniques, including primary closure and a bipedicle advancement flap, had failed.

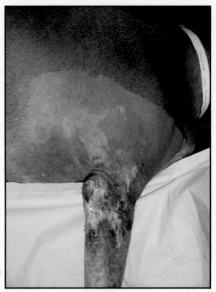

The wound on presentation.

Assessment
The wound was covered with chronic granulation tissue. There was scarring around the wound, consistent with previous attempts at reconstruction. There was also a small area of granulation tissue overlying the lateral epicondyle, where second intention healing of the bipedicle flap donor site was not complete. Options for reconstruction included: an axial pattern flap (thoracodorsal, superficial cervical and lateral thoracic); and an axillary fold flap. A thoracodorsal axial pattern flap was selected, as it is the most robust and reliable of the flaps available.

Treatment
Preoperative planning was performed to determine the length of flap needed to close the defect. The anatomical landmarks and flap margins were drawn on to the skin. The flap was harvested to the dorsal midline. Dissection of the flap using careful blunt and sharp dissection was performed from the dorsal aspect of the flap until the direct cutaneous vessels were visualized; care was taken not to damage them. Blood vessels at the edge of the flap were electro-coagulated.

A bridging incision was made from the caudal edge of the

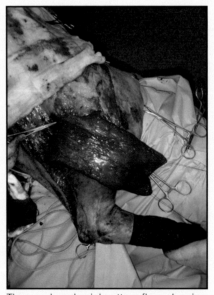

Thoracodorsal axial pattern flap, showing direct cutaneous vessels (forceps).

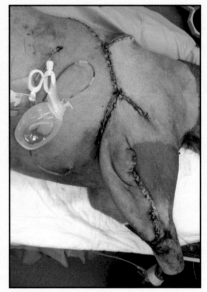

Active suction drain in place.

flap to the dorsal aspect of the wound. The chronic granulation tissue and thin epithelium at the wound edges were excised. The skin around the wound and on each side of the bridging incision was undermined. The flap was rotated through 180 degrees into the defect. Active suction drains were placed under the flap and the donor site, exiting the skin caudal to the flap.

Case Example 2 continues ▶

CASE EXAMPLE 2 continued:
Thoracodorsal axial pattern flap for an elbow wound in a dog

The flap was sutured to the skin margins of the bridging incision and the wound, using subcutaneous sutures and skin staples. The donor site was closed by undermining the skin under the cutaneous muscle and performing primary closure. The wounds were covered with non-adherent dressings and the limb was left undressed.

Complications and measures taken
Despite the presence of the drains, fluid accumulated under the distal aspect of the flap with discharge of fluid from the distal aspect of the wound. There was minor bruising of the distal 2 cm of the flap, though this resolved within a few days. The active suction drains were removed after 3 days and a Penrose drain inserted under the flap via a stab incision in the skin distal to the flap.

A small area of dehiscence occurred at the distal aspect of the flap 6 days postoperatively, at the site of wound discharge.

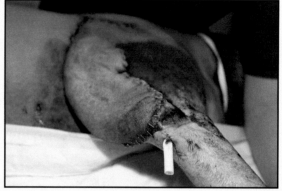

Penrose drain in place.

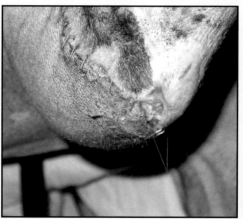

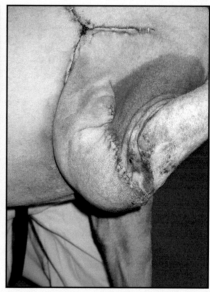

Discharge and dehiscence
6 days after surgery.

The staples were removed 14 days postoperatively and the small distal wound was allowed to heal by second intention.

OPERATIVE TECHNIQUE 7.1:
Axial pattern flap

Patient positioning
Depends on position of wound and flap to be harvested. The surgeon needs to position the patient so that both can be accessed, preferably without moving the patient. Patients are positioned with the limbs relaxed and with skin under no tension, to avoid distorting local anatomy. Failure to do this may result in raising a flap of skin that does not contain the direct cutaneous vessels.

> **PRACTICAL TIP**
> **Positioning aids placed underneath the thoracic or pelvic limb girdles may maximize local skin available for closure of donor sites on the trunk and neck.**

Assistant
Preferred.

Equipment extras
Skin hooks (optional).
Stay sutures.
Skin staples.

Surgical technique
A wide surgical clip is performed – including around the defect, the surface of the flap, the skin between the flap and the defect, and sufficient skin to allow undermining and closure of the donor site without hair impinging on the surgical site. In some cases enough hair is clipped to allow other reconstructive techniques to be performed if they may be necessary, e.g. musculocutaneous flaps. If a flap is to be rotated from the trunk on to a limb, the surgical preparation includes all skin between the defect and the donor site and the limb is hung in a routine manner.

The wound or defect is covered with moistened surgical swabs to avoid desiccation whilst the flap is being raised.

Before surgical preparation, a permanent marker pen is used to draw on the skin:

- Anatomical landmarks for the chosen flap
- The origin of the direct cutaneous artery and vein
- The flap pivot point
- The outline of the flap
- A bridging incision if there is skin interposed between the flap and the defect.

> **PRACTICAL TIP**
> **Pull together the skin along the edges of the flap (i.e. the width of the flap) preoperatively to check that the donor site can be closed. In animals with poor skin elasticity and a paucity of loose skin, such as Greyhounds, flaps of smaller width than those based on anatomical landmarks may have to be raised to allow closure of the donor site without tension.**

> **WARNING**
> **If an axial pattern flap is used to close a defect created after tumour excision, surgical gowns, gloves and instruments must be changed after removing the mass and before raising the flap to avoid contaminating the flap donor site with tumour cells.**

1. Make an incision through the skin, subcutaneous tissues and cutaneous musculature along the outline of the flap. Peninsular flaps and island flaps where the defect and the flap pedicle share a common border have incisions on three sides; other island flaps have incisions on four sides and only the direct cutaneous vessels attach the flap to the underlying tissues.

OPERATIVE TECHNIQUE 7.1 continued:
Axial pattern flap

If a long flap that includes a secondary angiosome is raised, the direct cutaneous artery and vein supplying the secondary angiosome must be ligated and divided at the distal tip of the flap.

L-shaped flaps are raised using the same principles as peninsular flaps.

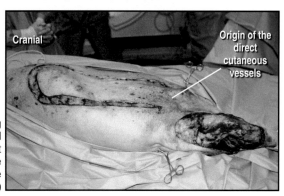

Caudal superficial epigastric axial pattern flap incised along an outline drawn on the skin. The flap is peninsular and includes mammary glands 3–5. The pedicle of the flap is not adjacent to the defect. In male dogs the incision includes the dorsal base of the preputial sheath to avoid damaging the vessels. (© Alison L Moores)

2. Place stay sutures in the subcutaneous tissues at the distal end of the flap, i.e. furthest from the origin of the blood vessels. These are used to manipulate the flap to avoid tissue trauma that can lead to vasospasm and poor flap survival. Alternatively, skin hooks can be used to manipulate the skin.

3. Use a combination of sharp and blunt dissection to undermine the flap, starting at the distal end. Take care to ensure that the cutaneous musculature (cutaneous trunci, platysma, sphincter colli superficialis, supramammaricus or preputialis) has been identified and that dissection is performed deep to the muscle. In the limbs, where there is no cutaneous muscle, the flap is undermined in the subcutaneous fat deep to the dermis or deep to fascia. Continue dissection towards the pedicle of the flap. Small blood vessels of the subdermal plexus will be encountered at the edge of the flap and should be ligated or electrocoagulated. If large aberrant vessels are encountered, such as branches of the cranial epigastric artery, they should not be divided, as they may be a major vascular supply to the skin in some individuals. In thin dogs and cats the direct cutaneous vessels may be visible running parallel to the long axis of the flap (see Case Example 2). Illumination of the flap may aid in vessel identification. However, in animals with a large amount of subcutaneous fat it may not be possible to visualize the vessels. Intraoperative fluid rates should be increased while the flap is being raised and until the donor site is closed, as fluid loss from the wound bed may cause hypovolaemia. The distal end of the flap should be covered with warm moistened swabs if increased time is needed to harvest the flap, to avoid spasm in the blood vessels.

WARNING
The exact location of a vessel may differ between individual animals and may be closer to one edge of the flap. Care must be taken not to sever or damage the vessels inadvertently, particularly during dissection close to the pedicle of the flap where the vessels emerge.

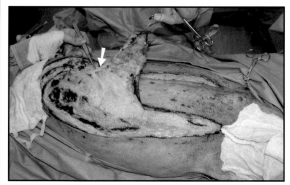

Flap elevated deep to supramammaricus muscle and mammary glands. Branches of the subdermal plexus located at the edge of the flap are ligated or electrocoagulated (shown in forceps). Note the use of stay sutures for flap manipulation. (© Alison L Moores)

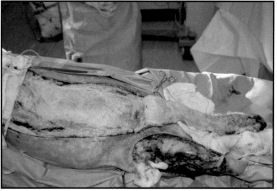

Flap elevated to the pedicle. The direct cutaneous vessels cannot be visualized. A bridging incision is made between the defect and the flap pedicle. (© Alison L Moores)

→

OPERATIVE TECHNIQUE 7.1 continued:
Axial pattern flap

4. Rotate the flap away from the pivot point into the defect. Rotation through 180 degrees to reach defects is usually tolerated in more durable flaps but limiting rotation to 90 degrees has been suggested to limit flap failure in flaps with small vessels, e.g. superficial temporal flaps (Fahie and Smith, 1999). To ease rotation, particularly through 180 degrees, a back cut into the flap can be created. Severing the pedicle completely to create an island flap (see Figure 7.8) will also aid rotation and may allow flaps to reach further, e.g. allowing a deep circumflex iliac flap (ventral branch) to reach the sacrum. Care must be taken not to damage the direct cutaneous vessels.

5. If the flap and defect are not adjacent, create a bridging incision between the corner of the pedicle opposite the pivot point and the defect, and undermine the edges.

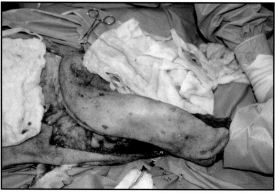

A bridging incision has been made between the pedicle of the flap and the defect, and the flap has been rotated through 180 degrees into the defect. (© Alison L Moores)

In rare instances the flap is tubed by suturing the free edges of the proximal part of the flap together where they pass over the skin between the pedicle of the flap and the defect . Care must be taken to ensure that damage to the vessels does not occur whilst tubing the flap. A second surgical procedure will be required to remove the tube when the flap has healed.

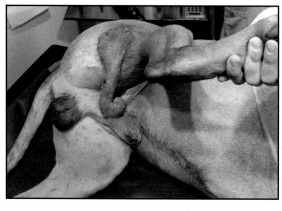

A caudal superficial epigastric flap has been tubed to bridge the skin between the base of the flap and the defect on the lateral aspect of the thigh. (© Richard Coe)

6. Place a surgical drain under the flap, exiting the skin adjacent to the flap. If using a passive drain, the drain must exit in a dependent position. Suture the drain in position.

> **WARNING**
> **The drain must not exit the skin through the flap as it might damage the direct cutaneous vessels.**

OPERATIVE TECHNIQUE 7.1 continued:
Axial pattern flap

7. Suture the edges of the flap to the edges of the skin wound/defect and the bridging incision. Interrupted or continuous sutures may be used in the subcutaneous tissues, and skin sutures or staples in the skin. Sutures are not placed through the middle of the flap, and tension-relieving incisions are not made through the flap, to avoid damaging the vessels.

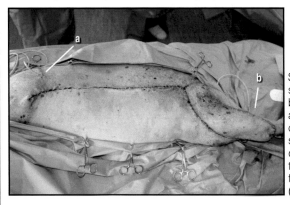

Subcutaneous sutures and skin staples between flap, defect and bridging incision. Donor site closed after undermining local skin deep to cutaneous trunci muscle. Active suction drains in dead space under donor site (a) and flap (b). Note that the drain exits the skin caudal to the flap and not through the flap.
(© Alison L Moores)

8. Close the donor site, undermining the wound edges deep to the cutaneous musculature where present. Place a surgical drain if there is dead space. Wound closure of the donor site is routine but take care to avoid tension along wound edges that may increase the risk of wound dehiscence.

Postoperative care

• Wounds are covered with a dressing in the immediate postoperative period. Bandaging may be done, depending on surgeon preference, but care must be taken to avoid pressure on the flap which could damage the direct cutaneous vessels. Occasionally limb immobilization using bandages or external skeletal fixation is employed.
• Active suction drain exit sites are covered with a dressing, and drains are attached to the animal using sutures or stockingettes (see Chapter 5). Elizabethan collars are worn whilst drains are in place.
• Dressings are changed as soon as they become soiled. The wound is monitored for common postoperative complications including: seroma formation, which may occur if wound drains become blocked or after drains have been removed; wound dehiscence; and total or partial flap necrosis. The owner is provided with detailed written postoperative care instructions, including information on identifying these problems and advice on when to contact the veterinary surgeon.
• Strict hygiene practices are used in handling the patient and the wound to decrease the risk of postoperative wound infection (see Chapter 12).
• Careful attention to analgesia is required, particularly in cases when large oncological resections have been performed. Analgesic techniques that may be employed include opioids (repeated doses, infusions, patches), lidocaine and/or ketamine infusions, application of local anaesthetic through wound catheters and NSAIDs. (See *BSAVA Manual of Canine and Feline Anaesthesia and Analgesia*.)
• Antibiotics are not given prophylactically but may be used if there is clinical evidence of infection postoperatively.
• Animals are housed on padded beds, especially if the flap overlies a bony prominence that may damage the vasculature, e.g. a thoracodorsal flap over the olecranon.
• Aspiration of fluid through the flap, or puncturing the flap in any way, is to be avoided to prevent damage to the direct cutaneous vessels.
• Complications should be addressed as soon as they are identified.
• The average hospital stay for animals having caudal superficial epigastric axial pattern flap reconstruction of skin wounds is 5 days.
• Sutures or staples are removed after 10–14 days, assuming the wound has healed uneventfully.

OPERATIVE TECHNIQUE 7.2:
Thoracodorsal axial pattern flap

Used to close defects of the:
Neck, thorax, axilla, shoulder, proximal thoracic limb/brachium, elbow, antebrachium, carpus (cats only), flank.

Anatomical landmarks
Scapular spine.
Acromion.
Caudal shoulder depression/caudal border of the scapula.
Axilla.
Dorsal midline.

Vessel origin
Caudal shoulder depression adjacent to the dorsal point of the acromion.

Planning

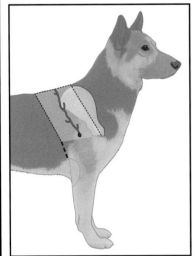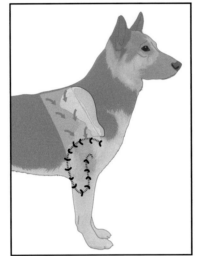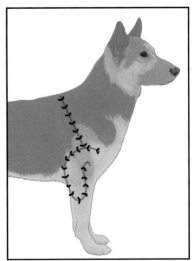

Planning a thoracodorsal axial pattern flap.

Flap pedicle
Perpendicular to the scapular spine: cranial aspect overlies acromion; caudal aspect at the axilla.

Incisions
Cranial and caudal incisions are parallel to the scapular spine and continue to the dorsal midline. The cranial incision overlies the scapular spine. There is an equal distance between the caudal shoulder impression/caudal border of the scapula and the cranial and caudal incisions.

Undermine
Deep to the cutaneous trunci muscle.

Modifications
* In dogs the flap can be continued over the dorsal midline to the contralateral scapulohumeral joint or a shorter L shape can be created on the dorsal midline.
* Flaps in cats are limited to the dorsal midline only.
* Wider flaps can be raised if the donor site can be closed but there is a greater risk of partial flap necrosis if flaps are very wide.
* An island graft is created by severing the flap pedicle.

Surgical procedure
For Patient positioning, Assistant, Equipment extras, Surgical technique and Postoperative care, see Operative Technique 7.1.

OPERATIVE TECHNIQUE 7.3:
Superficial cervical (omocervical) axial pattern flap

Used to close defects of the:
Maxillofacial area, orbit, pinna, neck, shoulder, axilla, oesophagus.

Anatomical landmarks
Scapular spine.
Acromion.
Cranial shoulder depression/cranial border of the scapula.
Prescapular lymph node.
Dorsal midline.

Vessel origin
Cranial shoulder depression adjacent to the prescapular lymph node.

Planning

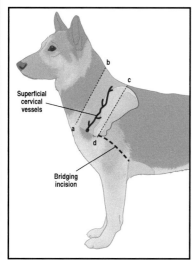 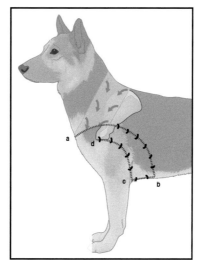 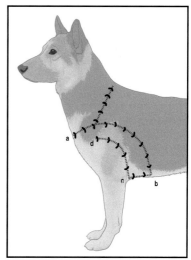

Planning a superficial cervical flap to close a wound in an axilla.

Flap pedicle
Perpendicular to the scapular spine: caudal aspect overlies acromion.

Incisions
Cranial and caudal incisions are parallel to the scapular spine and continue to the dorsal midline. The caudal incision overlies the scapular spine. There is an equal distance between the cranial shoulder impression/cranial border of the scapula and the cranial and caudal incisions.

Undermine
Deep to the sphincter colli superficialis muscle.

Modifications

* In dogs the flap can be continued over the dorsal midline to the contralateral scapulohumeral joint or a shorter L-shape can be created on the dorsal midline
* Flaps in cats are limited to the dorsal midline only
* An island graft is created by severing the flap pedicle

Surgical procedure
For Patient positioning, Assistant, Equipment extras, Surgical technique and Postoperative care, see Operative Technique 7.1.

OPERATIVE TECHNIQUE 7.4:
Caudal superficial epigastric axial pattern flap

Used to close defects of the:
Flank, inguinal region, perineum, prepuce, medial and lateral thigh, stifle, crus, hock (depends on conformation in dogs), metatarsus/phalanges (cats only).

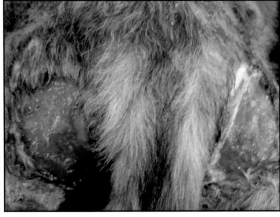

Dorsal view of bite wounds over the ischial tuberosities in a cat. (Courtesy of John M Williams)

Anatomical landmarks
Ventral abdominal midline.
Mammary glands and nipples.
Base of prepuce.
Inguinal region.

Vessel origin
Inguinal ring

Planning

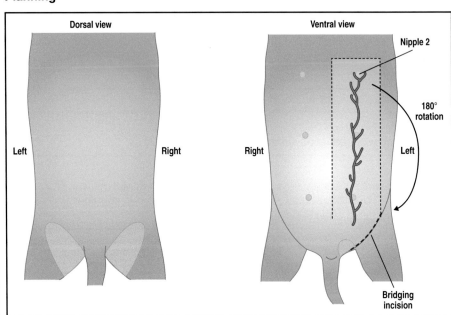

Planning a left-sided caudal superficial epigastric axial pattern flap in a cat to close the left side of the wound. A bridging incision is planned between the pedicle of the flap and the wound. The flap will be rotated through 180 degrees and sutured into the ischial wound dorsally.

OPERATIVE TECHNIQUE 7.4 continued:
Caudal superficial epigastric axial pattern flap

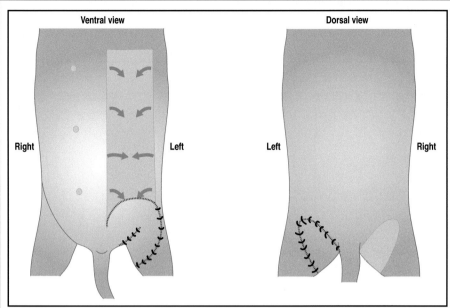

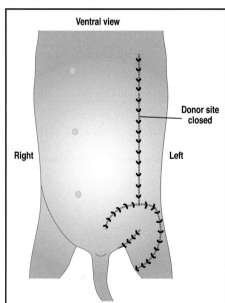

Planning a left-sided caudal superficial epigastric axial pattern flap to close the left side of the wound. A bridging incision is planned between the pedicle of the flap and the wound. The flap will be rotated through 180 degrees and sutured into the ischial wound dorsally

Flap pedicle
Perpendicular to the ventral midline; 3–5 cm caudal to the most caudal nipple.

Incisions
Medial and lateral incisions are parallel to the midline on the ventral abdomen and extend cranially from the flap pedicle. The medial incision is located on the ventral midline. There is an equal distance between the nipples and the medial and lateral incisions. In dogs the cranial border is a horizontal line cranial to the first or second mammary gland. In cats the cranial border is a horizontal line cranial to the first mammary gland. In male dogs the incision includes the dorsal base of the preputial sheath to avoid damaging the vessels.

OPERATIVE TECHNIQUE 7.4 continued:
Caudal superficial epigastric axial pattern flap

Undermine
Deep to the supramammaricus or preputialis muscles, just superficial to the aponeurosis of the external abdominal oblique muscle.

Flap transposition and closure

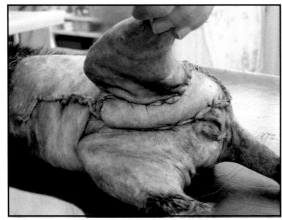

The flap is seen in the inguinal area ventrally and passes dorsally to close the ischial wound. (Courtesy of John M Williams)

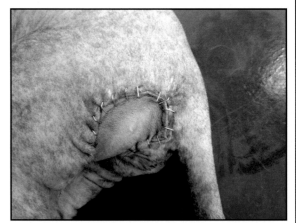

The distal end of the flap has been used to close the ischial wound dorsally. The right wound was closed using a right deep circumflex iliac (dorsal branch) flap. (Courtesy of John M Williams)

Modifications
An island graft can be created by severing the flap pedicle.

Surgical procedure
For Patient positioning, Assistant, Equipment extras, Surgical technique and Postoperative care, see Operative Technique 7.1.

OPERATIVE TECHNIQUE 7.5:
Lateral thoracic axial pattern flap

Used to close defects of the:
Caudal humerus; elbow.

Anatomical landmarks
Caudal shoulder depression/origin of the thoracodorsal artery.
Axillary skin fold.
Second mammary gland nipple.
Costal arch.
Dorsal border of the deep pectoral muscle.

Planning

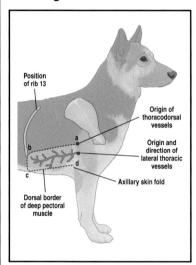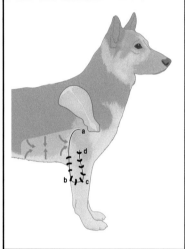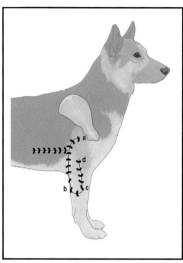

Planning a lateral thoracic axial pattern flap. The origin of the thoracodorsal and lateral thoracic vessels are close to each other. The flap will be rotated into an elbow wound.

Vessel origin
Adjacent to the first rib and cranioventral to the thoracodorsal artery.

Flap pedicle
Parallel to the scapular spine: ventral aspect at axillary skin fold; dorsal aspect at origin of thoracodorsal artery.

Incisions
The incisions are at an angle to the long axis of the body in a craniodorsal to caudoventral direction. The ventral incision overlies the dorsal aspect of the deep pectoral muscle. The dorsal incision starts at the origin of the thoracodorsal artery and is parallel to the ventral incision. The flap extends in a slightly ventral direction towards the second mammary gland nipple and ends at the costal arch.

Undermine
Deep to the cutaneous trunci muscle.

Surgical procedure
For Patient positioning, Assistant, Equipment extras, Surgical technique and Postoperative care, see Operative Technique 7.1.

OPERATIVE TECHNIQUE 7.6:
Deep circumflex iliac (ventral branch) axial pattern flap

Used to close defects of the:
Lateral abdomen; pelvic region (island flap); sacrum (island flap).

Anatomical landmarks
Cranial edge of the wing of the ilium.
Greater trochanter.

Vessel origin
Cranioventral to the wing of the ilium (see Figure 7.1a).

Planning

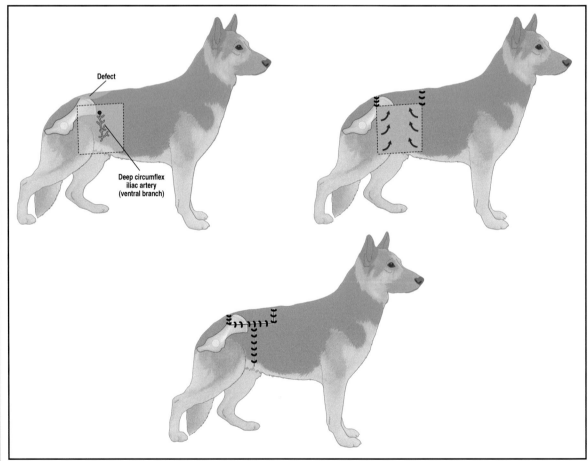

Planning a right-sided deep circumflex iliac (ventral branch) axial pattern flap to close a sacral wound. The flap is planned as an island.

Flap pedicle
Parallel to the long axis of the body; cranial to the greater trochanter.

OPERATIVE TECHNIQUE 7.6 continued:
Deep circumflex iliac (ventral branch) axial pattern flap

Incisions
Cranial and caudal incisions are perpendicular to the long axis of the body and extend ventrally. The caudal incision is halfway between the cranial edge of the wing of the ilium and the greater trochanter and extends distally along the flank and the lateral thigh parallel to the femur to a point proximal to the patella. The cranial incision extends distally, cranial and parallel to the cranial edge of the femur. There is an equal distance between the cranial edge of the wing of the ilium and the cranial and caudal incisions.

Undermine
Deep to the cutaneous trunci muscle.

Modifications
An island graft that can reach defects over the sacrum is created by severing the flap pedicle.

Surgical procedure
For Patient positioning, Assistant, Equipment extras, Surgical technique and Postoperative care, see Operative Technique 7.1.

OPERATIVE TECHNIQUE 7.7:
Deep circumflex iliac (dorsal branch) axial pattern flap

Used to close defects of the:
Caudal thorax; lateral abdomen; flank; lateral lumbar region; pelvic region; lateral and medial thigh; greater trochanter.

Anatomical landmarks
Cranial edge of the wing of the ilium.
Greater trochanter.

Vessel origin
Cranioventral to the wing of the ilium (see Figure 7.1a).

Planning

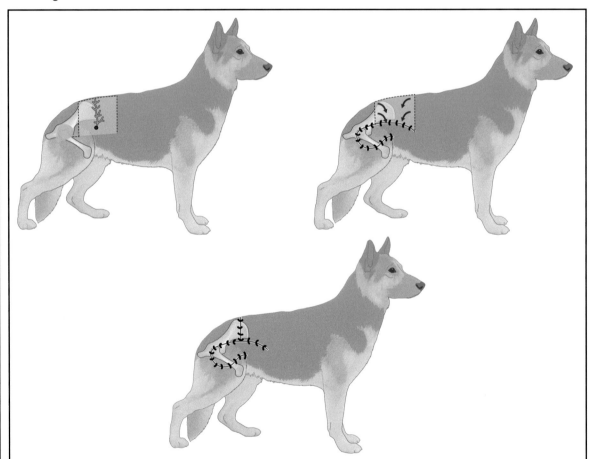

Planning a right-sided deep circumflex iliac (dorsal branch) axial pattern flap to close a right ischial wound.

Flap pedicle
Parallel to the long axis of the body; cranial to the greater trochanter.

Incisions
Cranial and caudal incisions are perpendicular to the long axis of the body and extend dorsally. The caudal incision is halfway between the cranial edge of the wing of the ilium and the greater trochanter. There is an equal distance between the cranial edge of the wing of the ilium and the cranial and caudal incisions.

OPERATIVE TECHNIQUE 7.7 continued:
Deep circumflex iliac (dorsal branch) axial pattern flap

Undermine
Deep to the cutaneous trunci muscle.

Transposition and closure

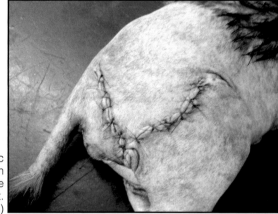

A deep circumflex iliac (dorsal branch) axial pattern flap has been used to close an ischial wound in this cat.
(© John M Williams)

Modifications
Flaps can be extended to the dorsal midline or continue to the contralateral flank fold.
An island graft can be created by severing the flap pedicle.

Surgical procedure
For Patient positioning, Assistant, Equipment extras, Surgical technique and Postoperative care, see Operative Technique 7.1.

OPERATIVE TECHNIQUE 7.8:
Cranial superficial epigastric axial pattern flap

Used to close defects of the:
Lateral abdomen; ventral thorax/sternum.

Anatomical landmarks
Ventral abdominal midline.
Mammary glands and nipples.
Xiphoid process.

Vessel origin
Lateral to the xiphoid process at the third mammary gland nipple (dogs).

Planning

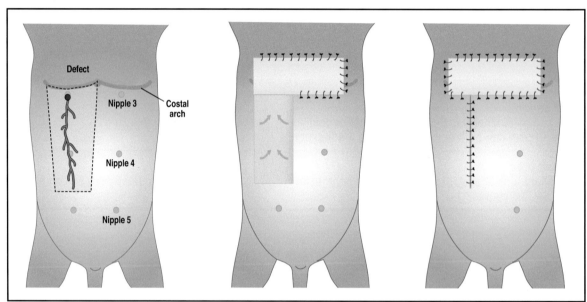

Planning a right-sided cranial superficial epigastric axial pattern flap to close a sternal wound. The flap is planned as an island incorporating nipples 3 and 4.

Flap pedicle
Perpendicular to the midline, level with the xiphoid process.

Incisions
Medial and lateral incisions parallel to the midline on the ventral abdomen extend caudally. The medial incision is located on the ventral midline. There is an equal distance between the nipples and the medial and lateral incisions. The caudal border is a horizontal line at the level of the fourth mammary gland so that the flap contains the third and fourth (and occasionally the fifth) mammary glands.

Undermine
Deep to the supramammaricus muscle.

Modifications
An island graft can be created by severing the flap pedicle.

Surgical procedure
For Patient positioning, Assistant, Equipment extras, Surgical technique and Postoperative care, see Operative Technique 7.1.

OPERATIVE TECHNIQUE 7.9:
Superficial brachial axial pattern flap

Used to close defects of the:
Elbow; antebrachium.

Anatomical landmarks
Elbow.
Humerus.
Greater tubercle.

Vessel origin
3 cm proximal to the elbow on the medial aspect.

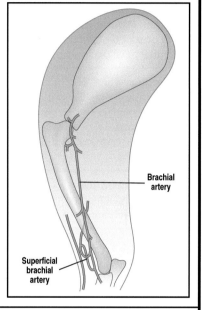

Planning

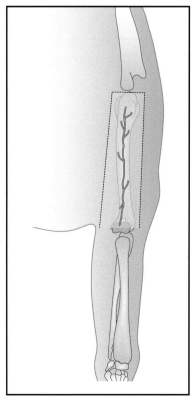

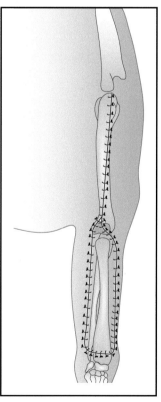

Planning a left-sided superficial brachial axial pattern flap to close an antebrachial wound.

OPERATIVE TECHNIQUE 7.9 continued:
Superficial brachial axial pattern flap

Flap pedicle
Perpendicular to the long axis of the limb on the flexor surface of the elbow.

Incisions
Medial and lateral incisions are on the cranial aspect of the limb parallel to the humerus and extend proximally to the proximal aspect of the greater tubercle. The incisions converge to create a flap 2 cm wide at the apex. The proximal incision is perpendicular to the long axis of the limb.

Undermine
In loose areolar fascial plane.

Modifications
A wider apex can be created to reconstruct wider defects but extensive undermining may be required to close the donor site.

Surgical procedure
For Patient positioning, Assistant, Equipment extras, Surgical technique and Postoperative care, see Operative Technique 7.1.

OPERATIVE TECHNIQUE 7.10:
Genicular axial pattern flap

Used to close defects of the:
Lateral and medial tibia; hock (depends on conformation in dogs).

Anatomical landmarks
Patella.
Tibial tuberosity.
Femoral shaft.
Greater trochanter.

Vessel origin
Medial aspect of the stifle.

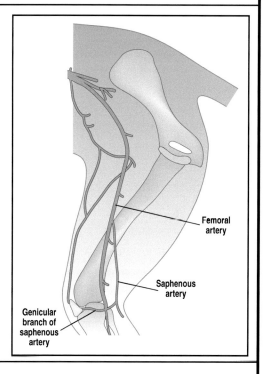

Planning

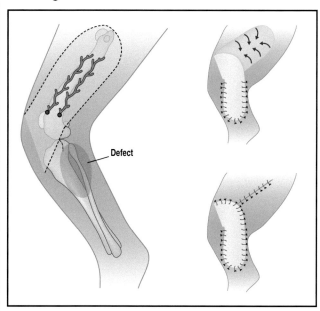

Planning a left-sided genicular axial pattern flap to close a
lateral crural wound in a dog after radical resection of a tumour.

→

OPERATIVE TECHNIQUE 7.10 continued:
Genicular axial pattern flap

Flap pedicle
On the lateral surface of the stifle diagonal to the long axis of the limb in a proximocranial to caudodistal direction. Proximocranial end is located 1 cm proximal to the patella. Distocaudal end lies 1.5 cm distal to the tibial tuberosity.

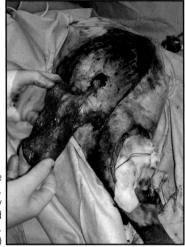

The flap has been raised to the level of the greater trochanter. The vessels are very susceptible to damage and should be handled with care. (Courtesy of Jane Ladlow)

Incisions
Cranial and caudal incisions are on the lateral aspect of the thigh parallel to the long axis of the femoral shaft and extend caudoproximally to the base of the greater trochanter. Incisions converge to create an apex 2 cm narrower than the pedicle. The proximal incision is perpendicular to the long axis of the femur.

Undermine
In loose areolar fascial plane.

Transposition and closure

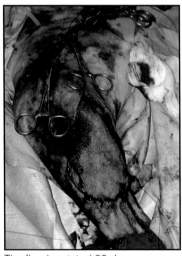

The flap is rotated 90 degrees distally into the wound. (Courtesy of Jane Ladlow)

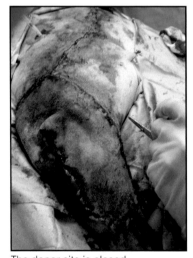

The donor site is closed. (Courtesy of Jane Ladlow)

Surgical procedure
For Patient positioning, Assistant, Equipment extras, Surgical technique and Postoperative care, see Operative Technique 7.1.

OPERATIVE TECHNIQUE 7.11:
Reverse saphenous conduit axial pattern flap

Used to close defects of the:
Dorsal, medial and plantar metatarsus.

Anatomical landmarks
Medial aspect of the thigh.
Tibial shaft.
Tibiotarsal joint.

Vessel origin
Saphenous artery arises on the medial aspect of the stifle but it is not a direct cutaneous artery; rather, the saphenous artery gives off a number of small direct cutaneous arteries.

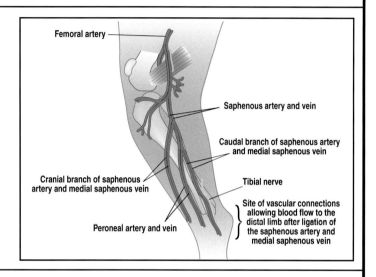

Planning

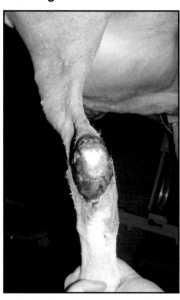

Chronic wound over the calcaneus secondary to rupture of the gastrocnemius tendon in a dog. (Courtesy of John M Williams)

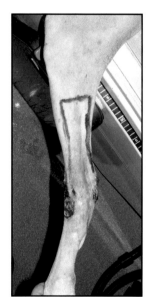

The outline of the flap is drawn on to the skin prior to surgery. The cranial and caudal lines are pulled together to ensure there is sufficient skin to close the donor site as there is little spare skin over the medial aspect of the crus. Flaps of smaller width must be raised in some cases. (Courtesy of John M Williams)

OPERATIVE TECHNIQUE 7.11 continued:
Reverse saphenous conduit axial pattern flap

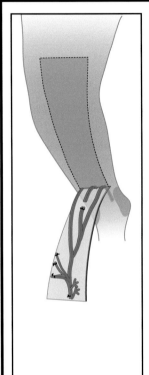
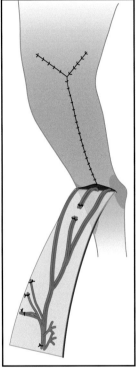
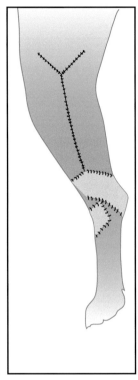

Planning a reverse saphenous conduit axial pattern flap to cover a defect on the lower leg.

Flap pedicle
Perpendicular to the long axis of the limb at the tibiotarsal joint.

Incisions
An incision perpendicular to the long axis of the limb is made in the central third of the medial thigh, at or just above the patella. Deep to this incision the saphenous artery, the medial saphenous vein and saphenous nerve are ligated and divided distal to the origin from the femoral vessels.

Two incisions are made in a distal direction, parallel to the long axis of the limb, 0.5–1 cm cranial to the cranial branch of the saphenous artery and medial saphenous vein (cranial incision) and 0.5–1 cm caudal to the caudal branch of the saphenous artery and medial saphenous vein (caudal incision). The incisions converge distally to allow closure of the donor site.

To protect the caudal branch of the saphenous artery and medial saphenous vein, part of the fascia of the medial gastrocnemius muscle is included in the dissection.

Division of the tibial nerve (before it merges with the caudal branches of the saphenous vessels) and peroneal artery and vein distal to the stifle is performed to allow the flap to be raised. It may be possible to dissect the tibial nerve from the saphenous vessels instead of dividing it, although there are no effects on limb function of severing the nerve.

Raising the flap terminates at the tibiotarsal joint to prevent damage to the vascular anastomoses located in the mid-metatarsal region.

Undermine
In loose areolar fascial plane.

OPERATIVE TECHNIQUE 7.11 continued:
Reverse saphenous conduit axial pattern flap

Transposition and closure

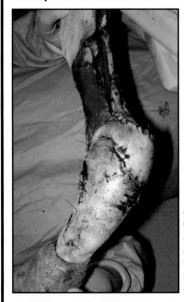

Caudomedial view of the flap, which has been rotated 180° distally into the wound over the calcaneus. The donor site on the medial aspect of the crus has not yet been closed. (Courtesy of John M Williams)

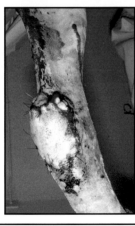

Postoperative appearance of the distal end of the flap over the calcaneus, viewed from the caudolateral aspect. (Courtesy of John M Williams)

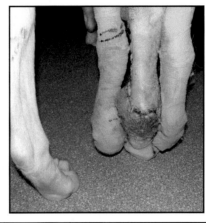

Appearance 2 weeks postoperatively. There is some oedema and bruising of the flap but this is within normal limits. (Courtesy of John M Williams)

Surgical procedure
For Patient positioning, Assistant, Equipment extras, Surgical technique and Postoperative care, see Operative Technique 7.1.

OPERATIVE TECHNIQUE 7.12:
Superficial temporal axial pattern flap

Used to close defects of the:
Maxillofacial region; orbit.

Anatomical landmarks
Zygomatic arch
Lateral aspect of the orbit

Vessel origin
Cranial to the base of the auricular cartilage.

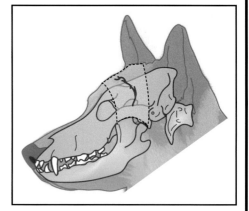

Planning

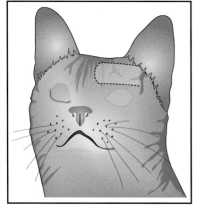 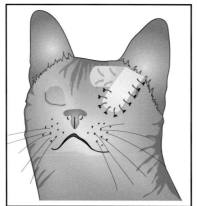 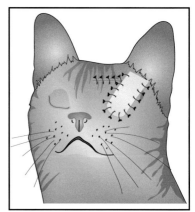

Planning a superficial temporal axial pattern flap to cover a defect on the face of a cat.

Flap pedicle
Parallel to the long axis of the face on the lateral aspect. Caudal end at the caudal aspect of the zygomatic arch. Rostral end at lateral orbital rim. Flap is therefore no wider than the zygomatic arch and lies between the eye and the ear.

Incisions
Cranial and caudal incisions are perpendicular to the long axis of the face and extend to the contralateral mid-dorsal orbital rim. The superficial branch of the rostral auricular nerve plexus located at the cranial edge of the flap by the flap pedicle must be divided to allow flap rotation but does not affect eyelid function.

Undermine
Deep to the frontalis muscle.

OPERATIVE TECHNIQUE 7.12 continued:
Superficial temporal axial pattern flap

Transposition, closure and outcome

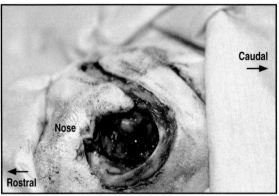

Enucleation wound in a cat. The flap has been raised adjacent to the wound. (Courtesy of Jane F Ladlow)

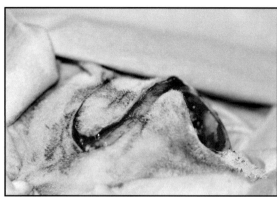

The length of the flap that is raised is sufficient to reach the distant end of the defect, but shorter than the maximum length that can be raised without significant distal necrosis. The flap is rotated through 90 degrees into the defect. (Courtesy of Jane F Ladlow)

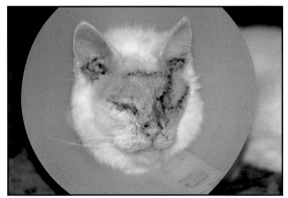

Donor site closed. (Courtesy of Jane F Ladlow)

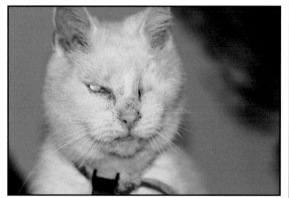

About 3 months after surgery, the flap has healed without complication and hair growth gives a good cosmetic appearance. (Courtesy of Claudia Hartley)

Surgical procedure
For Patient positioning, Assistant, Equipment extras, Surgical technique and Postoperative care, see Operative Technique 7.1.

OPERATIVE TECHNIQUE 7.13:
Caudal auricular axial pattern flap

Used to close defects of the:
Maxillofacial region; orbit; ear.

Anatomical landmarks
Base of the vertical ear canal.
Occipital protuberance.
Wing of atlas vertebra.
Scapular spine.
Dorsal midline (cats).

Vessel origin
Caudal to the base of the pinna, in a depression between the lateral ear canal and the lateral aspect of the wing of atlas.

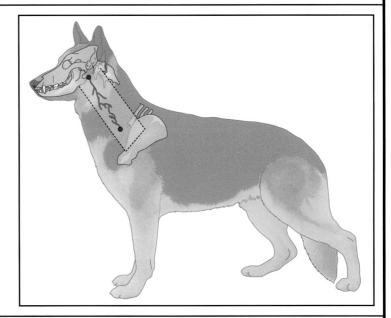

Flap pedicle
Perpendicular to the long axis of the neck overlying the lateral aspect of the wing of atlas.

Incisions
Ventral and dorsal incisions are parallel to the long axis of the neck. In dogs the flap is in the central third of the neck with the ventral incision starting at the base of the vertical ear canal and the dorsal incision commencing at the occipital protuberance. In cats flaps can be made wider, with the dorsal border on the dorsal midline and an equal distance between the vessel and the dorsal and ventral incisions. The caudal incision can be as far caudal as the scapular spine.

Undermine
Deep to the platysma muscle.

→

OPERATIVE TECHNIQUE 7.13 continued:
Caudal auricular axial pattern flap

Transposition, closure and outcome

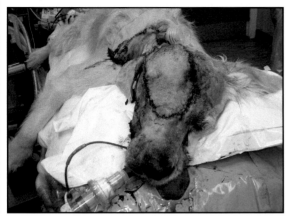

Use of a caudal auricular flap to close a wound over the right orbit in a dog after radical resection of a mass. The flap has been raised to the level of the scapular spine, therefore including the secondary angiosome of the superficial cervical vessels, and rotated 180 degrees rostrally into the defect. (Courtesy of Jane F Ladlow)

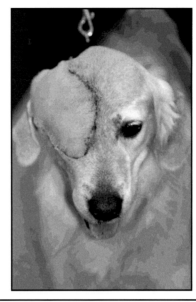

Appearance of the flap 10 days postoperatively. (Courtesy of Jane F Ladlow)

Surgical procedure
For Patient positioning, Assistant, Equipment extras, Surgical technique and Postoperative care, see Operative Technique 7.1.

OPERATIVE TECHNIQUE 7.14:
Lateral caudal axial pattern flap

Used to close defects of the:
Perineum; dorsal pelvic region.

Anatomical landmarks
Coccygeal vertebrae.

Vessel origin
Ventral to the transverse processes of the coccygeal vertebrae.

Planning

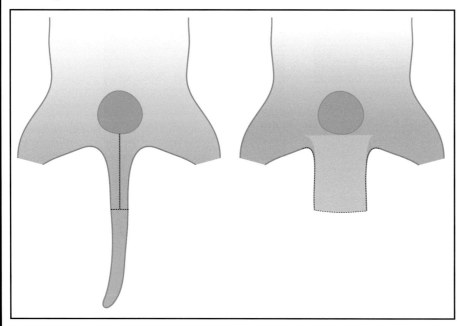

Planning a lateral caudal axial pattern flap to close a sacral wound. A dorsal incision is made over the tail, the coccygeal bones are removed and the distal two-thirds of the tail is amputated.

Flap pedicle
Perpendicular to the long axis of the tail at the junction of the tail and the trunk. The pedicle is ventral for treatment of dorsally located defects, and dorsal for ventral defects.

Incisions
A midline incision is made dorsally for treating dorsal defects or ventrally for ventral defects and extends to the proximal third of the tail. Dissection is performed between the subcutaneous tissues and the deep caudal fascia to protect the laterally located vessels. The bone and fascia of the tail is amputated between the second and third coccygeal vertebrae leaving the skin attached to the pedicle. Skin of the proximal third of the tail is used in the flap.

OPERATIVE TECHNIQUE 7.14 continued:
Lateral caudal axial pattern flap

Transposition and closure

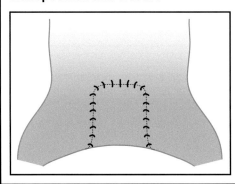

The flap is rotated dorsally into the wound and sutured. There is no donor site to close as the tail has been removed.

Surgical procedure

For Patient positioning, Assistant, Equipment extras, Surgical technique and Postoperative care, see Operative Technique 7.1.

8

Free skin grafting

Richard A.S. White

Introduction

Free skin grafts involve the transfer of variable thicknesses of dermis, with the epidermis, from a donor site to the recipient wound site. In veterinary wound management, grafts are exclusively autografts (i.e. donor and recipient are the same patient). Free grafts find occasional application in the reconstruction of full-thickness skin defects involving the extremities of the dog and cat. However, by comparison with other reconstruction techniques, grafting has a number of limitations:

- Grafting is time-consuming, especially in terms of the care necessary in the post-grafting period when regular and careful management is essential to ensure graft take
- Even after initial take, the grafted skin may still require prolonged ongoing care over several weeks until it is robust enough to become fully functional
- Although most grafting techniques employ full-thickness grafts, the outcome may be somewhat disappointing as regards both the functional and the cosmetic outcome.

For these reasons, skin grafting has fallen from favour as other reconstruction techniques (e.g. primary closure, flaps, etc.) have improved, and it is usually only considered where other techniques are not feasible.

Indications for skin grafting

Free skin grafts are used primarily in the management of large skin deficits involving the lower limb that present unique reconstruction challenges.

Elsewhere on the body a number of more suitable options may be considered:

- Simple *primary closure* of a wound (see Chapter 3) is the preferred technique for dealing with most skin deficits, but the lack of adjacent mobile skin often precludes this option when dealing with larger lesions involving particularly the distal limb
- It may be feasible in some cases to allow skin deficits to heal satisfactorily by *second intention* (see Chapter 4). However, this option should be reviewed carefully in the case of wounds involving the limbs that may develop excessive scar tissue in the vicinity of joints, which can impair function
- The use of *local pedicle flaps* (see Chapter 6) for reconstructing deficits over limbs is similarly restricted by the limited availability of adjacent skin used to create the pedicle
- For those patients that will tolerate adduction of the limb to the flank during the healing period, *distant direct flaps* (see Chapter 6) may prove a viable option
- *Axial pattern pedicle flaps* based on a single direct cutaneous arteriovenous supply (see Chapter 7) are often useful in the reconstruction of proximal limb deficits but can rarely make a contribution to distal limb lesions
- *Orthotopic axial pattern pedicle* grafts using microvascular anastomosis (see Chapter 10) provide greater flexibility for grafting near the distal limb and solve the problem of lack of skin close to the defect. They are limited, however, by the relatively small area covered by the pedicles and the complexity of the surgical procedures.

In increasingly rare circumstances, therefore, free skin grafts can sometimes provide a viable alternative solution to the problem of reconstructing skin deficits involving the distal limb.

How skin grafts 'take'

The process whereby dermal and, less importantly, epidermal cells survive from the point of being harvested at the donor site until they become fully revascularized by the ingrowth of capillaries in the recipient site is often termed graft take. The ease with which take occurs is determined largely by the nutritional requirement of the grafted tissue; this, in turn, is dictated by the volume of viable tissue (dermis) used in the graft (see Figure 8.1). In practice, grafts that contain the smallest volume of dermal tissue (i.e. thin split-thickness) are inherently more viable than grafts with a large dermal tissue component (i.e. full-thickness grafts) since their nutritional demand is less during the take period.

Graft take is a complex process involving more than the simple ingrowth of new capillaries from the recipient bed. Two separate but interrelated processes are important: adherence and nutrition.

Adherence

The development of a fibrin seal that literally 'sticks' the graft to the underlying recipient surface is termed adherence. The fibrin is exuded from the recipient surface; maximal adhesion strength occurs as early as 8 hours after grafting. Adherence is an important process that serves not only to hold the graft in close proximity to the underlying tissue but also to provide a 'scaffold' across which the subsequent ingrowth of new capillaries from the recipient tissue occurs. Leucocytes and fibroblasts marginate into the fibrin, which is progressively replaced by fibrous tissue, further adding to the stability of the grafted skin during the first week. The success of the early fibrin adherence is essential for the subsequent processes that contribute to graft nutrition.

Nutrition

This comprises three separate processes.

Plasmatic imbibition

Sometimes referred to as 'plasmatic circulation', this occurs during the first 2–3 days. The graft behaves like blotting paper at this stage and absorbs the fibrinogen-free serum proteins and erythrocytes exuded from the recipient surface. As a result it takes on an oedematous appearance and is often darkly pigmented through absorption of haemoglobin products. Plasmatic imbibition, however, is thought to be important in providing early nutritional support until capillary ingrowth begins to develop.

> **WARNING**
> **The rather unhealthy appearance of the graft at this stage can often be mistaken for early rejection of the graft.**

Inosculation

Inosculation is the development of a rudimentary vascular circulation within the graft and begins by the second or third day. It is the result of new capillary buds from the recipient tissue crossing the fibrin scaffold and connecting directly with the old redundant vessels in the graft. This process of re-anastomosis between new capillaries and old blood vessels is thought to provide some sluggish and disorganized movement of blood. It is not clear how important this process is in contributing to the long-term survival of the graft, but it may be responsible for the more viable appearance that successful grafts take on after the first week.

Revascularization

Revascularization, or vascular penetration, is the final process and may take a further 1–2 weeks to complete, by which time the healthy appearance of the graft underlines the re-establishment of circulation in the skin.

Types of skin graft

Skin grafts can be classified according to the depth of skin harvested (Figure 8.1) or the wound coverage provided by the graft (see Figure 8.2).

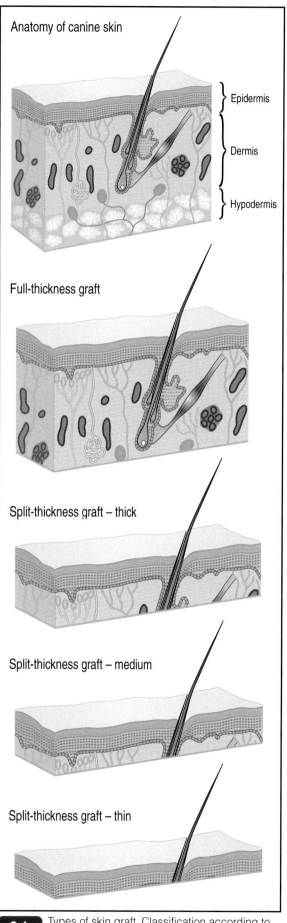

Anatomy of canine skin

Epidermis

Dermis

Hypodermis

Full-thickness graft

Split-thickness graft – thick

Split-thickness graft – medium

Split-thickness graft – thin

8.1 Types of skin graft. Classification according to skin depth.

Full-thickness grafts

Full-thickness grafts contain the entire dermal layer with the epidermis (see Figure 8.1) and are generally considered to be the most suitable type of graft for use in small animal reconstructive surgery, since:

- They are robust and capable of withstanding considerable handling during harvesting and positioning at the recipient site
- They retain all the adnexal dermal elements (e.g. hair follicles, elastin fibres, apocrine and sweat glands) that are essential for the ultimate functionality and cosmetic success of the graft.

The single major disadvantage of the full-thickness graft, however, is its comparatively greater nutritional need during take.

Split-thickness grafts

Split-thickness grafts contain a variable depth of the upper dermal layers and the epidermis. They can be further subclassified as thin, medium or thick, depending on the depth of the dermal contribution (see Figure 8.1).

Despite their widespread use in human plastic reconstruction, split-thickness grafts have a number of important disadvantages in small animal surgery and are only rarely used. Split-thickness grafts are normally harvested as sheets of skin by means of a Brown oscillating dermatome; although extremely time-consuming, they can also be hand-harvested using a Humby or Silva knife. They are rather fragile by comparison with full-thickness grafts and require considerable care during collection and placement. Depending on the depth of dermal collection, the harvesting process divides the adnexal components between the graft and the donor skin. The result is that both sites eventually have poor durability, a greater tendency to contracture, and sparse hair regrowth. In addition, the donor site is not amenable to surgical closure and therefore heals secondarily by epithelialization and contraction. There is consequently a considerable requirement for open wound management of this area too, which often causes the patient more discomfort than the recipient wound.

The major advantage of split-thickness grafts is their less fastidious nutritional requirement but the additional equipment costs, significant donor site care requirement, ultimate lack of hair coverage and poor skin functionality all tend to argue strongly against their use in small animals and they will not be discussed further.

Sheet grafts

Sheet grafts provide for complete wound coverage and are collected by removal of full-thickness skin cut to the shape of a template of the wound; the resulting defect requires primary closure.

Pinch, punch, stamp or strip grafts

Pinch, punch, stamp or strip grafts (Figure 8.2) provide partial wound coverage and can only be used to contribute to wounds that are intended to heal by secondary intention. They promote secondary healing by increasing the surface area of epithelialization

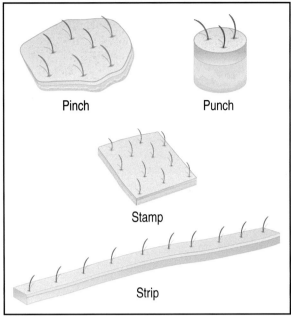

8.2 Types of skin graft: Classification according to wound coverage.

within the wound. Their collection and placement is very labour-intensive and they provide such a poor functional and cosmetic result that they have very few indications in small animals.

Harvesting the graft

Donor site

The donor site for the graft should be chosen bearing the following in mind:

- It should be capable of providing an area of skin sufficiently large for the intended reconstruction
- It should be readily accessible and amenable to simple reconstruction
- The harvested skin should be durable enough to provide resistance capable of coping with the anticipated 'wear' at the recipient site. This requires consideration not only of the hair density but also the quality of the dermal layer. Skin from the flank usually provides a balance of good hair density with reasonable quality dermal tissue. Skin from the ventrum, on the other hand, although containing a more robust dermal layer contains comparatively few hair follicles and is usually avoided
- Whilst some consideration may be given to 'matching' the appearance of the donor skin to that surrounding the recipient site, this is of relatively little importance compared to the general imperative of the reconstruction.

PRACTICAL TIP
In most patients, the most commonly used donor site that can usually fulfil all the criteria is the flank. The neck and the ventrum are possible, but inferior, options that might be considered if the flank were to be unavailable.

Graft collection

Sheet grafts are normally collected by dissecting between the loose adipose tissue below the hypodermal layer and the underlying panniculus muscle. This can be achieved more easily by means of skin hooks (or, more simply, hypodermic needles with bent-over tips) or using fine monofilament stay sutures strategically placed around the periphery of the graft as it is elevated. Sheet grafts can be collected by cutting around the shape of a gauze or paper template of the wound for reconstruction; however, since the resulting defect needs primary closure it may be easier simply to remove an adequately large area of skin for the graft in a shape that simplifies reconstruction (e.g. ellipse; Figure 8.3).

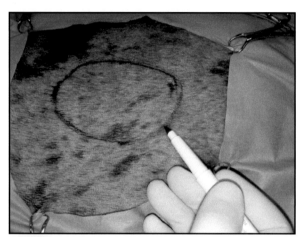

8.3 Skin graft harvesting: rather than use a template of the wound, it may be easier simply to remove an adequately large area of skin in a shape that simplifies reconstruction, such as an ellipse. (© RAS White)

PRACTICAL TIP
Grafts should be collected with an additional few millimetres of overlap to ensure collection of an adequate area.

Pinch grafts are collected by the rather laborious method of tenting small areas of skin with a hypodermic needle or skin hook, and then incising a circular shape. Pinch graft donor sites are left to heal secondarily.

Punch grafts are more easily and efficiently collected by means of a Keyes skin biopsy instrument; the donor sites require surgical closure.

Stamp and strip grafts are both collected by surgical resection; strip grafts are collected as 0.5 cm wide strips of full-thickness skin of lengths measured to that of the recipient site.

Preparing the graft

Removing hypodermal tissue

Full-thickness grafts are normally prepared with little or no hypodermal tissue, since the inclusion of any tissue interposed between the dermal tissue and the recipient wound merely serves to impede vascular access to the more important dermal cells, without contributing to the graft. The underlying hypodermal adipose tissue should be removed from the graft as far as possible in order to improve vascular access to the viable cells of the dermis. This is best achieved for sheet grafts by laying the graft on a graft board, or folding it over the forefinger with the hypodermal layer upwards, and carefully trimming off the adipose tissue with fine scissors (Figure 8.4). The tension that can be created by rolling the graft over the surgeon's finger can make adipose tissue easier to remove. An alternative method is to harvest the graft using a scalpel blade, separating the hypodermal adipose tissue from the dermis as the graft is harvested (Figure 8.5).

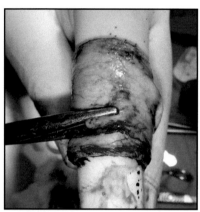

8.4 Skin graft preparation: removal of hypodermal tissue. The graft is draped over the surgeon's finger to permit removal of the unwanted tissue by careful trimming with scissors. (© RAS White)

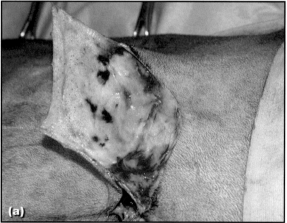

(a)

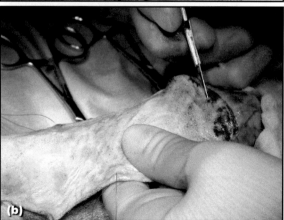

(b)

8.5 An alternative method to remove hypodermal tissue. **(a)** The graft is harvested using a scalpel blade. **(b)** Hypodermal adipose tissue is separated from the dermis as the graft is harvested. (© Alison L. Moores)

WARNING
Scraping hypodermal tissue away with a scalpel blade can cause considerable damage to the dermal layer and should be avoided.

All grafts should be collected under aseptic conditions and rolled in saline- or antibiotic-soaked sponges to prevent desiccation pending application to the recipient site. Harvested skin can be preserved for some days in a refrigerator at +4°C, although this is hardly ever required or practical.

Provisions for drainage

Recipient sites will produce a considerable volume of exudate below the graft during the first few days until adherence is complete. This exudate provides an important contribution to the early nutritional requirements of the graft but its excessive accumulation can separate sheet grafts from the recipient bed and may lead to their ultimate failure. It is essential, therefore, that some provision is made for drainage of this fluid.

Drains

Active suction drains (see Chapter 5) can be placed beneath the graft to aspirate the fluid. It is essential that the fenestrated tube component of the drain should be of the smallest diameter, to avoid interfering with the adherence of the graft, and that the drain is left *in situ* for no more than 24–48 hours.

'Pie-crusting'

Pie-crusting describes the process of making a small number of full-thickness stab incisions through the graft at strategic points to permit drainage of the exudate (Figure 8.6). The use of firm bandaging and daily cleansing to keep the pie-crust perforations open will promote ongoing drainage at these points.

Meshing

Meshing the graft involves increasing the number of perforations to provide increased opportunity for drainage. Grafts may be partially or fully meshed.

Partial meshing simply involves adding additional handmade stab incisions, as for pie-crusting, to increase the opportunity for drainage.

Full meshing of the graft is usually performed mechanically by means of a meshing table (Figure 8.7) or roller mesher and confers a number of additional qualities on the graft, including:

- The potential for expansion of the graft by 'opening' the meshes to allow it to cover larger wounds where donor skin is at a premium. The maximal expansion of the meshed graft is usually two to four times the original width of the graft but this is achieved at the expense of some reduction in graft length
- Precontouring the graft to a wound template is unnecessary, since meshed grafts can be expanded to meet irregular wound outlines
- Convex surfaces (e.g. over an elbow joint) are more easily covered (Figure 8.7c).

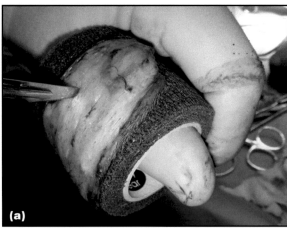
(a)

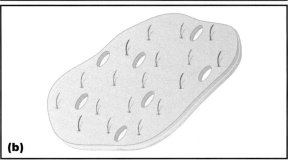
(b)

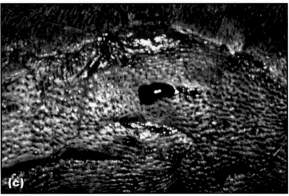
(c)

8.6 Skin graft preparation – 'pie crusting'. **(a)** Full-thickness stab incisions being made in a free skin graft draped over a sterilized roll of conforming bandage. **(b)** Diagrammatic representation of end result. **(c)** Pie-crust skin graft *in situ* 48 hours after grafting. Note the blue/red coloration and oedematous appearance due to plasmatic imbibition. Fluid can be seen exuding from below the graft through one of the pie-crust incisions. (© RAS White)

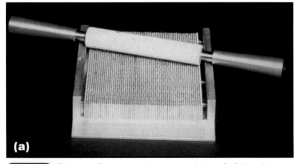
(a)

8.7 Skin graft preparation – meshing. **(a)** A table meshing instrument. The graft is laid over the table, which consists of parallel rows of blades, and then firmly rolled with the Teflon rolling pin to produce a fully meshed graft. (© RAS White) (continues) ▶

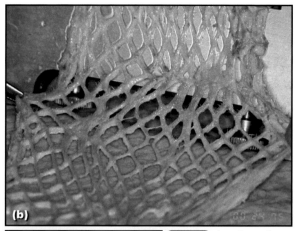

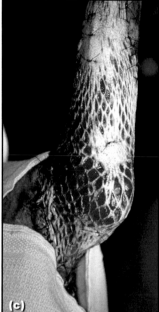

8.7 (continued) Skin graft preparation – meshing. **(b)** A mechanically prepared fully meshed full-thickness sheet graft. **(c)** Graft *in situ* over an elbow wound. Note how the graft can be expanded to cover wider areas of the wound and also Its capacity to mould to the convex surface of the joint. (© RAS White)

- Healthy granulation tissue
- Fresh surgical wounds
- Surgically 'clean' wounds.

Granulation tissue

This is an ideal recipient tissue for grafted skin because it contains an abundant supply of vascular capillaries in a matrix of collagen, with significant growth factor stimulation. It normally appears in clean open wounds within 3–4 days of the original injury (Figure 8.8); although the presence of necrotic debris or infection can slow its formation, its very presence is a good indication that any wound sepsis process has been controlled and grafting can proceed. Grafting is best performed at the earliest opportunity – when the granulation tissue first appears – despite what may be the absence of complete wound coverage by it; this ensures that there is both a wealth of vascular support and maximal stimulation from growth promoting factors. In open wounds in which the granulation tissue has become well established, the vascular support for the graft diminishes progressively as capillaries are replaced by increasing components of connective tissue.

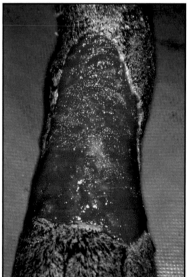

8.8 Fresh granulation tissue – an ideal site for skin grafting. There is evidence of early peripheral epithelial tissue; this should be incised prior to surgery to prevent it under-running the graft. (© RAS White)

It must be borne in mind, however, that expansion of the graft through meshing sacrifices the final functional and cosmetic result, since the 'open' areas of the mesh heal secondarily without any dermal contribution. Overall, less wound coverage is provided and hence the functional and cosmetic outcome suffers. Fully meshed grafts are therefore usually limited to patients where there is a need to cover very large wounds.

For most cases where adequate skin is available and the ultimate functional and cosmetic outcome is the priority, drains or pie-crusting remain the most employed solutions.

Recipient sites

Preparation

The recipient site for a skin graft should be free of tissue debris and major bacterial contamination. It should also be capable of providing a vascular supply and nutritional support to the graft. Suitable recipient tissues for skin grafting therefore include:

> **PRACTICAL TIP**
> Recent wounds covered with granulation tissue can be stimulated to produce further vascularization by mechanical debridement using dressings for 24–48 hours prior to grafting.

More chronic granulation tissue (Figure 8.9) often does not provide sufficient nutritional support for a graft, however, and more established wounds are best managed by the complete resection of chronic tissue to permit the development of a further fresh granulation bed. In wounds in which the process of secondary wound healing has progressed to the point that epithelialization is occurring at the wound periphery, the wound edges should be excised with a scalpel to interrupt this process, which will otherwise progress to undermine the graft.

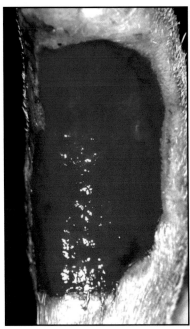

8.9
Established granulation tissue: the less active appearance of the granulation tissue and the presence of significant peripheral epithelial tissue indicates that a graft is less likely to take. (© RAS White)

Surgical wounds

Surgically 'clean' and fresh surgical wounds are frequently overlooked as potential sites for skin grafting but they are very suitable recipient sites provided the wound remains well vascularized. The development of haematomas or serous exudate below the graft is, however, a more frequent problem in the fresh wound, and it is essential that some kind of provision is made for drainage (Figure 8.10). Delaying the graft by 24–48 hours to encourage early granulation is often considered to improve the chances of success.

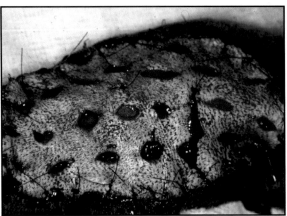

8.10 A fresh surgical wound covered by a sheet graft. There is extensive meshing to accommodate the anticipated additional exudate under the graft. Note the presence of sutures between the centre of the graft and the wound bed to provide greater graft contact. (© RAS White)

> **WARNING**
> **Skin grafts are unlikely to be successful in wounds that are still grossly infected, contain necrotic tissue debris or have previously epithelialized surfaces.**

Applying the graft

Sheet grafts can be applied to both granulation tissue and fresh surgical wounds.

- Non-meshed or unexpanded sheet grafts should be trimmed to the outline of a template of the wound shape, allowing a few millimetres overlap on all edges to accommodate any contracture as the graft takes.
- The graft is then sutured in place with loosely applied simple interrupted 2 metric (3/0 USP) monofilament nylon around its periphery.
- An unmeshed graft will require some form of active drainage so as to prevent the accumulation of fluid interfering with its take. Meshed grafts conform more readily – depending on the extent of the meshing – to irregular wound surfaces and shapes.

Stamp grafts are anchored into place with minimal numbers of fine monofilament sutures as for sheet grafts.

Pinch and **punch grafts** need to be firmly embedded in the recipient bed to prevent movement or their loss and cannot be attached to the wound surface. They are only suitable, therefore, for application to wounds that have an established bed of granulation tissue. They should be implanted as deeply as practical into stab incisions made with a scalpel into the surface of the wound.

Strip grafts are likewise difficult to attach firmly to the wound surface. They are implanted in grooves cut in the surface of the granulation tissue before being anchored at each end with monofilament sutures.

Care of the graft

The processes of preparing a recipient bed, harvesting a graft and anchoring it in place are comparatively easy. However, the subsequent care of the graft to the point at which it has not just become established but is capable of functioning adequately, is considerably more complex and calls for a clear understanding of the graft 'take' process (see above), combined with meticulous and frequent wound care.

The survival of a skin graft depends upon:

- Careful asepsis
- Immobilization of the graft on the recipient surface
- The accumulation of minimal quantities of fluid below the graft.

Asepsis

Infection associated with skin grafting is not common if routine aseptic techniques are observed during surgery and subsequent wound management. Where infection does occur, *Pseudomonas* spp. or *Klebsiella* spp. are the organisms most often implicated, and can lead to rapid and disastrous graft loss. Bacterial toxins are released and, together with the associated cell death, inhibit vascularization and activate the fibrinolytic system, dissolving the all-important fibrin attachment between recipient bed and graft. The septic process may also result in sufficient exudation from the wound to separate it from the graft.

The incidence of sepsis can be minimized by attention to aseptic technique at both the donor and recipient sites. Presoaking the graft in antibiotic solutions is reported to reduce the incidence of sepsis, although the role of systemic antibiotics is probably more important. Topical antibiotics are best delivered by spray and should be active against both *Pseudomonas* and β-lactamase-producing organisms.

Immobilization
Movement of the graft in the first few hours after placement can interfere with the initial development of the fibrin attachment; any subsequent movement of the graft during the first week can still shear this fibrin attachment and interfere with graft contact, delaying or even preventing graft take.

- Adequate placement of sutures around the periphery of the graft helps to minimize this problem.
- For large grafts covering irregular surfaces, additional mattress sutures can be placed through the graft to the underlying granulation tissue at strategic points.
- Alternatively, bandage support should be used comprising:
  - *a non- or low-adherent contact layer* usually consisting of a commercially available perforated silicone sheet (Figure 8.11) or plastic sheet backed with an absorbent material, which allows the dressing to be removed with minimal risk of the graft being disrupted during dressing changes
  - *an absorbent intermediate layer* (e.g. cotton wool) to remove any exudate from the wound and to provide support to limit movement of the limb
  - *an outer protective layer* into which a gutter splint can be incorporated for further immobilization if necessary.

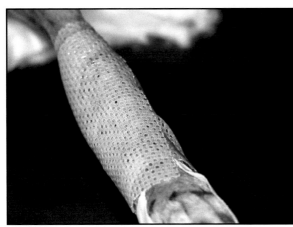

8.11 A non-adherent silicone contact layer is positioned over a full-thickness graft over the hock prior to placement of a compressive dressing. Great care should be taken to prevent detachment of the graft when re-dressing during the first 3–4 days. (© RAS White)

Dressings should be changed regularly to prevent exudate from accumulating in the vicinity of the graft and to prevent ingress of any soiling materials. The first dressing change is normally undertaken 48 hours after grafting; since graft adherence is only partially developed at this stage, great care should be taken to avoid disturbing the graft as the contact layer is peeled away from its surface. The frequency of subsequent changes will depend on the amount of exudate produced by the graft site but changes every 24–48 hours are usually appropriate during the first 2 weeks. Fresh surgical wounds are the most productive, and require almost daily changes during the first week.

Prevention of fluid accumulation
Firm contact between the graft and recipient bed is essential for the development of the fibrin scaffold that permits the ultimate vascular ingrowth. Haematoma or seroma development below the graft can quickly separate it from the recipient bed, breaking down the fibrin seal.

- Good graft contact begins with a properly prepared recipient surface, which is free of debris and any surface irregularities.
- Careful preparation of the wound, to ensure that all vascular oozing is controlled with diathermy, will help to minimize the accumulation of blood or exudate.
- Provision should be made for drainage (e.g. drains, mesh graft; see above), particularly in cases where pronounced exudation is anticipated, such as after grafting a fresh wound.
- Suturing the graft in place under a little peripheral tension helps to improve wound contact and prevents it from rolling up or moving over the wound. The use of tie-over or bolus dressings (see Chapter 4) to create firm uniform downward pressure across the graft surface is also a very efficient way of tackling this problem; these dressings can be held in place by means of monofilament skin loops.
- Regular inspection of the graft should enable any exudate accumulation or haematoma formation to be recognized. Fluid can be removed by gentle pressure over graft mesh sites with cotton buds (Figure 8.12) or aspirated by fine hypodermic needle as soon as possible to preserve the graft.

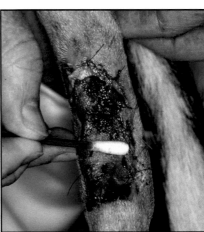

8.12 Management of sub-graft exudate (day 5) by careful pressure with a cotton bud over the mesh openings. (© RAS White)

Ongoing care

Once a graft has reached the point of revascularization, it will still require ongoing bandaging to ensure that it remains protected from normal 'wear'; this may be for a period of a further 3–4 weeks. The return of full dermal function requires contribution from sweat and apocrine gland secretions and, again, it may be several weeks before this function returns. In the meantime, the skin is often dry and likely to be pruritic; topical application of emollient creams (e.g. E45, lanolin) will alleviate these signs and some provision should also be made to protect the skin from self-trauma.

Interpreting graft appearance

What to expect

- From **day 1** onwards the graft will be surprisingly well fixed to the recipient bed and capable of resisting reasonable disturbance or even firm digital pressure during dressing changes, although this should be avoided where possible.
- From **day 1 to day 3** the graft will become engorged and oedematous as plasmatic imbibition peaks. The graft colour will darken and regions of the graft will take on a range of blue to brown hues. At this point, areas of blue coloration should be regarded as a healthy sign and not as an indicator of graft failure!
- Towards the **end of week 1**, the graft will become less oedematous and assume a pinker appearance as modest circulation begins. It will be several days yet before it takes on a pink, well vascularized colour.
- Signs of hair growth may appear during **weeks 2 to 3** but this is variable and may take several weeks.

What NOT to expect

- Any indication of **graft movement** during dressing changes, even from the earliest stages of grafting, is a concerning development. It is perhaps potentially less disastrous during the first 24–48 hours, whilst there is still potential for continuing plasmatic imbibition provided the graft is adequately stabilized. Beyond this period, any graft instability will result in shearing of the fibrin bed and failure of angiogenesis.
- Separation of the graft is usually seen in cases of total failure; however, partial or complete **epidermal sloughing** can sometimes occur (Figure 8.13). Despite the graft site appearance most cases go on to success as the deeper, dermal layer embeds in the wound and continues to be viable.
- Whereas blue is an encouraging early colour change, other colours are not:
  - **white** (blanching) (Figure 8.14) usually indicates graft ischaemia
  - **black** is always indicative of necrosis; affected areas should be resected as soon as this is recognized so that any unaffected areas can be salvaged.

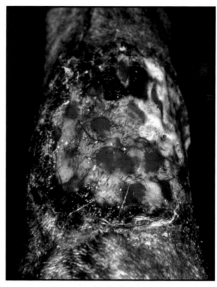

8.13

Epidermal sloughing. Although there is apparent necrosis of the graft peripherally, only the superficial epidermal layer is affected. The deeper dermal layer remained viable and progressed to a complete take. (© RAS White)

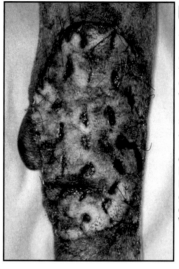

8.14

A full-thickness partially meshed graft on day 3. In addition to the expected colour changes associated with plasmatic imbibition, there are significant areas that are blanched white – in this case due to overly firm bandaging. Less constrictive bandaging allowed the graft to go on to complete take. (© RAS White)

- Some grafts may show signs of minor superficial infection, but any evidence of **purulent exudate** under the graft is usually indicative of imminent failure, and graft salvage proves impossible in most cases.

The functional and cosmetic result

The functional and cosmetic outcome of a free skin graft depends ultimately on two main factors:

- The amount of dermis and associated adnexal structures contained in the graft
- The proportion of the wound covered by grafted dermis.

Thus, the more dermal tissue grafted into the wound, the greater the likelihood of a good functional and cosmetic result.

- Split-thickness grafts contain comparatively few adnexal structures, including hair follicles, and hence regrowth is sparse and the skin is poorly lubricated.

- Full-thickness grafts retain most of their adnexal structures, including hair follicles, but even these can be significantly reduced in number where the graft is extensively meshed and is accompanied by some secondary healing.
- Epithelialized areas contain no adnexal structures and hence are less functional and cosmetic.
- Techniques that cover the wound completely (e.g. unmeshed sheet grafts) achieve the best result because of minimal secondary healing.
- Widely expanded mesh grafts heal with a greater proportion of epithelialized skin and hence have a sparser hair/adnexal contribution (Figure 8.15).

- The most inferior results are achieved with strip and pinch grafts, which heal with large areas of the wound containing no adnexal structures at all.

For most practical purposes, a full-thickness sheet graft with minimal or no perforation will provide the best outcome. It will, however, dictate more careful management in the take period.

Trouble shooting

Figure 8.16 lists the problems associated with skin grafting and suggests how they can be managed.

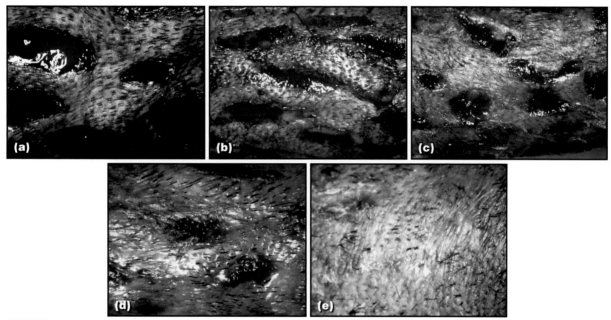

8.15 Take in a fully-meshed full-thickness graft. **(a)** Day 3: plasmatic imbibition is the major nutrition process and is responsible for the blue/brown coloration in the grafted skin. **(b)** Day 5: coloration through imbibition is less evident; pinker appearance is consistent with beginnings of vascular flow through inosculation. **(c)** Day 8: vascular circulation is increasingly evident; secondary healing in 'open' mesh area progressing. **(d)** Day 14: graft take now established with circulation through revascularization complete; secondary healing in ungrafted areas progressing rapidly. **(e)** Day 21: hair growth now evident in grafted areas; secondary healing with epithelialization now complete in ungrafted areas. (© RAS White)

Problem	Pathophysiology	Management
Fluid accumulation below the graft		
All recipient beds exude some fluid but excessive fluid may be produced after: • poor haemostasis in wound preparation • grafting over fresh wounds	Fluid separates the graft from the recipient bed • removes the serum nutritional source • the fibrin scaffold is broken down preventing in-growth of new capillaries	Drainage can be achieved by: • using a meshed graft • placing an active suction drain below the graft • using 'tie over' bolus dressing • aspirating fluid with a hypodermic needle daily
Graft movement		
Inadequate immobilization of the graft: • poor suture placement • insufficient/inadequate bandaging to prevent movement at graft site	Some minor movement of the graft in the first 24 hours is acceptable and does not necessarily lead to graft failure Subsequent movement will lead to shearing of the new capillaries and failure of revascularization	The graft should be sutured with a little tension: mattress sutures can be placed through the graft and recipient surface An appropriate three-layer Robert Jones bandage should be employed during the first week (see Chapter 4)

8.16 Trouble shooting for skin grafting. (continues) ▶

Problem	Pathophysiology	Management
Infection		
Poor aseptic technique Pre-existing infection in the graft bed	Toxin release and cell death cause lysis of fibrin Scaffold and failure of revascularization	Good aseptic technique during graft surgery Pre-soak graft in antibiotic solution Systemic antibiotic therapy Rapid resection/drainage at infected sites
Graft necrosis		
Early (Days 1–4) Inadequate debridement of the dermal aspect of the graft Poorly vascularized recipient bed (e.g. indolent granulation tissue)	Failure of early nutrition due to impaired serum exudate/imbibition	Resect non-viable areas as soon as apparent Start over again if grafting on to chronic granulation tissue
Late (days 4 – onwards) Graft dressings applied too tightly Impaired systemic health of the patient	Failure of inosculation/revascularization	Check dressing construction Investigate general patient health (e.g. endocrine disease)

8.16 (continued) Trouble shooting for skin grafting.

Further reading

Pavletic M (1998) *Atlas of Small Animal Reconstructive Surgery, 2nd edn.* WB Saunders, Philadelphia

Pope ER (1998) Mesh skin grafting. In: *Current Techniques in Small Animal Surgery, 4th edn*, ed. MJ Bojrab, pp.603–605. Willliams and Wilkins, Baltimore

Swaim SF (2002) Skin grafting. In: *Textbook of Small Animal Surgery, 3rd edn*, ed. D Slatter, pp.321–338. WB Saunders, Philadelphia

CASE EXAMPLE 1:
Free skin grafting for a chronic open wound

History
A 7-year-old female Collie was presented with a chronic open wound over the distal forelimb and non-weightbearing thoracic limb lameness. She had sustained a degloving injury to the distal limb more than 4 weeks before in a road traffic trauma. Reconstructive surgery was initially declined by the owner and the wound had undergone open wound management in an attempt to promote secondary healing.

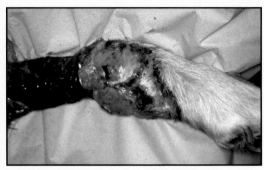

The wound on presentation. (© RAS White)

Assessment
The lameness was found to be the consequence of the development of exuberant chronic granulation tissue around the carpus, limiting the range of movement. Imaging ruled out any underlying orthopaedic complications.

Management options
In view of the complications of secondary healing, a reconstructive procedure of the cutaneous defect was considered to be essential and the only likely means of permitting return of function for the limb. Options for reconstruction were considered to include the following:

- Distant direct flap
- Orthotopic microvascular transfer
- Free skin graft.

The patient's temperament was considered to be unsuited to the postoperative wound maintenance necessary for distant direct flap management. It was felt that an orthotopic transfer was not feasible in view of the extent of the wound. A free skin graft was therefore selected as the only remaining option.

Treatment
Assessment of the wound showed the granulation tissue to be indolent and poorly vascularized; it was considered highly unlikely that this would support a skin graft.

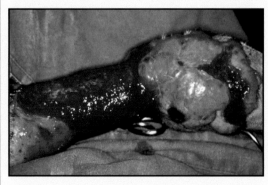

Indolent and poorly vascularized granulation tissue. (© RAS White)

The granulation tissue was therefore resected and open wound management performed until fresh granulation tissue was re-established in the wound.

Case Example 1 continues ▶

CASE EXAMPLE 1 continued:
Free skin grafting for a chronic open wound

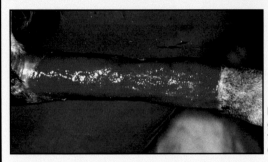

Fresh granulation tissue. (© RAS White)

A full-thickness sheet graft was harvested from the patient's flank and prepared by removal of the hypodermal tissue and partial meshing to ensure adequate drainage. The graft was attached to the recipient wound at its periphery and also with mattress sutures at strategic points through its surface.

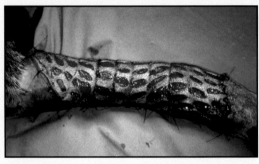

Partially meshed full-thickness graft in place. (© RAS White)

The limb was managed in a Robert Jones dressing for 1 week before progressive reduction in bandaging support; ongoing dressing and graft management was continued for a further 2 weeks.

Outcome
There was successful take of the entire graft; assessment at 21 days post-grafting showed early hair regrowth and, importantly, a return to a completely functional weightbearing limb.

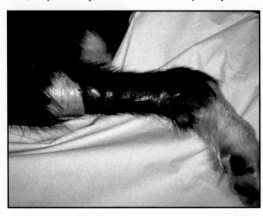

21 days post-grafting. (© RAS White)

Drainage was thought to be the most important priority for this graft in view of its large circumferential area and hence extensive meshing was performed. In retrospect, the result, although very functional, could have been more cosmetic through limited meshing.

CASE EXAMPLE 2:
Free skin grafting for a burn wound

History
A 5-year-old male Dalmatian was presented with an open wound over the lateral aspect of the distal hindlimb and hock, 27 days after sustaining an arc burn as the result of close proximity to a high-voltage rail line.

Assessment
The burn had removed the full thickness of the soft tissue covering the lateral aspect of the distal tibia. Secondary healing was underway and a bed of healthy granulation tissue was beginning to cover the exposed bone.

Management options
Coverage of the tibia with vascularized tissue was considered to be an essential preliminary step prior to any reconstructive procedure. Options for subsequent reconstruction were considered to include the following:

- Distant direct flap
- Free skin graft.

A caudal superficial epigastric flap was thought unlikely to be sufficiently long to reach the wound area. The patient's temperament was considered to be unsuited to the postoperative wound maintenance necessary for distant direct flap management and hence a free skin graft was considered to be the most practical option.

Treatment
Open wound management was continued for a further week until the secondary healing process had covered the exposed bone.

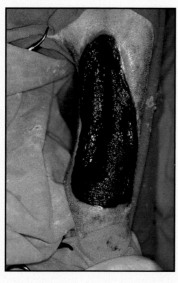

Granulation tissue covering the bone. (© RAS White)

Skin was harvested from the patient's flank and prepared as a pie-crust/partially meshed graft. The graft was attached at its periphery and also with mattress sutures through its surface.

Case Example 2 continues ▶

CASE EXAMPLE 2 continued:
Free skin grafting for a burn wound

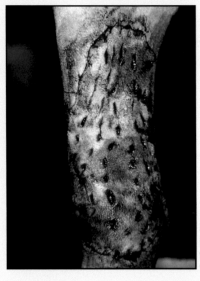

Pie-crust/
partially meshed
graft in place.
(© RAS White)

Outcome
The limb was managed in a compressive bandage and re-dressed daily. Inspection of the graft showed progressively less viable appearance and by day 5 there was evidence of complete graft failure.

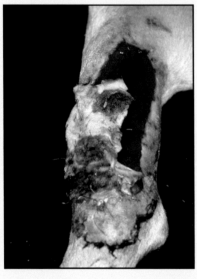

The graft has failed.
(© RAS White)

Following removal of the necrotic grafted skin, the wound was again managed by open wound management and eventually allowed to heal with an epithelialized covering.

The graft was thought to have failed in this case due to lack of vascular support from the recipient granulation tissue. The extended open wound management necessary for bone coverage meant that the granulation tissue was more than 5 weeks old at the time of grafting. In retrospect, aggressive debridement, or even resection, of the granulation tissue and detachment of the epithelializing margins would have induced a more active secondary healing likely to have supported the graft.

9

Pedicled muscle flaps

Stephen Baines

Introduction

A muscle flap involves elevating all or part of a skeletal muscle, whilst preserving sufficient vascular supply to allow it to remain viable, and transposing it into a recipient site.

Local transposition of a muscle flap is a useful and simple technique and does not require any special instrumentation. However, it does require a good knowledge of anatomy, an understanding of the indications and limitations of the technique, and careful dissection. A muscle flap is indicated when the specific benefits of transposed muscle tissue is needed. This is particularly the case when closing defects that are ischaemic, infected or irradiated, or when muscle bulk or physical support is needed.

Indications

Muscle flaps may provide the following functions:

* Support of tissue, such as in the repair of hernias or ruptures of the body wall, diaphragm or of internal organs, e.g. bladder, oesophagus
* Augmentation of vascular supply, e.g. chronic osteomyelitis, poorly healing or open fractures, traumatic tissue loss, areas of poor collateral circulation, and decubital or radiation ulcers
* Provision of early soft tissue coverage of exposed tissues, including open fractures, to protect against infection, trauma and desiccation
* Provision of substrates for wound healing, e.g. chronic wounds, radiation ulcers
* Enhancement of fracture healing through increased blood supply and enhanced callus formation
* Improvement in function when a muscle has been rendered non-functional by loss or denervation
* Provision of optimum cosmesis by structural filling and restoration of normal body contour
* Provision of a vehicle for the delivery of systemic antibiotics
* Improvement in function of another part of the body, e.g. augmentation of myocardial contractility with latissimus dorsi muscle
* Provision of a good surface for skin grafts.

The use of muscle flaps in traumatic wounds with large defects has many advantages over using skin alone. The rich blood supply allows the influx of host defence mechanisms (e.g. immunoglobulins, complement, leucocytes) and oxygen and nutrients. Compared to reconstruction with skin alone, muscle flaps allow earlier wound repair and a reduced incidence of wound infection.

PRACTICAL TIP
Muscle flaps may be transposed in their normal orientation, or inverted, since they do not have a normal 'face' which must face exteriorly as skin flaps do. This provides an additional degree of flexibility and arc of transposition for a given sized flap, compared to a skin flap.

Where closure of a cutaneous and subcutaneous defect is required, a number of options exist:

* Closure of the subcutaneous defect with a muscle flap and closure of the skin separately
* Closure of the defect with a myocutaneous flap
* Closure of the subcutaneous defect with a muscle flap, followed by an immediate or delayed free skin graft.

Types of muscle flap

A number of different types of muscle flap may be used.

* The flap may remain attached to the donor site via a vascular pedicle (pedicle or island flap), or may be completely detached and anastomosed to blood vessels in the recipient site (heterotopic free flap).
* The flap may be attached to the donor site by tissue, such as the tendon of origin or insertion, or may be free of all attachments apart from the blood vessels (pedicle or island flap).
* The flap may consist only of skeletal muscle (muscle flap) or may consist of other tissue (composite flap) such as skin (myocutaneous flap), fascia, peritoneum or bone.
* A myocutaneous flap may be created by including the overlying skin at the time of muscle flap elevation (primary myocutaneous flap) or may involve suturing skin to the muscle intended for the flap and elevating the muscle and skin at a later date (secondary myocutaneous flap).

Myocutaneous flap

In humans, the skin overlying the muscle receives its blood supply from perforating arteries that penetrate the surface of the muscle. In dogs and cats, the supply to the overlying skin is provided by a direct cutaneous artery. Although myocutaneous flaps are popular in human medicine because they are versatile and provide large areas of skin in a single procedure, in dogs and cats they are used less often and either random-pattern subdermal or axial pattern flaps are more commonly used for skin reconstruction.

Properties of an ideal muscle flap

These are summarized in Figure 9.1 and discussed below in detail.

- Reasonable size and bulk to provide coverage of the proposed area
- Available bilaterally
- Expendable function, or a function that can still be preserved
- Easily accessible, i.e. lies superficially
- Donor site can be closed with minimal morbidity
- Consistent vascular supply between individuals
- Favourable vascular supply, ideally a single pedicle, to allow transposition of the muscle. This should allow survival based on a single pedicle, ideally either of two for flexibility, and ideally a distal pedicle to allow use on the distal limb
- Wide arc of transposition
- Be sufficiently far from the recipient site to ensure that it is not compromised by the disease process
- Permit preservation of the motor supply if maintenance of muscle bulk is desired, i.e. avoid neurogenic atrophy

---

9.1 Properties of an ideal muscle flap.

Nature of the muscle

Size: The size of the muscle belly must be adequate to cover the defect.

Bulk: Aesthetically, if the muscle flap is used superficially it should be neither too bulky nor too thin, so as not to change the external contour of the patient. Excessive bulk should be avoided, since it is unsightly and it may be difficult to close the wound. However, some degree of muscle atrophy is inevitable and this must be allowed for.

Durability and pliability: The durability of a flap is important in areas subject to repeated wear and tear. Pliability may also be an important consideration when resurfacing a complex area, and is inversely proportional to the thickness of the muscle.

Reliability: Elevation of a muscle flap should be based on a reliable technique, which has been previously reported and well documented, with consistent results.

Location

The muscle and its vascular pedicle should be sufficiently far from the recipient site to ensure that neither is compromised by the disease process. The muscle should be close enough to the recipient site to allow its transposition. The site of the muscle flap should be as normal as possible, as previous trauma, disease or irradiation will adversely influence its survival.

Accessibility

The most useful muscles are located superficially and should be easily accessible through a standard surgical approach. In addition, dissection of the muscle free from surrounding tissue should be simple and easy, and the origin and insertion should be well defined. Ideally, the muscle should be available bilaterally, so that it may be used wherever the need arises, or both muscles may be used for large defects.

Function

The muscle should have an expendable function, or its function should be supplied by synergistic muscles. Alternatively, in some cases, the function may still be preserved, particularly if only part of the muscle is used as a flap. For example, this may be achieved by leaving the tendon of insertion intact and moving the origin (e.g. cranial tibial muscles) so that it still has a proximal location.

Donor site

The donor site should be closed with minimal morbidity. Effects of donor site morbidity include loss of function and increased likelihood of abdominal hernia following transposition of one of the muscles of the abdominal wall. Immediate primary closure of the donor site is desirable and usually achievable.

Vascular supply

The muscle should have a consistent vascular supply between individuals and it should allow a viable muscle flap to be developed. The most useful muscles have a single or dominant pedicle near the origin of the muscle. In the limb, muscles which survive based on a distally based pedicle are particularly useful. This is primarily because they allow distal defects to be covered and allow the proximal part of the muscle, which is usually more bulky, to be used as the flap.

The muscle should have venous drainage which runs with the arteries and preserving the venous supply should not place further constraints on muscle flap elevation. If there is overlying skin which obtains its blood supply via the vessels which supply the muscle, then a myocutaneous flap may be developed.

Nerve supply

Motor: The motor nerve normally enters the proximal part of the muscle, usually at the dominant pedicle, and may not be easily seen. The motor nerve supply should be preserved if retention of muscle bulk is desired, i.e. to avoid neurogenic atrophy, or if the purpose of the muscle is to provide a functional outcome. The motor nerve supply may be divided if its preservation would limit the arc of transposition or if neurogenic atrophy of the muscle is desirable.

Sensory: If the muscle is elevated as a myocutaneous flap, then preservation of the sensory nerve supply is important to preserve superficial sensation of the skin after transposition. Deep sensation may be preserved if a muscle flap is elevated and subsequently covered with a free skin graft. However, protective sensitivity is not routinely achieved even in innervated muscle and myocutaneous flaps.

Blood supply to skeletal muscles

Vascular supply to tissue may be defined in terms of angiosomes (see Chapter 7). An angiosome is a composite of muscle, nerve, bone, connective tissue and skin supplied by a source artery and drained by a satellite vein. Adjacent angiosomes are linked by small terminal anastomoses. These may be 'choke' anastomoses, where the diameter of the anastomosing arteries is smaller than the parent arteries, or 'true' anastomoses, where the diameter is the same.

All tissues within an angiosome can be separated from the adjacent tissue and elevated from the body and will survive as long as the vascular pedicle remains intact. Design of a muscle flap is normally restricted to a single angiosome, since survival of tissue beyond the boundaries of the angiosome is less predictable. It is therefore essential to know the vascular supply to the muscle and the number of angiosomes within it.

Although an entire muscle may be contained in a single angiosome, muscles generally span two or more angiosomes. Knowledge of the number, size and orientation of the angiosomes in the muscle is critical in muscle flap design.

Classification according to vascular supply

A classification system has been developed based on the vascular anatomy of the skeletal muscles (Figure 9.2). This system correlates well with the clinical survival of a muscle flap.

- Regional source of the arterial pedicle(s) entering the muscle
- Size of pedicle(s)
- Number of pedicle(s)
- Location of vascular pedicle(s) in relation to anatomical attachments
- Pattern of vessel distribution in the muscle

9.2 Elements of muscle flap classification according to vascular supply.

Vascular pedicles supplying a muscle may be described as dominant (major) or minor (Figure 9.3).

- **Dominant or major vascular pedicles** are of relatively large diameter, enter the muscle at consistent locations and are major contributors to the blood supply of the muscle. If a dominant pedicle is divided, ischaemic necrosis of the muscle may occur, since blood flow through choke anastomoses is not sufficient to maintain complete survival of the muscle (Figure 9.4).

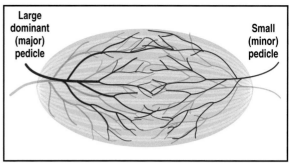

9.3 Typical vascular supply to a skeletal muscle. Note that it is composed of a combination of large and small pedicles, and the pedicle systems often share small anastomotic channels at their borders.

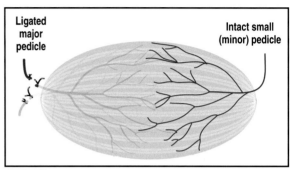

9.4 The probable consequence of basing muscle flap perfusion on a minor pedicle system. The volume of blood that can be forced through and returned via anastomotic channels is insufficient, and a large portion of muscle becomes severely ischaemic, if not necrotic.

- **Minor vascular pedicles** are small, inconsistent in their location and presence, and may be divided with minimal necrosis if the other vessels supplying the muscle are intact (Figure 9.5). Blood flow to the angiosome of a minor vascular pedicle is maintained by choke anastomoses from adjacent angiosomes.

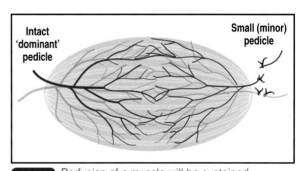

9.5 Perfusion of a muscle will be sustained throughout after ligation of minor pedicles because the remaining dominant pedicle is sufficiently large to maintain arterial and venous flow.

Anatomical dissection and vascular perfusion studies have shown five major vascular patterns (Figure 9.6). Classification of the vascular anatomy of the muscle helps to dictate whether it is likely to be of use as a flap and which pedicles should be retained. However, because it is based on anatomical studies using cadavers, it may not reflect the true physiological status and these studies must be used together with experimental and clinical studies. Confirmation of the

Type I: One vascular pedicle

One vascular pedicle supplies the entire muscle. This muscle can be elevated completely and transposed, based entirely on its dominant vascular pedicle

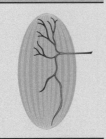

Type II: Dominant vascular pedicles with minor pedicles

One or more dominant vascular pedicles enter the muscle near its origin or insertion, and minor vascular pedicles enter the belly of the muscle. This type of muscle may be elevated based on its dominant pedicles(s) even if the minor pedicles are ligated. Note: only limited transposition of the muscle is possible based on the minor pedicles

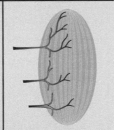

Type III: Two dominant pedicles

Two dominant pedicles from regional arteries are each responsible for approximately half of the vascular supply of the muscle. A muscle flap may be elevated based on preservation of one dominant pedicle and ligation of the other, but survival of the muscle may be inconsistent

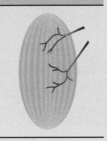

Type IV: Segmental vascular pedicles

Several minor pedicles enter the belly of the muscle between its origin and insertion. This type of muscle has a limited range of transposition because each minor pedicle supplies a small region of muscle. One or two minor pedicles can generally be ligated safely, but survival is inconsistent if more pedicles are ligated

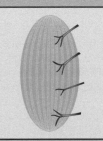

Type V: One dominant vascular pedicle and secondary segmental pedicles

The blood supply is provided by two connected vascular systems, consisting of a single dominant vascular pedicle which enters near the insertion, and segmental pedicles which enter near the origin. The entire muscle will survive based on either the single dominant pedicle or the secondary segmental pedicles. However, flap transposition based on preservation of the segmental pedicles is limited because of the broad base of the flap

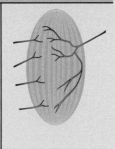

9.6 Patterns of vascular anatomy of skeletal muscles.

vascular pattern *in vivo* for all muscles, apart from type I, would require assessment of the blood flow after selective division of the vascular pedicles and flap elevation.

Using muscle flaps

PRACTICAL TIP
As with all reconstructive surgery, an alternative plan for reconstruction should be prepared in case the proposed method is found to be unsuitable intraoperatively.

Planning and preparation
A list of the closure techniques that might be used to close the defect should be made, and the most appropriate technique chosen for the patient (see Chapter 3).

Surgical technique
General principles to be followed when raising a muscle flap are outlined in Operative Technique 9.1.

Common flaps
The key features of a number of commonly used muscle flaps are summarized in Figures 9.7 to 9.9 and procedures described in Operative Techniques 9.2 to 9.23.

Flap	Type of pedicle	Indicated for defects of:	Operative Technique
Humeral head of the flexor carpi ulnaris	II	Antebrachium, carpus, manus	9.2
Ulnaris lateralis	I	Proximally based: proximal and mid antebrachium Distally based: distal limb	9.3

9.7 Common muscle flaps of the thoracic limb.

Flap	Type of pedicle	Indicated for defects of:	Operative Technique
Superficial gluteal	II	Dorsal perineal hernia, perianal area	9.4
Internal obturator	I	Ventral perineal hernia	9.5
Cranial sartorius	II	Greater trochanter, caudal abdomen, femoral region	9.6
Caudal sartorius	IV	Distal crus	9.7
Rectus femoris	I	Thigh, greater trochanter	9.8
Semitendinosus	III	Perineal hernia, perianal area	9.9
Cranial border of the lateral head of the gastrocnemius	IV	Crus, stifle	9.10
Cranial tibial	IV	Crus	9.11

9.8 Common muscle flaps of the pelvic limb.

Flap	Type of pedicle	Indicated for:	Operative Technique
Temporalis	II/III	Defects of orbit, paranasal sinus	9.12
Cranial portions of the sternocephalicus, sternothyroideus and sternohyoideus	II	Patching oesophagus, trachea, larynx	9.13
Caudal portions of the sternocephalicus, sternothyroideus and sternohyoideus	II	Local wounds; patching viscera, oesophagus, trachea; stenting or augmenting repair of local structures, e.g. larynx	9.14
Cervical portion of the trapezius	II	Defects of neck, shoulder, brachium	9.15
Deep pectoral	V	Defects of cranial and ventral thoracic wall	9.16
Latissimus dorsi	V	Defects of thoracic wall; patching intrathoracic structures; augmentation of myocardium	9.17
Cranial portion of the external abdominal oblique	III	Defects of trunk, abdominal and caudal thoracic walls	9.18
Rectus abdominis	III	Abdominal wall defects	9.19

9.9 Common muscle flaps of the head, neck and trunk.

Complications

Along with all reconstructive surgery, general complications, such as haemorrhage, infection, seroma formation, delayed wound healing and dehiscence, may be encountered (see Chapter 12).

Complications specific to the use of muscle flaps may be seen, and are generally due to errors in judgement, surgical technique and patient management. Although major complications such as muscle flap necrosis are uncommon, poor flap design is the usual cause. This may be amplified by technical error during surgery, such as excessive tension on the muscle or its vascular pedicle, or direct damage to the vascular pedicle. Partial dehiscence of a large flap is not uncommon.

Gross examination of the muscle flap during elevation is a reasonable predictor of muscle flap viability and survival. Keeping the flap moist, to reduce the depth of tissue loss, and warm, to prevent cold-induced vasoconstriction, will increase the chance of flap survival.

Flap necrosis is usually caused by venous outflow occlusion rather than arterial insufficiency. This is a slow phenomenon, and may require a few days to become apparent. In this case, tissue loss is likely to occur centrally where the blood flow is most compromised. Because necrosis is slow, there is time to salvage the flap if there are signs of impending failure, e.g. removing sutures and staples to reduce tension and reducing congestion with periodic needle sticks.

Myocutaneous flaps

Myocutaneous flaps based on the platysma, latissimus dorsi, cutaneous trunci, gracilis, semitendinosus and trapezius muscles have been described. These muscles are all superficial, allowing easy access and elevation, and have direct cutaneous arteries exiting the surface of the muscle to supply the overlying skin.

Any random-pattern subdermal plexus flap (see Chapter 6) which lies above one of the divisions of the panniculus carnosus muscle (platysma, sphincter colli, cutaneous trunci, supramammarius and preputialis), which includes the majority of the head, neck and trunk, is developed by undermining the skin below this muscle. Hence, these flaps may be regarded by definition as myocutaneous flaps. However, named myocutaneous flaps (Figure 9.10) are usually developed to include the entirety of that muscle.

Flap	Indicated for defects of:
Platysma	Head and neck
Cutaneous trunci	Proximal thoracic limb
Latissimus dorsi	Lateral thoracic wall, proximal and mid antebrachium (depends on conformation of patient)
Trapezius	Neck, cranial thorax, proximal thoracic limb
Gracilis	Perineum

9.10 Common myocutaneous flaps.

Further reading

Alexander LG, Pavletic MM and Engler SJ (1991) Abdominal-wall reconstruction with a vascular external abdominal oblique myofascial flap. *Veterinary Surgery* **20**, 379–384

Baines SJ, Gardner J, Allnutt R *et al.* (2000) The deep pectoral muscle flap in the cat: its vascular supply and potential use. *Veterinary and Comparative Orthopaedics and Traumatology* **13**, 141–145

Basher AWP and Presnell KR (1987) Muscle transposition as an aid in covering traumatic tissue defects over the canine tibia. *Journal of the American Animal Hospital Association* **23**, 617–628

Bennett D and Vaughan LC (1976) Use of muscle relocation techniques in treatment of peripheral-nerve injuries in dogs and cats. *Journal of Small Animal Practice* **17**, 99–108

Bentley JF, Henderson RA *et al.* (1991) Use of a temporalis muscle flap in reconstruction of the calvarium and orbital rim in a dog. *Journal of the American Animal Hospital Association* **27**, 463–466

Berger D, Bright RM and McCrackin MA (1995) Use of a pedicled rectus-abdominis muscle flap for repair of a failed vesicourethral anastomosis in a dog. *Journal of Small Animal Practice* **36**, 330–332

Chambers JN, Purinton PT, Allen SW *et al.* (1990) Identification and anatomic categorization of the vascular patterns to the pelvic limb muscles of dogs. *American Journal of Veterinary Research* **51**, 305–313

Chambers JN, Purinton PT, Allen SW *et al.* (1990) Treatment of trochanteric ulcers with cranial sartorius and rectus femoris muscle flaps. *Veterinary Surgery* **19**, 424–428

Chambers JN, Purinton PT, Moore JL *et al.* (1998) Flexor carpi ulnaris (humeral head) muscle flap for reconstruction of distal forelimb injuries in two dogs. *Veterinary Surgery* **27**, 342–347

Chambers JN and Rawlings CA (1991) Applications of a semitendinosus muscle flap in 2 dogs. *Journal of the American Veterinary Medical Association* **199**, 84–86

Degner DA, Bauer MS, Steyn PF *et al.* (1994) The cranial rectus-abdominus muscle pedicle flap in the dog. *Veterinary and Comparative Orthopaedics and Traumatology* **7**, 21–24

Gregory CR, Gourley IM, Snyder JR *et al.* (1988) Experimental definition of latissimus dorsi, gracilis, and rectus abdominus musculocutaneous flaps in the dog. *American Journal of Veterinary Research* **49**, 878–884

Hardie EM, Kolata RJ, Early TD *et al.* (1983) Evaluation of internal obturator muscle transposition in treatment of perineal hernia in dogs. *Veterinary Surgery* **12**, 69–72

Mathes SJ and Eshima I (1988) Muscle flaps in the management of vascular grafts in contaminated wounds – an experimental study in dogs – discussion. *Plastic and Reconstructive Surgery* **82**, 484–485

Mathes SJ and Nahai F (1981) Classification of the vascular anatomy of muscles – experimental and clinical correlation. *Plastic and Reconstructive Surgery* **67**, 177–187

Pavletic MM, Kostolich M, Koblik P *et al.* (1987) A comparison of the cutaneous trunci myocutaneous flap and latissimus dorsi myocutaneous flap in the dog. *Veterinary Surgery* **16**, 283–293

Philibert D and Fowler JD (1993) The trapezius osteomusculocutaneous flap in dogs. *Veterinary Surgery* **22**, 444–450

Philibert D and Fowler JD (1996) Use of muscle flaps in reconstructive surgery. *Compendium on Continuing Education for the Practicing Veterinarian* **18**, 395–404

Philibert D, Fowler JD *et al.* (1992) The anatomic basis for a trapezius muscle flap in dogs. *Veterinary Surgery* **21**, 429–434

Puerto DA and Aronson LR (2004) Use of a semitendinosus myocutaneous flap for soft-tissue reconstruction of a grade IIIB open tibial fracture in a dog. *Veterinary Surgery* **33**, 629–635

Purinton PT, Chambers JN and Moore JL (1992) Identification and categorization of the vascular patterns to muscles of the thoracic limb, thorax, and neck of dogs. *American Journal of Veterinary Research* **53**, 1435–1445

Smith MM, Shults S, Waldron DR *et al.* (1993) Platysma myocutaneous flap for head and neck reconstruction in cats. *Head and Neck* **15**, 433–439

Sylvestre AM, Weinstein MJ, Popovitch CA *et al.* (1997) The sartorius muscle flap in the cat: an anatomic study and two case reports. *Journal of the American Animal Hospital Association* **33**, 91–96

Tomlinson J and Presnell KR (1981) Use of temporalis muscle flap in the dog. *Veterinary Surgery* **10**, 77–79

Weinstein MJ, Pavletic MM, Boudrieau RJ *et al.* (1988) Caudal sartorius muscle flap in the dog. *Veterinary Surgery* **17**, 203–210

Weinstein MJ, Pavletic MM, Boudrieau RJ *et al.* (1989) Cranial sartorius muscle flap in the dog. *Veterinary Surgery* **18**, 286–291

Wood MB (1987) The influence of muscle flap coverage on the repair of devascularized tibial cortex – an experimental investigation in the dog. *Plastic and Reconstructive Surgery* **79**, 957–958

ASE EXAMPLE 1:
Repair of a perineal hernia with a semitendinosus muscle flap

History
A 7-year-old castrated male cross-bred dog presented with a recurrence of a right-sided perineal hernia. A bilateral repair had been performed using an internal obturator muscle flap prior to presentation, along with castration.

Surgical planning
The surgical plan consisted of exploration of the muscles of the pelvic diaphragm, with a view to re-using an internal obturator muscle flap if the condition of the muscles of the pelvic diaphragm allowed this. If this was not possible, a semitendinosus muscle flap was planned and the dog was prepared and positioned to allow this decision to be made intraoperatively. Consideration was given to performing a colopexy and vas deferens pexy and cystopexy, but it was elected not to perform these procedures at this time.

Surgical procedure
The dog was positioned in sternal recumbency, with the left hindlimb extended caudally. The perineal region and the entire left hindlimb were draped. Exploration of the muscles of the pelvic diaphragm on the right side revealed marked atrophy, so a semitendinosus flap was selected.

The incision made for exploration of the perineal hernia was continued ventrally below the anus at the level of the ischium and then continued along the caudomedial aspect of the left hindlimb, directly over the semitendinosus muscle, to immediately proximal to the stifle joint. The superficial fascia was dissected to expose the semitendinosus muscle. The muscle was elevated to identify the distal insertion and the distal vascular pedicle. The distal vascular pedicle was ligated and divided and the tendon of insertion transected. The muscle flap was then dissected free of the surrounding tissues and reflected proximally to allow the proximal vascular pedicle to be identified. The muscle was transposed to cover the defect in the pelvic diaphragm and sutured to the external anal sphincter medially, and to the levator ani, coccygeus and internal obturator muscles and sacrotuberous ligament laterally. The subcutaneous tissues and skin were closed routinely.

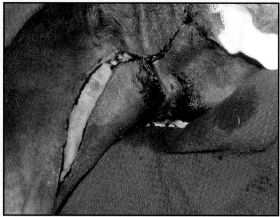
Incision.

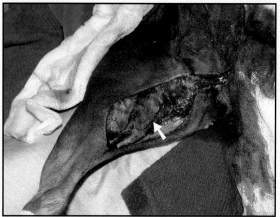
Semitendinosus muscle exposed.

CASE EXAMPLE 1 continued:
Repair of a perineal hernia with a semitendinosus muscle flap

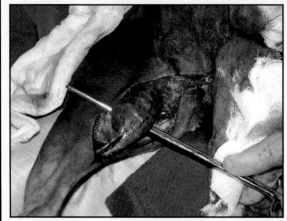
Muscle elevated.

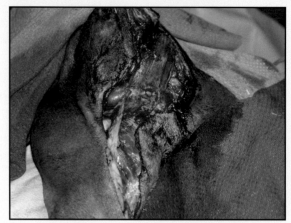
Muscle flap dissected free and reflected to show vascular pedicle.

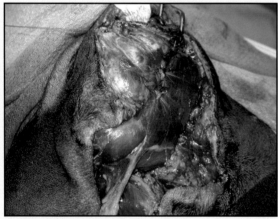
Muscle flap transposed.

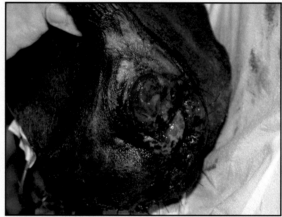
Wound closed. There is a prolapsed rectum.

Outcome
The dog made an uneventful recovery and was clinically normal with no recurrence of a perineal hernia at 6 weeks and 6 months postoperatively.

CASE EXAMPLE 2:
Reconstruction of a thoracic wall deficit (following tumour resection) with a latissimus dorsi myocutaneous flap

History and assessment
A 7-year-old spayed German Shepherd bitch was presented with a large firm, fixed mass over the ventral right thoracic wall. An incisional biopsy indicated low-grade chondrosarcoma. Dorsoventral and lateral radiographs showed a large, well demarcated soft tissue opacity, with patchy mineralization, arising from the distal aspect of the right 7th rib; the mass extended to the 6th rib cranially and the 8th rib caudally. A thoracic CT scan confirmed the nature of the mass and did not show any evidence of pulmonary metastases. Reconstruction of the CT images showed the extent of the bony lesion.

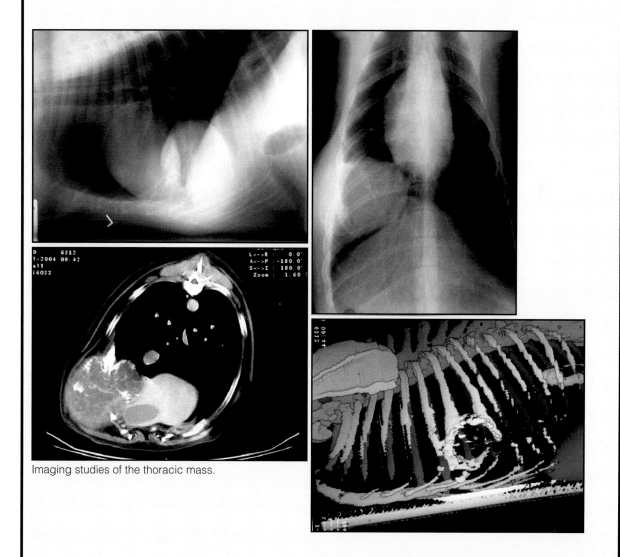

Imaging studies of the thoracic mass.

Surgical planning
Radical local excision of the mass comprising *en bloc* chest wall resection was planned, with 3 cm cutaneous margins and including one unaffected rib either side of the mass, i.e. resection of ribs 5 to 9. Plans for reconstructing the resulting deficit included: synthetic polypropylene mesh with omentalization; a latissimus dorsi muscle flap; and a latissimus dorsi myocutaneous flap.

Case Example 2 continues ▶

CASE EXAMPLE 2 continued:
Reconstruction of a thoracic wall deficit (following tumour resection) with a latissimus dorsi myocutaneous flap

Prior to surgery, the margins of the tumour, proposed margins of resection, borders of rib 6 to 8 and the borders of the latissimus dorsi myocutaneous flap were outlined. Although the proposed margins of excision encroached on the cutaneous borders of the latissimus dorsi myocutaneous flap, the thoracodorsal artery was likely to stay intact, and so the remaining tissue in the angiosome would still be viable. The cutaneous landmarks do not exactly outline the underlying muscle in all cases, so a larger flap can be harvested once the borders of the muscle are inspected following resection of the primary tumour.

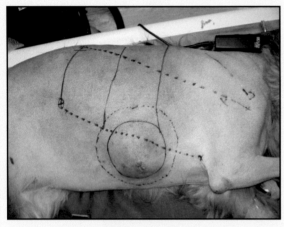

Anatomical landmarks and flap margins outlined.

Surgical procedure

Resection of the mass via *en bloc* chest wall resection was performed, to leave a large tissue deficit.

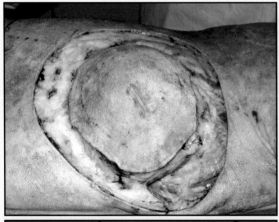

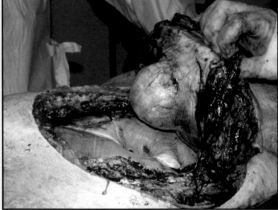

Tumour resection.

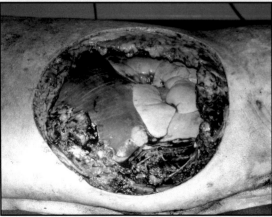

Case Example 2 continues ▶

CASE EXAMPLE 2 continued:
Reconstruction of a thoracic wall deficit (following tumour resection) with a latissimus dorsi myocutaneous flap

The patient was redraped and the instruments and gloves were changed. Examination of the local skin showed that local skin mobilization was unlikely to provide closure of the cutaneous defect.

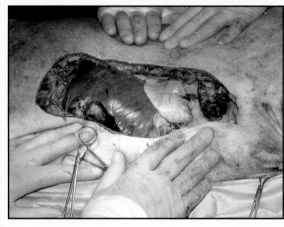

There is insufficient local skin to close the defect.

A one-step procedure using the latissimus dorsi myocutaneous flap to close the thoracic wall and cutaneous defect was chosen. The ventral border of the flap was made by continuing an incision from the caudodorsal aspect of the excisional wound. The ventral aspect of the latissimus dorsi muscle was elevated from the underlying tissue. The caudal border of the flap was incised and the skin elevated to allow incision of the caudal border of the latissimus dorsi muscle. The skin of the flap was sutured to the underlying latissimus dorsi muscle to avoid shear trauma to the vessels supplying the skin. Stay sutures were placed to manipulate the flap. The dorsal border of the flap was incised and the flap was transposed cranioventrally to cover the chest wall defect. A chest drain was placed.

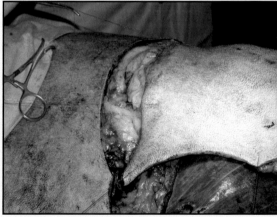 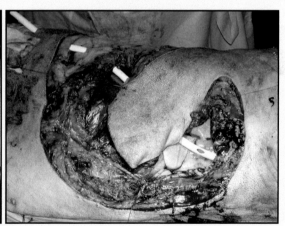

Latissimus dorsi myocutaneous flap raised and transposed.

Case Example 2 continues ▶

CASE EXAMPLE 2 continued:
Reconstruction of a thoracic wall deficit (following tumour resection) with a latissimus dorsi myocutaneous flap

The muscular edges of the latissimus dorsi myocutaneous flap were sutured to the surrounding remaining muscles of the thoracic wall with simple interrupted sutures of 3.5 metric (0 USP) polydioxanone. Closure of the subcutaneous tissue of the recipient and donor sites was routine. An active suction drain was placed at the caudoventral aspect of the wound.

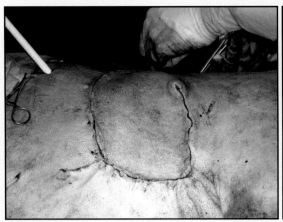 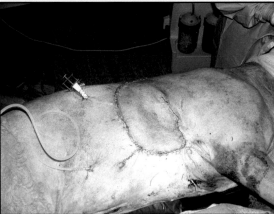

Wound closed and drain in place.

Outcome
At 14 days postoperatively the wound had healed. A concavity, which exhibited mild paradoxic movement, was present at the site of chest wall resection. The appearance of the concavity improved over the following months.

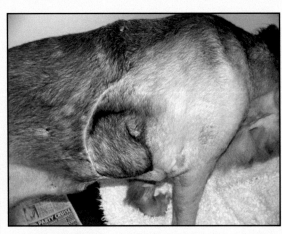

Obvious concavity at 14 days postoperatively.

OPERATIVE TECHNIQUE 9.1:
Raising a muscle or myocutaneous flap

Patient positioning
The patient should be positioned to allow surgical access to the donor site and the recipient site at the same time, during a single procedure. Limbs are in a relaxed position without flexion or extension. Consider placing sandbags under the thoracic or pelvic limb girdle or head to allow loose skin to be used to close the donor site.

Assistant
Ideal but not essential.

Equipment extras
None.

Surgical technique
A wide surgical clip is performed – including the defect, the skin of the flap, the skin between the flap and the defect, and sufficient skin to allow undermining and closure of the defect without hair impinging on the surgical site. In some cases enough hair is clipped to allow other reconstructive techniques to be performed should they prove necessary.

The regional anatomy is reviewed and a defined plan made for reconstruction using a muscle flap. If a myocutaneous flap is planned, the borders of the flap may be marked on the skin using a surgical marker pen. Preoperative measurements should be made to ensure that the muscle flap is of sufficient size and proximity to perform the intended function once transposed.

The surgeon should plan to use the entire muscle and its tendon, and the entire muscle should be exposed. The muscle will contract following division of the origin or insertion but will relax once the nerve supply is transected. The muscle can be trimmed to fit once it is transposed into the recipient site.

WARNING
Ensure that the muscle flap chosen can reach the defect. Check that the defect is in an area that the flap has been shown to cover and perform surgical planning to determine that this is possible in the individual patient, as differences in conformation/size may affect how far a flap can reach.

1. The muscle may be accessible via the primary wound, or an extra incision may be required to expose the muscle. Begin dissection away from the vascular pedicle that is to be retained and take care as the pedicle is approached.
2. Tendons of origin or insertion may be sectioned to relieve tension and increase the arc of transposition. Muscular or tendinous attachments at the vascular pedicle may be left intact to prevent tension disrupting the vascular supply.
3. Ligate and divide small blood vessels between the muscle and surrounding tissue as dissection proceeds.
4. If the incision to elevate the muscle does not lie adjacent to or within the recipient wound, make a bridging incision between the donor and recipient sites to allow transposition of the muscle. (The bridging incision is closed when the recipient site is closed.)
5. Take care to avoid kinking, twisting, or placing excessive tension on the vascular pedicle.
6. The epimysium may be removed from the muscle without adversely affecting its blood supply.
7. The muscle flap and pedicle should be inspected during elevation and at closure of the wound for evidence of ischaemia. Normal colour is a good indicator of normal blood flow. Arterial supply may be assessed by bleeding from a cut edge, intraoperative Doppler ultrasonography or oximetry, but these are not good indicators of venous obstruction.
8. A tension-free skin closure over the flap should be obtained. If this is not possible, then leave the wound open for immediate or delayed free skin grafting.

Postoperative care
Dead space at the donor and recipient sites should be managed with drains, ideally closed active suction drains.

OPERATIVE TECHNIQUE 9.2:
Humeral head of the flexor carpi ulnaris muscle flap

Indications
Open wounds of the distal antebrachium, carpus and manus.

Anatomy

- Origin: medial epicondyle of the humerus.
- Insertion: accessory carpal bone.
- The muscle body lies cranial to the ulnar head, except distally, where the tendon lies caudally.

Vascular pedicles (Type II)

- Proximally: branches of the recurrent ulnar, ulnar and deep antebrachial arteries.
- Distally: the caudal interosseous vessels that enter on the deep face of the muscle, near the tendon of insertion.
- Anastomoses between these two vascular domains are present within the muscle and the muscle will survive based on its distal pedicle.

Raising the flap

1. Make a skin incision over the caudomedial aspect of the antebrachium, from the medial epicondyle proximally to just distal to the accessory carpal bone.
2. Incise the antebrachial and carpal fascia to expose the humeral head of the muscle lying between the ulnar head caudally and the ulnaris lateralis laterally.
3. Transect the distal tendon of the ulnar head to expose the humeral head.
4. Divide the fascial attachments of the humeral head.
5. Divide the proximal aspect of the muscle between the proximal and middle thirds.

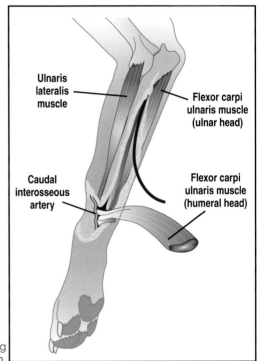

Raising the flap.

Area of transposition
Adjacent areas of the distal antebrachium and carpus, distally to the metacarpophalangeal junction.

The muscle may be transposed or inverted in either direction around the antebrachium or carpus.

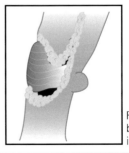

Flap transposed, based on its distal interosseous pedicle.

OPERATIVE TECHNIQUE 9.3:
Ulnaris lateralis muscle flap

Indications

- Proximally based flap: open wounds of the proximal and mid antebrachium.
- Distally based flap: to provide cover of wounds of the distal limb if the inconsistent distal pedicle is present.

WARNING
Since the distal pedicle is not always present, the humeral head of the flexor carpi ulnaris muscle is a better choice for distal thoracic limb wounds.

Anatomy

- Origin: lateral epicondyle of the humerus, behind the lateral collateral ligament of the elbow joint.
- Insertion: proximal end of metacarpal V.

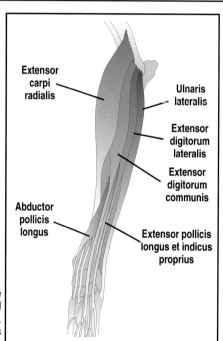

Muscles of the superficial antebrachium, showing ulnaris lateralis.

Labels: Extensor carpi radialis; Ulnaris lateralis; Extensor digitorum lateralis; Extensor digitorum communis; Abductor pollicis longus; Extensor pollicis longus et indicus proprius

Vascular pedicles (Type I)

- Proximally: on the deep aspect of the muscle, the cranial interosseous artery and vein provide a consistent pedicle.
- Distally: a second inconsistent pedicle, the caudal interosseus artery and vein, enters near the musculotendinous junction, on the deep aspect of the muscle.

Raising the flap
The muscle is exposed with a skin incision over the caudolateral aspect of the antebrachium.

Area of transposition
Adjacent areas of the antebrachium.

OPERATIVE TECHNIQUE 9.4:
Superficial gluteal muscle flap

Indications
Augmentation of the dorsal part of a perineal hernia and perianal wounds.

Anatomy

- Small, flat, almost rectangular muscle.
- Origin: the gluteal fascia, and thereby from the tuber sacrale, caudal fascia, lateral sacrum and proximal sacrotuberous ligament.
- Insertion: third trochanter of the femur (tendon runs over the greater trochanter).

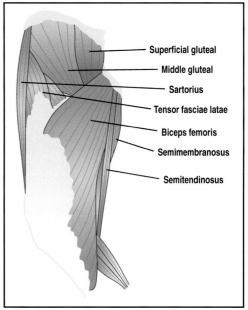

Superficial muscles of the lateral thigh, showing the superficial gluteal muscle.

Vascular pedicles (Type II)

- Proximally: the caudal gluteal artery and vein, which enter the deep face of the muscle near the sacral origin and sacrotuberous ligament.
- Distally: there are consistent small pedicles from the caudal gluteal artery, which enter the dorsal border, and from the lateral circumflex femoral artery, at the tendon of insertion.

Raising the flap

1. Make a curved skin incision from the caudal aspect of the ischium, extending craniodorsally over the ilium to end at the tuber coxae.
2. Dissect subcutaneous fat from the underlying muscles to expose the superficial gluteal and proximal biceps femoris muscles and the fascia lata.
3. Transect the tendon of insertion of the superficial gluteal muscle and transpose the distal portion of the muscle caudally.

→

OPERATIVE TECHNIQUE 9.4 continued:
Superficial gluteal muscle flap

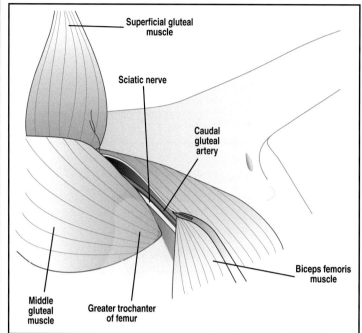

Tenotomy of the tendon of insertion and dorsal reflection of the muscle.

4. The tendon of origin may be partially sectioned, taking care to avoid the vascular pedicle, to increase the caudal mobility of the muscle.

Area of transposition
Caudally to the external anal sphincter.

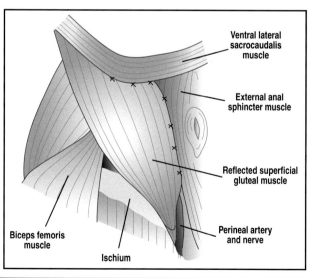

Transposition of the superficial gluteal muscle to augment perineal hernia repair.

OPERATIVE TECHNIQUE 9.5:
Internal obturator muscle flap

Indications
Augmentation of the ventral part of a perineal hernia repair.

Anatomy

- Fan-shaped muscle.
- Origin: medially on the dorsal surfaces of the pubis and ischium and from the ischiatic arch.
- Insertion: via a strong flat tendon which runs over the lesser sciatic notch to the trochanteric fossa (combines with the tendon of the gemelli muscle).

Vascular pedicles (Type I)
Obturator branch of the medial circumflex femoral artery and vein enter the muscle at its cranial border after passing from ventral to dorsal through the obturator foramen.

Raising the flap

1. Perform subperiosteal elevation of the origin of the muscle along the caudal dorsal ischium, leaving the origin cranial to the obturator foramen, and the blood supply, intact.
2. The tendon of insertion may be transected as it crosses the ischium to increase the mobility of the flap. Take care to avoid the blood vessel cranial to the tendon.

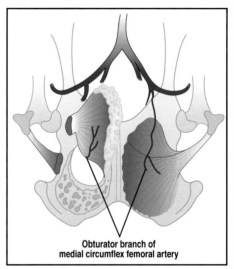

Obturator branch of
medial circumflex femoral artery

Flap elevated and inverted.

Area of transposition
Dorsomedially to the ipsilateral anal sphincter.

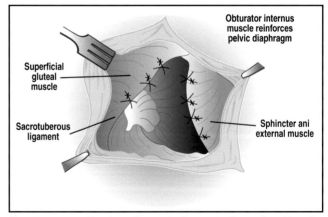

Obturator internus
muscle reinforces
pelvic diaphragm

Superficial
gluteal
muscle

Sacrotuberous
ligament

Sphincter ani
external muscle

Flap transposed to close the ventral aspect of a perineal hernia.

OPERATIVE TECHNIQUE 9.6:
Cranial sartorius muscle flap

Indications

- Craniodorsally and laterally: for defects in the region of the greater trochanter, such as pressure sores, wounds and oncological resections.
- Cranioventrally: to repair caudal abdominal hernias and ruptures, particularly chronic prepubic tendon ruptures and femoral hernias where local tissue loss prevents simple anatomical re-apposition. The pectineus muscle tendon can be cut to mobilize this muscle to augment a repair in this location.

Anatomy

- A long, flat, strap-like muscle.
- Origin: the iliac crest and lumbodorsal fascia.
- Insertion: the patella, after joining the medial femoral fascia with the rectus femoris.

Vascular pedicles (Type II)

- The superficial circumflex iliac artery supplies all but the proximal and distal tips of the muscle. This vessel divides into a proximal and distal branch immediately before entering the muscle at the junction of the proximal and middle thirds, on the caudal aspect of the muscle.
- A branch of the femoral artery may enter the muscle slightly more distal to the superficial circumflex iliac and should be preserved.
- A minor contribution from the descending genicular artery may enter near the insertion.
- The blood supply to the single sartorius muscle in the cat is similar.

Raising the flap

1. Make a skin incision over the medial aspect of the thigh, from the inguinal region to the stifle.
2. Identify the borders of the muscle by dissection.

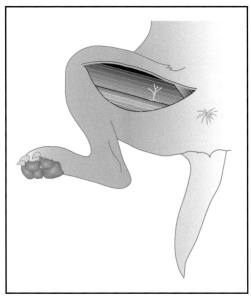

Skin incision over the medial aspect of the thigh to expose the cranial sartorius.

OPERATIVE TECHNIQUE 9.6 continued:
Cranial sartorius muscle flap

3. Sever the insertion of the muscle at its tibial insertion and continue dissection of the flap proximally.

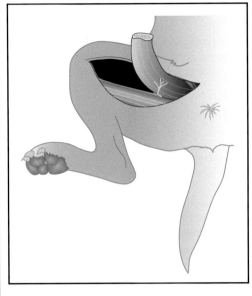

Transection of the muscle at the tibial insertion and dissection up to the proximal vascular pedicle.

- Dissection of the vascular pedicle towards the femoral artery and ligation of smaller blood vessels supplying the tensor fasciae latae and caudal sartorius increases the arc of transposition. The muscle may also be passed under the tensor fasciae latae to increase its caudal reach.
- Subperiosteal elevation of the muscle's origin allows the development of an island flap.

Area of transposition

- Distal portion: may be transposed to the lateral thigh or hip and will reach the midline dorsally and the umbilicus cranially in dogs of standard conformation.
- Proximal portion: may be transposed to the hip region.

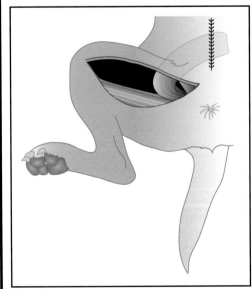

Transposition of the cranial sartorius muscle through 180 degrees to augment the repair of a caudal abdominal hernia.

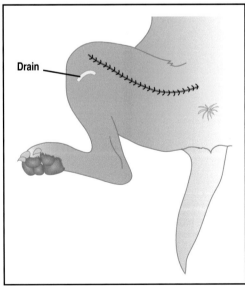

Drain

Wound closed.

OPERATIVE TECHNIQUE 9.7:
Caudal sartorius muscle flap

Indications
Reconstruction of defects over the distal crus and open fractures or osteomyelitis of the tibia.

Anatomy

- A long, narrow, thin muscle, which lies close to the cranial belly of the sartorius on the medial aspect of the thigh.
- Origin: cranioventral iliac spine and ventral border of the ilium and extends distally, immediately caudal to the cranial sartorius, over the medial surface of the vastus medialis and the stifle joint.
- Insertion: cranial border of the tibia via the aponeurosis which blends with that of the gracilis muscle.

Vascular pedicles (Type IV)

- The muscle has a segmental supply from a dominant vascular pedicle supplied by the saphenous artery and medial saphenous vein at the distal third of the muscle belly.
- In some dogs, the vascular supply resembles a type V, with the saphenous vessels being the dominant pedicle.

Raising the flap

1. Make a skin incision over the medial aspect of the thigh to the mid crus.

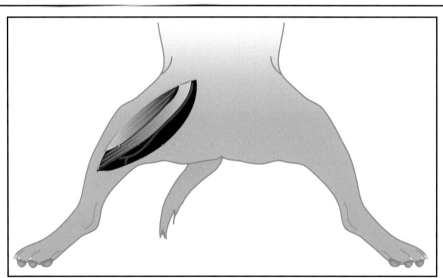

Skin incision over the medial aspect of the thigh to expose the caudal sartorius.

2. Sever the proximal origin of the muscle, approximately 4 cm distal to its origin on the ilium.

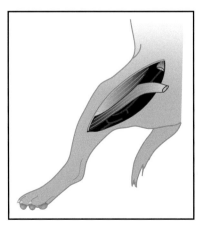

Transection of the muscle 4 cm distal to its origin.

OPERATIVE TECHNIQUE 9.7 continued:
Caudal sartorius muscle flap

3. Ligate the saphenous artery and medial saphenous vein and transect them where they join the femoral artery and vein. Take care to preserve the saphenous vessels in the midtibial region and more proximally where they are associated with the caudal border of the muscle.
4. The muscle may be transposed based on its distal insertion, or its insertion may be severed to give an island muscle flap.

Area of transposition

- Isolated segments, based on segmental vessels, may be transposed locally.
- The entire muscle may be elevated based on the more distal pedicle, with a reversal of saphenous blood flow, but this requires the blood flow to be intact across a number of angiosomes. In cases of trauma, consideration should be given to performing a preoperative angiogram to ensure that the other vessels, e.g. cranial tibial, are still intact and that the saphenous artery is not the primary source of blood flow to the distal limb. Trauma to the saphenous vessels or a previous medial approach to the tibia in which these vessels were ligated prevent this flap being used.
- A flap based on a distal pedicle may extend as far as the dorsal metatarsus.

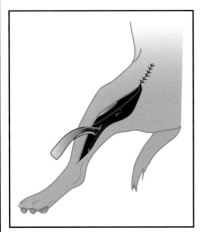

Transposition of the muscle flap distally.

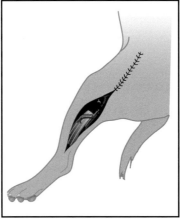

Transection of the muscle insertion to give an island flap.

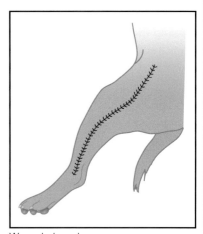

Wound closed.

OPERATIVE TECHNIQUE 9.8:
Rectus femoris muscle flap

Indications
Defects in the region of the thigh and greater trochanter, such as traumatic wounds, oncological resections and pressure sores. It is an alternative to the cranial sartorius flap.

Anatomy

- A relatively long, narrow, bulky muscle enclosed between the vastus muscles.
- Origin: iliopubic eminence of the ilium and runs between the vastus lateralis and vastus medialis.
- Insertion: tibial tuberosity (patella within the tendon).

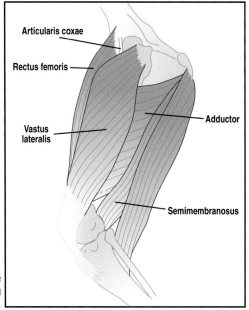

Deep muscles of the lateral thigh, showing the rectus femoris.

Vascular pedicles (Type I)

- A branch of the lateral circumflex femoral artery and vein enters the proximal aspect of the muscle on the caudal surface.
- The muscle occasionally receives a minor branch from the descending genicular artery near its insertion, making it a type II muscle.

Raising the flap

1. Make a skin incision over the craniolateral surface of the thigh, directly over the muscle.
2. Dissect the muscle free from the other members of the quadriceps femoris group and transect its insertion in the distal quarter. Elevation of the muscle origin further increases the mobility of the muscle.

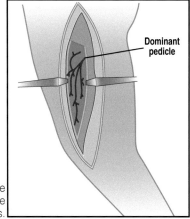

Skin incision over the lateral thigh to expose the rectus femoris.

OPERATIVE TECHNIQUE 9.8 continued:
Rectus femoris muscle flap

Area of transposition
The distal part of the muscle may be transposed to
the lateral thigh and hip. Transpose the flap based
on the proximal dominant vascular pedicle.

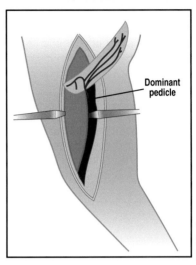

Dominant
pedicle

Transposition of
the muscle flap
proximally.

OPERATIVE TECHNIQUE 9.9:
Semitendinosus muscle flap

Indications

- A proximally based flap may be used to augment a perineal hernia repair or reconstruction of perianal wounds.
- A distally based flap may be used to close defects of the crus. However, this is a rather bulky flap and the cranial tibial flap or lateral gastrocnemius flap may be considered for this purpose.

Anatomy

- A long, narrow bulky muscle, which runs in the caudal thigh between the biceps femoris and semimembranosus muscles.
- Origin: ischial tuberosity and ventral surface of the ischium.
- Insertion: medial surface of the tibia, with the gracilis muscle, plus a strand with the medial gastrocnemius to the common calcaneal tendon.

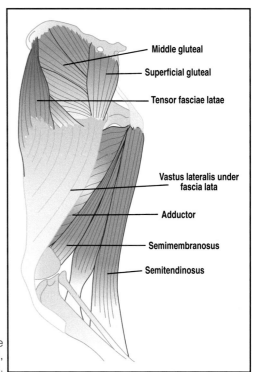

Deep muscles of the lateral thigh and crus, showing semitendinosus.

Vascular pedicles (Type III)

Two codominant pedicles enter the muscle and comprise a branch from the caudal gluteal artery proximally and a branch from the distal caudal femoral artery distally. The muscle will survive based on either pedicle.

Raising the flap

1. Make a skin incision over the caudal aspect of the thigh, from the caudal border of the ischium to the caudal aspect of the stifle joint.
2. Transect the distal portion of the muscle or the tendon of insertion.
3. Ligate and divide the distal vascular pedicle.

OPERATIVE TECHNIQUE 9.9 continued:
Semitendinosus muscle flap

Area of transposition
The muscle flap will extend dorsally to the midline or just beyond, cranially to the junction of the iliac body and wing, caudomedially to the contralateral tuber ischii and distally to the tarsus, depending on the animal's conformation. The muscle may be transposed proximally as a proximally based muscle flap. When used to augment a perineal hernia, the contralateral semitendinosus muscle is used.

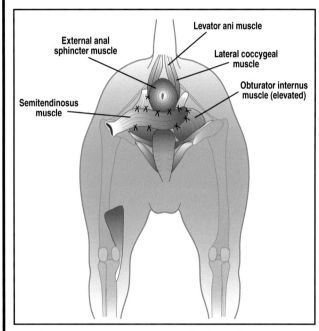

Transposition of the contralateral semitendinosus muscle, based on the proximal caudal gluteal pedicle, to augment a perineal hernia repair.

OPERATIVE TECHNIQUE 9.10:
Cranial border of the lateral head of the gastrocnemius muscle flap

Indications
Wounds of the crus and stifle region.

Anatomy

- Origin: large tendon, containing the lateral fabella, on the lateral supracondylar tuberosity of the femur.
- Insertion: calcaneus after fusing with the medial head of the gastrocnemius.

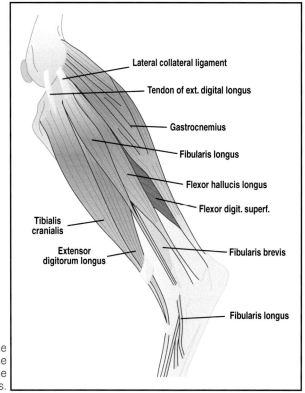

Superficial muscles of the lateral crus, showing the lateral head of the gastrocnemius.

Vascular pedicles (Type IV)
A long pedicle of the popliteal blood vessels supplies the muscle and runs superficially from proximal to distal.

Raising the flap

1. Make a skin incision over the caudolateral crus, immediately distal to the stifle joint.
2. Dissect the cranial border of the lateral head of the gastrocnemius from the surrounding tissue.

Area of transposition
This muscle will cover adjacent regions of the crus.

OPERATIVE TECHNIQUE 9.11:
Cranial tibial muscle flap

Indications
Wounds of the crus, particularly open tibial fractures.

Anatomy

- A superficial, strong, flat muscle on the lateral aspect of the crus (see Operative Technique 9.10).
- Origin: cranial and lateral tibia and passes over the craniomedial surface of the crus.
- Insertion: the extensor retinaculum of the pes.

Vascular pedicles (Type IV)
Segmental branches of the cranial tibial artery and vein perfuse the muscle.

Raising the flap

1. Make a skin incision over the craniolateral crus.
2. Transect the tendon of insertion.

Area of transposition
This muscle will cover adjacent areas of the mid and distal crus. The distal end of the muscle may be transposed based on a short pedicle supplied by the proximal segmental branches. Given the arrangement of the blood supply, the proximal part of the muscle might be transposed based on a distal pedicle, although no clinical reports of this exist.

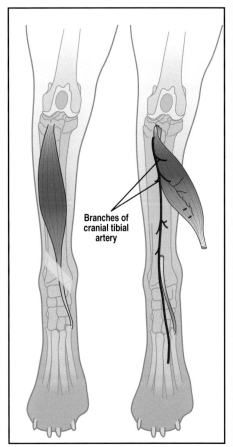

Branches of cranial tibial artery

Transposition of the distal end of the cranial tibial muscle to cover adjacent wounds of the crus.

OPERATIVE TECHNIQUE 9.12:
Temporalis muscle flap

Indications

- Defects of the orbit and paranasal sinuses.
- Improved cosmesis after orbital exenteration.

Anatomy

- A thick, fan-shaped muscle.
- Origin: temporal fossa of the skull.
- Insertion: the mandibular coronoid process.
- The temporalis and masseter muscles fuse between the zygomatic arch and the coronoid process.

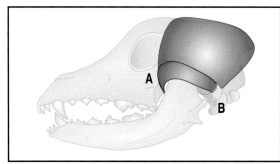

Lateral aspect of the skull showing the temporalis muscle. The zygomatic arch has been removed from A to B.

Vascular pedicles (Type II/III)

The temporal branches of the superficial, cranial deep and caudal deep temporal arteries. The blood supply enters the muscle near its mandibular insertion and runs ventrodorsally, parallel with the muscle fibres.

Raising the flap

1. Make a skin incision rostrocaudally, centred over the orbit and temporalis muscle, preserving the superficial temporal artery.
2. Dissect the temporalis fascia from the zygomatic arch and incise and subperiosteally elevate the muscle. The overlying temporalis fascia is included in the flap to avoid damage to the superficial pedicles. Flap mobility in a rostral direction is improved with resection of the orbital ligament and rostral zygoma.

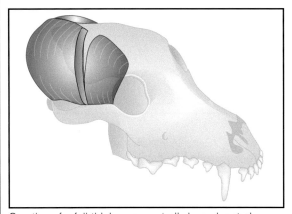

Creation of a full-thickness, ventrally based rostral muscle flap with an incision in the transverse plane.

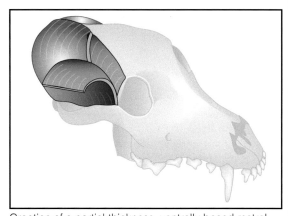

Creation of a partial-thickness, ventrally based rostral muscle flap with an incision in the sagittal plane.

Area of transposition
Immediately adjacent areas.

OPERATIVE TECHNIQUE 9.13:
Cranial portions of the sternocephalicus, sternothyroideus and sternohyoideus muscle flaps

Indications
Patching defects of the oesophagus, trachea and larynx.

Anatomy

Sternohyoideus:

- A strap-like muscle.
- Origin: deep surface of the manubrium and cranial border of the first costal cartilage. It extends up the neck, covering the ventral aspect of the trachea.
- Insertion: basihyoid.

At its origin and throughout its caudal third, the sternohyoideus is fused to the sternothyroideus. The caudal portion of the sternohyoideus is covered by the sternocephalicus.

Sternocephalicus:

- Origin: sternum.
- Insertion: mastoid part of the temporal bone and dorsal nuchal line of the occipital bone.

Vascular pedicles (Type II)
The cranial thyroid artery and vein provide a major pedicle at the cranial aspect of the muscles.

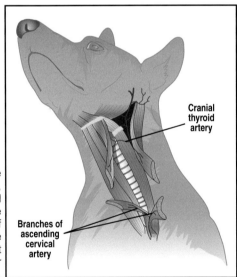

Vascular supply to the sternocephalicus, sternothyroideus and sternohyoideus muscles. The cranial or caudal portions of these muscles can be transposed to adjacent areas, based on their respective pedicles.

Raising the flap
Midline ventral cervical approach, incising skin from cranial to the larynx to the manubrium. The median raphé is incised and the muscle belly isolated. The muscle is transected in the distal third.

Area of transposition
Adjacent areas of the cranial neck and head.

OPERATIVE TECHNIQUE 9.14:
Caudal portions of the sternocephalicus, sternothyroideus and sternohyoideus muscle flaps

Indications
Local wounds, patching viscera, oesophagus and trachea, and stenting or augmenting repair of local structures, e.g. larynx. The cervical portion of the trapezius muscle is an alternative muscle flap in this region.

Anatomy
See Operative Technique 9.13.

Vascular pedicles (Type II)
The muscle is supplied by pedicles from the ascending branch of the superficial cervical artery and vein, which runs along the dorsal border of the muscles. These muscles have a type II supply, with contributions cranially from the vessels above.

Raising the flap
These three muscles share the same blood supply of the caudal pedicles and it is safer, and indeed easier, to transpose them as a complete unit.

Area of transposition
Adjacent areas of the neck.

OPERATIVE TECHNIQUE 9.15:
Cervical portion of the trapezius muscle flap

Indications

- Wounds of the neck, shoulder or brachium. (The caudal portions of the sternocephalicus, sternothyroideus or sternohyoideus are alternative flaps in this region.)
- The scapular spine may be included with the muscle, but this bone is primarily a source of osteogenesis, rather than structural bone.

Anatomy

- A thin, broad, triangular muscle, which may be divided into cervical and thoracic parts. The cervical part is overlapped by the cleidobrachialis muscle, and the thoracic trapezius is overlapped by the latissimus dorsi muscle.
- Origin: dorsal median raphé of the neck and supraspinous ligament, from the level of the third cervical vertebra to the ninth thoracic vertebra.
- Insertion: the scapular spine.

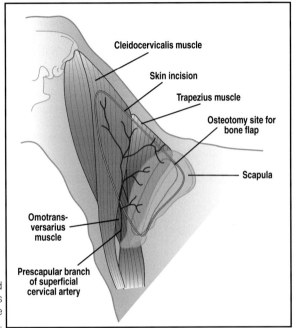

The anatomy and blood supply to the trapezius muscle and outline of the myocutaneous flap.

Vascular pedicles (Type II)
Branches of the prescapular division of the superficial cervical artery and vein enter the midcranial border, supplying the cranial half to two-thirds of the muscle. The caudal half is supplied by the subscapular artery.

Raising the flap

1. Make an incision over the trapezius muscle on the lateral aspect of the neck.
2. Transect the origin of the muscle along the dorsal raphé and supraspinous ligament and dissect the muscle from the cleidocervicalis and omotransversarius muscles.
3. Transect the insertion along the scapular spine to create an island flap tethered only by superficial cervical vessels.

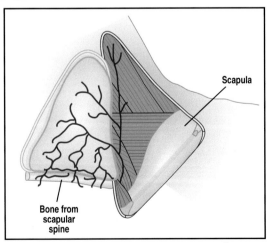

Elevation of a trapezius osteomyocutaneous flap.

OPERATIVE TECHNIQUE 9.15 continued:
Cervical portion of the trapezius muscle flap

Area of transposition
Adjacent neck, shoulder, brachium and cranial thorax.

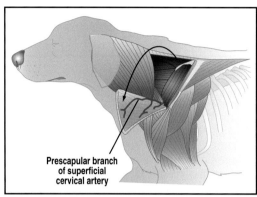

Prescapular branch
of superficial
cervical artery

Transposition of the cervical portion of the trapezius muscle, based on pedicles from the superficial cervical artery and vein.

OPERATIVE TECHNIQUE 9.16:
Deep pectoral muscle flap

Indications
A flap based on the lateral thoracic and external thoracic arteries may be used to reconstruct the cranial and ventral thoracic wall.

Anatomy

- A broad muscle on the ventral thorax.
- Origin: all the sternebrae and the deep fascia of the trunk and its fibres run cranially and laterally below the superficial pectoral muscle.
- Insertion: minor tubercle of the humerus, with an aponeurosis to the major tubercle.

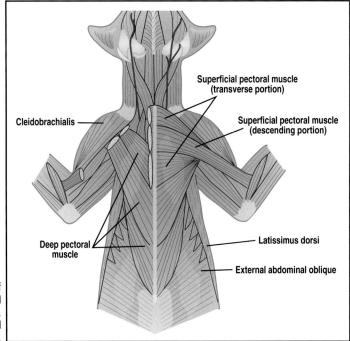

Ventral aspect of the thorax of a cat, showing the superficial and deep pectoral muscles. The right superficial pectoral muscle has been removed.

Vascular pedicles (Type V)
The lateral thoracic artery and external thoracic artery enter the muscle cranially, and a segmental supply from the internal thoracic artery enters the muscle along its origin on the sternum.

Raising the flap

- A craniolaterally based flap is created by dividing the segmental supply along the long sternal origin of the muscle.
- Alternatively, the tendon of insertion on the humerus and the lateral and external thoracic arteries may be divided to create a ventromedially based flap. The flap is limited cranially as it is covered by the superficial pectoral muscle.

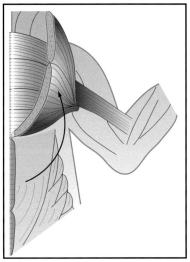

Incision of the origin of the deep pectoral muscle, and cranial transposition.

Area of transposition
Adjacent areas of the chest wall, sternum and trunk.

OPERATIVE TECHNIQUE 9.17:
Latissimus dorsi muscle flap

Indications

- Thoracic wall reconstruction following thoracic wall resection for neoplasia. (When used to close a chest wall defect, paradoxical movement of the flap may be seen for a few days postoperatively, and a shallow concavity may always be present).
- Patching of intrathoracic structures, e.g. the lung, trachea or oesophagus.
- Augmentation of myocardial blood supply and function.

Anatomy

- A large, flat triangular muscle overlying the dorsal thoracic wall.
- Origin: a wide leaf from the superficial leaf of the lumbodorsal fascia, associated with the spinous processes of the lumbar and last seven or eight thoracic vertebrae.
- Insertion: muscles fibres converge to an aponeurosis medially on the teres tuberosity of the humerus, dorsal to the deep pectoral and medial to the thoracic trapezius muscles.

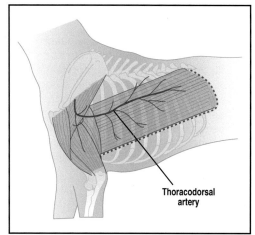

Landmarks for the latissimus dorsi and cutaneous trunci myocutaneous flaps.

Vascular pedicles (Type V)

The thoracodorsal and lateral thoracic arteries supply the dorsal and ventral portions of the latissimus dorsi, respectively. The intercostal arteries also supply segmental branches to the dorsal part of the muscle and overlying cutaneous trunci muscle.

Raising the flap

1. The muscle can usually be exposed through the primary surgical approach, but if this is not possible, make an incision over the muscle, parallel to the direction of the fibres.
2. Ligate the perforating intercostal arteries, which enter the muscle on the deep surface and exit on the superficial surface.
3. Free the dorsal, caudal and ventral borders.
4. Transpose the flap into the recipient site.

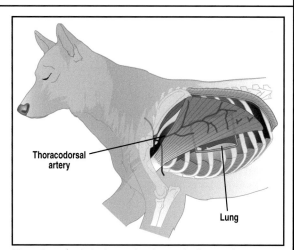

Elevation of a latissimus dorsi muscle flap and transposition to cover a thoracic wall defect.

Area of transposition

Adjacent areas of the thoracic wall, cranially to the lateral shoulder and brachium, distally to the antebrachium and transthoracically to the contralateral chest wall.

OPERATIVE TECHNIQUE 9.18:
Cranial portion of the external abdominal oblique muscle flap

Indications

- Reconstruction of wounds over the trunk.
- Hernias and ruptures of the abdominal wall and caudal thoracic wall and full-thickness defects following compartmental excision.

Anatomy

- A long, thin, flat muscle with fibres oriented caudoventrally.
- Origin: costal component originates segmentally from the 4th or 5th rib to the 13th rib and the lumbar component arises from the thoracolumbar fascia, along the iliocostalis muscle.
- Insertion: wide tendinous aponeurosis which inserts on the linea alba and contributes to the external rectus sheath, the external inguinal ring and the prepubic tendon.

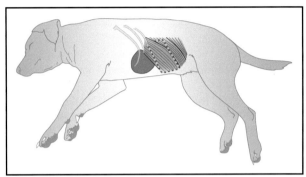

Lateral aspect of the thorax and abdomen illustrating the external abdominal oblique muscle.

Vascular pedicles (Type III)

- A pedicle of the cranial branch of the cranial abdominal artery and vein.
- The deep branch of the deep circumflex iliac artery anastomoses with the cranial and caudal abdominal arteries and is the main supply to the caudodorsal quarter of the abdominal wall.

Raising the flap

1. Make a paracostal incision from the level of the transverse processes to the midline, approximately 5 cm caudal to the 13th rib. If the surgical wound provides access to the cranial border of the muscle, the caudal border may be exposed with an incision parallel to the last rib, but situated further caudally in the flank.
2. Identify the aponeurosis of the muscle ventrally and caudally and make incisions in it, leaving a 5–10 mm rim of fascia attached to the muscle edge.
3. Undermine the muscle, taking care to preserve the vascular pedicle located craniodorsally, immediately caudal to the 13th rib.
4. Divide the dorsal fascial attachment and sever the remaining attachment at the level of the 13th rib.

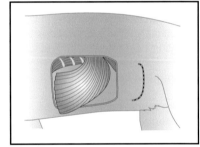

Creation of a muscle flap by division of the fascial attachments and cranial transposition.

Area of transposition
Adjacent portions of the thoracic and abdominal wall.

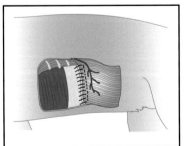

Closure of a caudal thoracic wall defect with the muscle flap, showing the neurovascular pedicle.

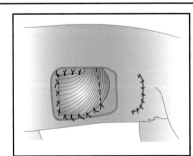

Wound closed.

OPERATIVE TECHNIQUE 9.19:
Rectus abdominis muscle flap

Indications
Reconstruction of wounds or full-thickness defects of the abdominal wall. The cranial part of the external abdominal oblique muscle, which is wider, thinner and more pliable, may also be used for this purpose.

Anatomy

- A long, wide, flat muscle, which extends either side of the linea alba on the ventral thoracic and abdominal walls, between the external and internal rectus sheath.
- Origin: the sternum and first costal cartilage and rib.
- Insertion: pecten of the pubis with the pectineus muscle and prepubic tendon.

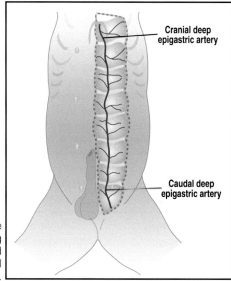

Ventral aspect of the abdominal wall, showing the rectus abdominis and the cranial and caudal deep epigastric vessels.

Vascular pedicles (Type III)
Two codominant pedicles enter at each end of the muscle, from the cranial and caudal deep epigastric vessels.

Raising the flap

1. Make a ventral midline skin incision and reflect the skin laterally to expose the linea alba, external rectus sheath and rectus abdominis.
2. Make an incision in the external rectus sheath and bluntly dissect the rectus abdominis from the internal rectus sheath.
3. Ligate the cranial or caudal superficial epigastric vessels.
4. Elevate and transpose the muscle flap.
5. Close the external rectus sheath.

Area of transposition
Adjacent areas of the trunk.

OPERATIVE TECHNIQUE 9.20:
Cutaneous trunci myocutaneous flap

Indications
This flap is similar to the latissimus dorsi myocutaneous flap but is considerably thinner. It is therefore less rigid but has increased pliability and mobility. These properties make it more suitable for reconstructing defects on the proximal thoracic limb rather than thoracic wall defects.

Anatomy

- A thin muscular sheet, which covers the dorsal, lateral and ventral walls of the abdomen.
- Origin: caudal gluteal region – muscle fibres fan out cranially and ventrally.
- Insertion: the axillary region, closely associated with the latissimus dorsi and deep pectoral muscles.
- Due to the intimate association of the muscle with the skin and subdermal plexus, this muscle is used primarily as a myocutaneous flap rather than a muscle flap.

Vascular pedicles
The blood supply is provided by small muscular branches and direct cutaneous arteries supplying the overlying skin. Two to four short direct cutaneous branches of the thoracodorsal artery perforate the latissimus dorsi muscle, caudal to the border of the triceps muscle, and supply the cutaneous trunci muscle and overlying skin.

Raising the flap
The general outline and landmarks of the cutaneous trunci myocutaneous flap are similar to the latissimus dorsi myocutaneous flap (see Operative Technique 9.21).

1. Outline and incise the cutaneous borders of the flap.
2. Dissect the flap in the loose areolar tissue between the cutaneous trunci and latissimus dorsi muscles.
3. Ligate the proximal lateral intercostal direct cutaneous arteries leaving the surface of the latissimus dorsi.

OPERATIVE TECHNIQUE 9.21:
Latissimus dorsi myocutaneous flap

Indications
Ideally suited to close defects of the lateral thoracic wall where simultaneous reconstruction of the thoracic wall and closure of the skin are required.

Anatomy
The latissimus dorsi myocutaneous flap is bulky because the muscle itself is thick, and because it also incorporates the overlying cutaneous trunci muscle and subcutaneous fat (see Operative Technique 9.17).

Vascular pedicles
Branches of the thoracodorsal and lateral thoracic arteries leave the muscle as direct cutaneous arteries, to supply the overlying cutaneous trunci and skin. The thoracodorsal artery also sends a large direct cutaneous artery to supply the skin caudal to the scapula. The intercostal arteries supply segmental branches to the dorsal part of the muscle and overlying cutaneous trunci muscle. These branches perforate the latissimus dorsi to supply the cutaneous trunci and overlying skin as the proximal lateral cutaneous branches of the intercostal arteries. The distal lateral cutaneous branches of the intercostal arteries emerge below the ventral border of the latissimus dorsi muscle to supply the overlying skin.

Raising the flap

Flap landmarks:

- Dorsal border: a line joining a point ventral to the acromion and caudal to the triceps muscle to the head of the 13th rib.
- Ventral border: a line extending from the axillary skin fold, caudal to the triceps at the level of the distal third of the humerus, to the 13th rib, keeping parallel to the dorsal border.
- Caudal border: by joining the dorsal and ventral borders along the length of the 13th rib.

The ventral border of the myocutaneous flap is incised first to allow the ventral border of the latissimus dorsi muscle to be elevated. As the skin incision is developed, a flap of latissimus dorsi of equal width is elevated. As the muscle flap is elevated, the perforating intercostal branches are ligated.

Area of transposition
May extend to the proximal or mid antebrachium, depending on the patient's conformation.

OPERATIVE TECHNIQUE 9.22:
Trapezius myocutaneous flap

Indications
Defects in the neck, cranial thorax and proximal thoracic limb.

Anatomy
See Operative Technique 9.15.

Vascular pedicles
Survival is based on a pedicle supplied by the prescapular branch of the superficial cervical vascular pedicle.

Raising the flap

1. Make a triangular incision over the cervical part of the trapezius.
2. Divide the origin of the muscle at the dorsal midline and dissect the trapezius free from the adjacent cleidocervicalis and omotransversarius muscles.

Myocutaneous flap: Divide the attachments of the muscle to the scapular spine.

Osteomyocutaneous flap: Dissect the attachments of the caudal half of the supraspinatus, deltoideus, thoracic trapezius and cranial half of the infraspinatus from the scapular spine. Create a bone flap (from scapular spine and body) with a saw or burr and remove the medial attachments of the subscapularis and serratus ventralis.

OPERATIVE TECHNIQUE 9.23:
Gracilis myocutaneous flap

Indications
Possible perineal repair or potentially for microvascular free transfer due to its robust vascular pedicle.

Anatomy

- A broad muscular sheet that lies superficially on the medial aspect of the thigh.
- Origin: the pelvic symphysis via a symphyseal tendon which also serves as the origin for the adductor muscle. The origin extends from the pecten of the pubis to the ischial arch.
- Insertion: via a wide flat tendon on to the cranial border of the tibia, as well as sending a tendinous band to the common calcaneal tendon.

Flap landmarks:

- Ventral border: a horizontal line, three-quarters of the way down the thigh
- Caudal border: the palpable recess between the semimembranosus and semitendinosus muscles
- Dorsal border: immediately ventral to the iliopectineal eminence
- Cranial border: the caudal border of the pectineus muscle and femur.

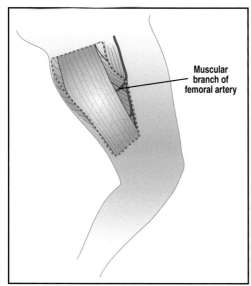

Muscular branch of femoral artery

Outline of the gracilis myocutaneous flap.

Vascular pedicles
The blood supply to the flap is from a muscular branch of the femoral artery. In some dogs a smaller muscular branch also enters the distal muscle, and thus the muscle may have a type I or II supply.

Raising the flap

1. Make the cranial and ventral incisions first.
2. Then make the caudal incision to allow the muscle and skin to be elevated as a unit. The skin may be sutured to the underlying muscle to prevent shear injury to the cutaneous blood supply.
3. Free the gracilis muscle from its fascial attachments and dissect it from its origin on the pubis and insertion on the medial tibia, taking care to preserve the vascular pedicle which enters the muscle along the cranial border at the junction of the proximal and middle thirds. If a distal vascular pedicle is present, it is ligated.
4. When elevating the craniodistal portion of the flap, take care to avoid the saphenous vessels.

10

Microsurgery

David Fowler and John Williams

Introduction

Microsurgery is defined as the use of magnification at some point during an operative procedure.

Although the use of operating loupes and surgical microscopes has been commonplace in human neurosurgery, ophthalmic surgery and reconstructive surgery for decades, experience with microvascular free tissue transfer is limited in veterinary surgery. Despite this fact, the utility of microvascular free tissue transfer for one-stage reconstruction of difficult problems, particularly of the distal limbs and the oral cavity, has been established. Early reconstruction of traumatic tissue loss using vascularized tissue is feasible, as is functional and cosmetic reconstruction after ablative cancer surgery. Tissues transferred in this manner are referred to as 'microvascular free tissue transfers', 'free flaps', 'microvascular free flaps' or 'autogenous vascularized grafts'.

Microvascular free tissue transfer involves:

1. The dissection of an 'island' of tissue based on a feeding artery and vein
2. Complete transection of the tissue from its donor site
3. Transfer of the tissue to a recipient wound bed
4. Revascularization of the tissue through microvascular anastomosis of the donor artery and vein to an appropriately sized recipient artery and vein.

Any tissue, or combination of tissues, may be used in the development of a microvascular free flap, as long as it meets several criteria (Figure 10.1).

Microvascular free flaps are identified according to the tissue type(s) included within the flap. Commonly used tissues/flaps include:

- Free cutaneous flaps
- Muscle flaps
- Omental flaps
- Bowel flaps
- Vascularized bone grafts.

Combinations of tissues may also be incorporated into flap designs, resulting in the formation of, for example:

- The tissue must be nourished by a single source artery and drained by a single vein; generally the artery and vein are parallel, but this is not an absolute requirement for a successful flap.
- The source artery and vein must be of sufficient size, usually **>1 mm** in diameter to accommodate successful microvascular anastomosis. Vessels <1 mm in diameter show progressively increased rates of thrombosis at the anastomosis site.
- The donor tissue must be dispensable. Reconstructive microsurgery has been referred to as 'the art of robbing Peter to pay Paul'; it is essential to ensure that 'Peter' will not miss the substance of which he is being robbed.
- The tissue flap and its associated vessels should be relatively easy to identify and dissect.

10.1 Criteria for the development of a microvascular free flap.

- Myocutaneous flaps
- Myo-osseous flaps
- Osteomusculocutaneous flaps.

Free flaps can be further identified according to the specific source of tissue. Examples include:

- Trapezius muscle flap
- Rectus abdominis muscle flap
- Latissimus dorsi myocutaneous flap
- Cranial abdominal myoperitoneal flap
- Free vascularized ulnar bone graft
- Free omental graft.

The overall success rate reported for veterinary microvascular free tissue transfer is approximately 93%, which compares quite favourably with reported success rates in human patients. Training in microvascular technique is becoming more commonplace in veterinary surgical training programmes, and microvascular reconstructive procedures are being performed in veterinary referral centres. Increasing levels of experience will lead to the use of microvascular tissue transfer as a reconstructive technique of choice for complex and difficult reconstructive problems. However, it is still accepted that there are clear disadvantages associated with free tissue transfer: the requirement for an operating microscope so that vascular anastomosis can be carried out; the need for specialized instrumentation and appropriate advanced training; and prolonged operating times.

Microvascular technique

Instrumentation

Equipment required for microvascular free tissue transfer is not extensive but is relatively expensive. The following are basic requirements.

Operating microscope

An operating microscope (Figure 10.2) is essential for successful harvest and anastomosis of the small vessels in microvascular reconstruction (typically 1–2 mm diameter). The microscope should have a foot control for adjustment of coarse focus, fine focus and magnification, leaving the surgeon's hands free for surgical manipulations The range of magnification used varies from approximately 5X to 30X. It is also beneficial to have a foot-controlled 'X–Y axis' on the microscope; this allows the surgeon to move the head of the operating microscope in two planes and is useful when dissecting along the length of a vessel or shifting between vessels. Ideally, the operating microscope has a beam-splitter that provides an identical stereoscopic visual field to two surgeons. Although microvascular anastomosis may be accomplished by one surgeon, it is greatly facilitated by a second.

Surgical instruments

The following instruments (Figure 10.3) are used:

- Jewellers' forceps are required for manipulation of small vessels. No. 3 and No. 5 jewellers' forceps are generally of greatest use
  - No. 3 forceps are used for handling the vessel during initial dissection
  - No. 5 forceps are used for final dissection, during anastomosis, or for handling very small vessels
  - Curved or angled jewellers' forceps are useful for grasping the 'back-side' of the vessel wall during vascular dissection

- Vessel dilators are similar to jewellers' forceps, but have a blunted tip to help prevent intimal injury. Vessel dilators are inserted into the vessel lumen prior to anastomosis and used to dilate the end of the vessel gently, thereby facilitating handling and suturing of the vessel end
- Very fine microsurgical scissors are required for adventitial dissection and vessel transection. It is beneficial to have both straight and curved scissors to facilitate vascular dissection in all planes
- Both straight and curved microsurgical needle drivers are available, with varying tip dimensions.

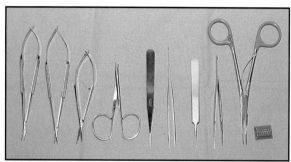

10.3 Fine microsurgical instruments are required for atraumatic handling and dissection of small vessels. An assortment of fine adventitial scissors, vessel dilators, jewellers' forceps and vascular clips is shown. Fine suture materials and needles are also required: the recommended sizes are shown in Figure 10.4.

- **The tunica intima or 'intima' is the innermost layer of an artery or vein and is composed of a single layer of endothelial cells supported by an elastic lamina.**
- **The tunica adventitia or 'adventitia' is the outer connective tissue covering of a vein or artery.**

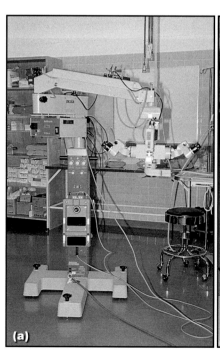
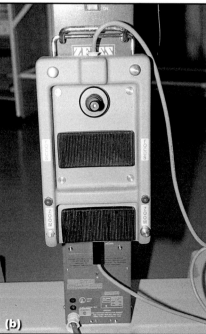

10.2 **(a)** An operating microscope is needed for successful microvascular surgery. This microscope is fitted with a 'beam splitter', allowing two surgeons to view the same surgical field with stereoscopic vision. **(b)** A foot pedal control facilitates adjustment of the microscope, leaving the surgeon's hands free. This foot pedal has adjustments for zoom, focus, and an 'X–Y' axis that allows repositioning of the field of vision.

Very fine suture material and needles are required for microvascular anastomosis (Figure 10.4).

Vessel diameter	Suture size	Needle size
< 1mm	0.1 metric (11/0 USP)	50 µm
1–2 mm	0.2 metric (10/0 USP)	70 or 100 µm
> 2 mm	0.3 or 0.2 metric (9/0 or 10/0 USP)	100 µm

10.4 Recommended suture and needle sizes for microsurgery.

Microvascular approximating clamps

Microvascular approximating clamps (Figure 10.5) may have several different features, depending upon the specific use and the preference of the surgeon. Approximating clamps are used to stabilize vessel ends in approximation and to block blood flow in the vessel and haemorrhage at the site during anastomosis.

- Double clamps consist of two clamps (one for each vessel end) connected on a sliding bar. After placing the donor and recipient vessel ends into opposing clamps, the clamps are adjusted on the sliding bar to bring the vessels into approximation.

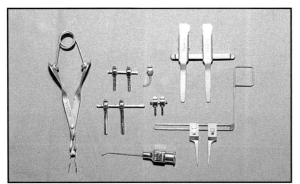

10.5 Vascular approximating clamps are available in various sizes and as single or double clamps. It is important that clamp size is matched to vessel size to ensure security of the vessel during anastomosis, but to avoid vessel injury from excessive clamp pressure.

- Double clamps can be provided with a wire frame. Long suture ends from previously placed sutures may be affixed to the wire frame to gain additional stability and to provide specific positioning of the vessel in preparation for the next suture. These are generally reserved for situations where an assistant surgeon is not available.
- Single clamps are used to control haemorrhage temporarily after vessel transection, but prior to anastomosis.
- Microvascular clamps are available in varying sizes. Each size will accommodate a specific range of vessel diameters. It is important that an appropriately sized clamp is used. Too large a clamp will produce a crush injury, while too small a clamp will allow the vessel end to slip out.

Flap dissection

It is advantageous, though not absolutely necessary, to have two surgical teams during microvascular free tissue transfer. One surgical team harvests the flap (Figure 10.6) while the second surgical team exposes recipient vessels and prepares the wound bed for transfer. The use of two surgical teams will significantly reduce operating time. When only one experienced team is available, the flap is dissected first, leaving the vascular pedicle intact. Following preparation of the recipient site, the vascular pedicle of the flap is transected and transferred.

It is imperative that the surgeon understands the vascular anatomy of the flap to be dissected. The surgical approaches to recipient vessels to the head and neck and to the limbs have recently been described to enable access to the most readily accessible recipient vessels (Degner *et al.*, 2004, 2005).

> **WARNING**
> **It must be remembered that microvascular free flaps are totally dependent upon a single vascular source for survival after transfer, and that inadvertent damage to the vascular supply during flap dissection can have disastrous consequences.**

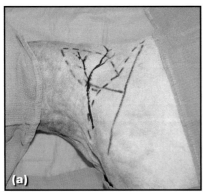
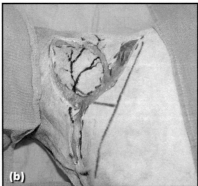
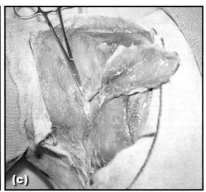

10.6 The surgical approach to flap harvest. **(a)** All pertinent anatomical landmarks are identified prior to incision. Landmarks and proposed incision for harvest of the trapezius myocutaneous flap are indicated. **(b)** Skin incision is made and small bleeding vessels are carefully controlled using electrocautery. Dissection is begun distant from and continued towards major vascular pedicles. **(c)** Vascular pedicles must be identified and preserved during flap dissection. (continues) ▶

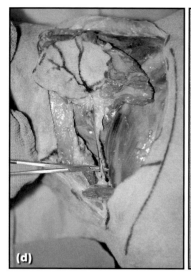
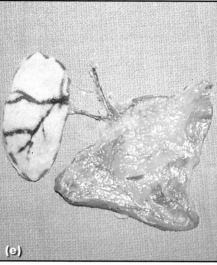

10.6 (continued) The surgical approach to flap harvest. **(d)** The vascular pedicle is skeletonized after its identification. As much length of the vascular pedicle as possible should be harvested. **(e)** Final appearance of the dissected myocutaneous flap, showing the vascular pedicle and its associated muscle and skin territories. (Illustrated using a cadaver specimen.)

Flap dissection is begun distant to the vascular pedicle, in a similar fashion to axial pattern flap dissection (see Chapter 7). The tissues should be handled gently. When multiple tissue planes are present, such as in a myocutaneous flap, sutures are placed as needed to prevent shearing of tissue planes during dissection (i.e. suturing the skin to the muscle rather than using stay sutures). Vascular branches that are encountered and isolated distant to the vascular pedicle may be controlled by traditional ligature or electrocautery techniques. As dissection approaches the vascular pedicle, great care must be taken to ensure a non-traumatic dissection of the vessels. Small vascular branches arising from the vascular pedicle may be carefully ligated using 0.3 or 0.2 metric (10/0 or 9/0 USP) suture material. Small vascular haemostatic clips may be used on larger vascular branches. Bipolar electrocautery may be used cautiously to coagulate vascular branches, but must be performed sufficiently distant to the parent artery that endothelial thermal injury is avoided.

The vascular pedicle is 'skeletonized' after its identification, by dissecting along the vessels' adventitial surfaces. The full thickness of the vessel wall must not be grasped during manipulation, since this will result in injury to the intimal surface. Instead, jewellers' forceps are used to grasp only the adventitial surface and to elevate the vessel gently to allow dissection. The artery and vein are dissected to a length beyond that estimated to be required, to ensure excess length of the vascular pedicle after transfer to the recipient site. The vessels are then trimmed to an appropriate length at the time of anastomosis. Once vascular dissection is complete, the flap is wrapped in moist swabs.

PRACTICAL TIP
The vascular pedicle should not be transected until the recipient site is prepared, in order to minimize flap ischaemic time. Flap ischaemia times will range from a minimum of 30 minutes to 1.5 hours. Anything less than 2 hours is acceptable, although this may extend up to 4 hours for skin or muscle.

Recipient site preparation

Appropriate preparation of the recipient wound bed is extremely important (see Chapter 4). Wound beds must be free of ongoing tissue necrosis and active infection. Infected wounds, especially those with osteomyelitis, may be managed with microvascular free flaps as part of a one-stage operation, but thorough debridement of all grossly infected tissue remains a necessity (Figure 10.7).

WARNING
Free flaps are not a solution to suboptimal wound management.

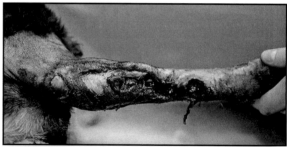
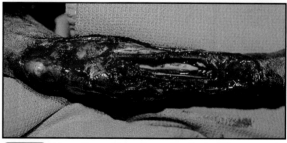

10.7 Necrotic and heavily contaminated tissue must be excised prior to wound reconstruction. Aggressive debridement and open wound management has converted this heavily contaminated forelimb injury to a clean contaminated state over a 3-day period.

Vessel selection and anastomosis

Consideration must be given to selecting an appropriate recipient artery and vein to be used in revascularizing the free flap. This requires a thorough knowledge of regional vascular anatomy. In cases of severe and extensive trauma, preoperative angio-graphy is indicated to document the integrity and location of regional vessels. There are several criteria that must be considered when selecting an appropriate recipient artery and vein:

- Recipient vessels should be dissected outside the margins of the 'zone of trauma' to ensure the use of vessels without pre-existing intimal injury
- Recipient vessels must approximate the diameter of flap vessels when performing end-to-end anastomosis
- A size discrepancy of approximately 1.5:1 may be accommodated fairly easily when performing end-to-end anastomosis, but a greater size discrepancy leads to an increasing incidence of thrombosis
- Recipient vessels should be larger than donor vessels when performing end-to-side anastomosis
- Incisions used to access recipient vessels are planned such that suture lines will not directly overlie the vascular pedicles. Curved incisions, resulting in the formation of a skin flap over the recipient vessels, are generally indicated.
- As with all reconstructive surgical procedures, preoperative surgical planning is essential. It is important to consider flap location and the position of donor vascular pedicles prior to starting dissection of recipient vessels. Anticipation of the exact location where anastomosis will be performed will limit the amount of recipient vessel dissection that needs to be done.

End-to-end anastomosis (see Operative Tech-nique 10.1) 'steals' the vascular supply of the recipi-ent artery from its terminal destination and diverts that blood supply into the microvascular free flap. This is an important consideration in situations involving compromised vascularity to structures distal to the reconstruction. In these instances, end-to-side ana-stomosis (see Operative Technique 10.2) should be performed in order to ensure vascular integrity of dis-tal structures (Figure 10.8).

The order of vascular repair – artery first or vein first – is largely a matter of personal preference. Flow should not be re-established through either anastomosis until both are completed. At that time, the venous anastomosis should be released, followed by the arterial anastomosis.

Assessing patency

Thrombosis at the anastomotic site, resulting from faulty technique such as intimal damage due to poor handling, is usually apparent within 15 minutes of re-establishing blood flow. Blood flow should be confirmed a few minutes after clamp release, and again at 15 minutes after clamp release. Several methods have been described for this purpose. Simple visual inspection of the vessel is not a reliable indicator of blood flow, since longitudinal pulsation may be seen in a thrombosed artery.

One of the simplest reliable tests for vascular patency is the venous occlusion test (Figure 10.9):

- The vein is visualized under magnification
- Jewellers' forceps are used to occlude the recipient vein gently, immediately 'downstream' from the anastomosis
- Progressive venous distension 'upstream' from the occlusion indicates a patent arterial anastomosis
- Once venous engorgement is seen (this requires only a few seconds) the jewellers' forceps are released; immediate relief of venous distension indicates a patent venous anastomosis.

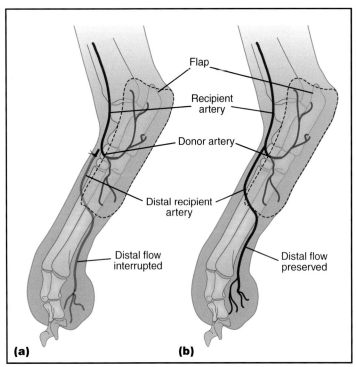

Flap

Recipient artery

Donor artery

Distal recipient artery

Distal flow interrupted

Distal flow preserved

(a)   **(b)**

10.8 **(a)** End-to-end arterial anastomosis results in diversion of arterial flow away from distal structures normally nourished by the recipient artery. **(b)** End-to-side arterial anastomosis allows revascularization of the transferred tissue while maintaining distal arterial flow.

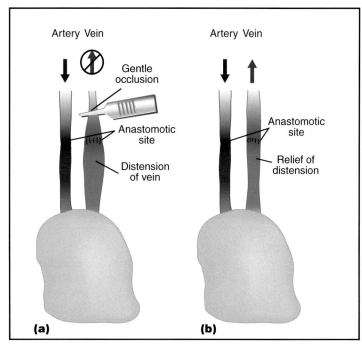

10.9 The venous occlusion test is a safe and reliable method to assess patency and the venous anastomoses. **(a)** Gentle occlusion of the recipient vein 'downstream' from the anastomosis results in distension of the vein 'upstream'. Rapid distension reveals a patent arterial anastomosis. **(b)** Rapid relief of venous distension following release of the vein is compatible with a patent venous anastomosis.

A second commonly used patency test for both artery and vein is the 'empty and refill' test (Figure 10.10), using two pairs of jewellers' forceps:

- The vessel is occluded with one pair of jewellers' forceps immediately 'downstream' from the anastomosis
- A second pair of jewellers' forceps is used to 'milk' blood gently from the vessel lumen, and subsequently occlude the vessel 1–2 cm further 'downstream'
- The 'upstream' forceps are released and the vessel is observed. Rapid refill of the emptied segment is indicative of a patent anastomosis.

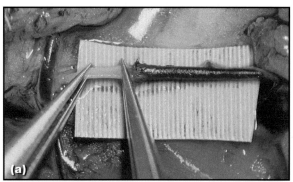

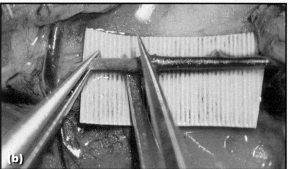

10.10 The empty and refill test can be used to test both arterial and venous patency. **(a)** The vessel is grasped gently using two jewellers' forceps 'downstream' from the anastomosis. Blood is 'milked' from a vessel segment. **(b)** Release of the 'upstream' forceps should result in rapid refill of the emptied segment.

Postoperative care

Astute postoperative care and monitoring are essential:

- Flaps are reliant upon the integrity of a single artery and vein for vascular flow. Restrictive bandages must be avoided and patient positioning must be planned to avoid compression of the vascular pedicle
- The patient's hydration is maintained by provision of intravenous balanced electrolyte solutions or colloids
- Flaps are kept warm by application of circulating warm water blankets, heat lamps, or loosely applied bandages.

Bandages are applied loosely to protect the flap from trauma or self-mutilation. A window is cut through the bandage to allow frequent visual inspection at least once a day. Cutaneous flaps should maintain a pink appearance. Blanching of the flap is a possible indication of arterial insufficiency, while congestion and purplish discoloration is consistent with venous insufficiency. Brisk flow of bright red blood following a pin-prick with a 20–22 gauge needle indicates adequate perfusion (with care taken not to do this over the known location of the donor vessels). Sluggish flow of dark blood is consistent with poor perfusion or arterial insufficiency. Transcutaneous Doppler flow transducers may be used to verify flow through a superficially located arterial pedicle.

Early detection and treatment of failing flaps often leads to successful salvage. Re-exploration of the vascular pedicle is indicated at the first suggestion of poor perfusion. Corrective action depends on the specific cause of failure but may necessitate repeat anastomosis, relocation of vascular pedicles, or additional vascular dissection. Medicinal leeches may be used for the management of venous insufficiency in the presence of adequate arterial inflow.

Antithrombotic and anticoagulant drugs are not routinely recommended. Patency rates >95% are expected, given proper planning and meticulous technique. Antithrombotic agents are not a substitute for accurate surgical technique. In animals at risk of developing thrombosis, low-dose aspirin or systemic heparin therapy may be beneficial.

Specific flaps in the dog and cat

Cutaneous flaps
Cutaneous angiosomes ('territories' of tissue that are supplied by a single source artery and vein) have been described thoroughly in the dog and cat, and this information has been used for the development of large axial pattern skin flaps (see Chapter 7). These flaps may also be used for free microvascular transfer, assuming adequate size of the vascular pedicle for successful anastomosis. Vessel diameters for most described cutaneous flaps in dogs of average size approach 1–2 mm. The superficial cervical (omocervical) axial pattern flap, the caudal superficial epigastric axial pattern flap, and the saphenous fasciocutaneous conduit flap have been used clinically for microvascular transfer.

Detailed anatomical descriptions of flap dissection are given in Chapter 7. Two points are worth emphasizing here:

- The microvascular supply to cutaneous flaps, in areas where superficial cutaneous musculature exists, courses deep to this muscular layer. Dissection must, therefore, be performed deep to the superficial cutaneous musculature. For example, the cutaneous trunci muscle must be included with the dissection of the thoracodorsal cutaneous flap
- During flap dissection, there is a tendency for tensile or shearing forces to cause a separation between tissue layers. Placement of occasional simple interrupted sutures between cutaneous musculature, subcutaneous tissue and dermis helps to stabilize these tissues and prevent trauma to the microvasculature.

Footpad flaps
Footpads are specialized cutaneous/subcutaneous structures designed for resistance to weightbearing stresses. Injury to large portions of the footpads inevitably results in compromised function. Reconstruction of such defects requires the use of 'like' tissue to replace lost tissue.

The fifth digital footpad has been described as a microvascular free flap based on the deep plantar metatarsal artery IV and the superficial metatarsal vein IV:

- The digital footpad and associated soft tissues are harvested following excision of the phalanges through a dorsal incision (Figure 10.11)
- Sensory re-innervation may be provided by repair of the deep plantar metatarsal nerve IV to an appropriate sensory nerve at the recipient site. However, the necessity of sensory re-innervation of transferred footpads has not been established.

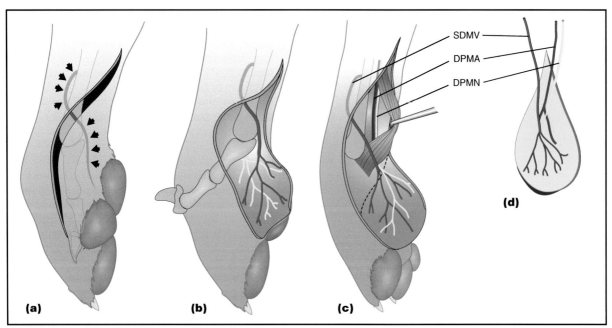

10.11 Harvest of the fifth digital footpad flap. **(a)** The incision is initiated laterally over the fifth metatarsal bone and curves distally to end on the dorsal aspect of the coronary band. **(b)** The phalangeal bones are dissected extraperiosteally. Care is necessary to avoid damage to neurovascular structures in the surrounding soft tissues. **(c)** The vascular pedicle, consisting of the superficial dorsal metatarsal vein (SDMV), the deep plantar metatarsal artery (DPMA) and deep plantar metatarsal nerve (DPMN), is identified. The broken line indicates the level of skin incision through the interdigital skin to complete flap formation. **(d)** Appearance of the dissected flap, as viewed from the deep surface.

The accessory carpal footpad has also been used as a microvascular free tissue transfer based on the caudal interosseous artery and the cephalic vein (Figure 10.12):

- A sensory branch of the ulnar nerve parallels the arterial pedicle through the carpal canal, and may be used for sensory re-innervation
- The carpal footpad is not situated in a weightbearing position, but it shares the physical characteristics of a weightbearing footpad. Loss of the carpal footpad is of no functional consequence.

Both the digital footpad and carpal footpad flaps are of limited size relative to most weightbearing defects requiring reconstruction. Careful positioning of footpad tissue is required at the recipient site, to ensure fixation in a central weightbearing position. Excessive shear forces and partial incisional dehiscence of the flap margins inevitably occur if the footpad becomes displaced (Figure 10.13). Several minor revisional procedures for flap repositioning are commonly required. Over time, the transferred footpads hypertrophy, thereby adopting a more functional weightbearing role at the recipient site.

Muscle flaps

Muscle is probably the most useful of any single tissue used for wound reconstruction. It facilitates re-vascularization of ischaemic wound beds, delivers nutrients to the wound and decreases the incidence of significant wound complications, such as infection and delayed healing. Muscle flaps are generally

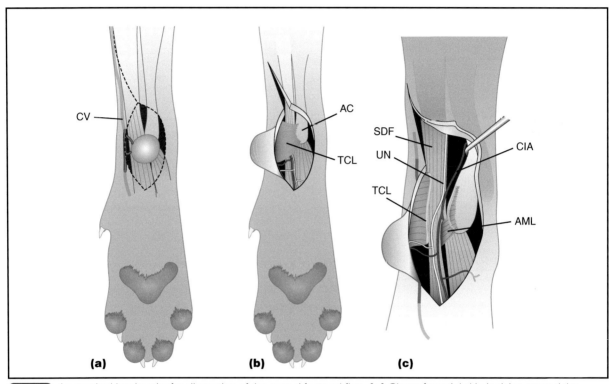

10.12 Anatomical landmarks for dissection of the carpal footpad flap. **(a)** Circumferential skin incision around the footpad is extended proximally, parallel to the cephalic vein (CV). **(b)** Deep subcutaneous dissection is initiated from the lateral aspect until the small arterial branch to the footpad is identified. The accessory carpal bone (AC) and the transverse carpal ligament (TCL) are shown. **(c)** After dissection through the carpal canal, the caudal interosseous artery (CIA) and a superficial branch of the ulnar nerve (UN) are identified as they course between the transverse carpal ligament and the accessory metacarpeum ligament (AML). The pedicle closely parallels the tendon of the superficial digital flexor muscle (SDF). Venous drainage is provided by the cephalic vein.

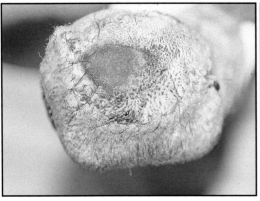
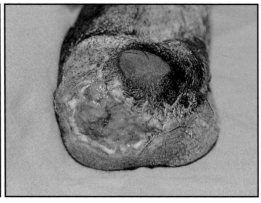

10.13

Shear stresses acting upon weightbearing incisions frequently result in partial dehiscence and flap migration. Minor revisional procedures are often required after footpad transfer.

dissected quite easily due to their enveloping fascial layers. Vascular pedicles are easily identified and protected. Most muscles may be harvested with little resulting donor site morbidity. In nearly all instances, synergistic muscle groups adapt to the loss of a single muscle with little functional consequence. When muscle alone is used for reconstruction of wounds, overlying cutaneous resurfacing is accomplished by immediate placement of a full-thickness skin graft on to the transferred muscle. The success of such grafts is consistently excellent.

The vascular supply to muscles may be divided into one of five basic types, based on the number and size of vascular pedicles nourishing the muscle. This classification system, and the specific vascular anatomy of commonly used muscles, is described in Chapter 9. Muscles with a Type I, II or V vascular pattern are preferred for microvascular transfer since their survival is expected, based entirely upon revascularization of only the dominant vascular pedicle. The trapezius and latissimus dorsi muscle flaps are most commonly used for microvascular transfer.

Trapezius muscle flap

The cervical portion of the trapezius muscle has a Type II vascular pattern, with the prescapular branch of the superficial cervical artery forming the dominant vascular pedicle (Figure 10.14). Survival of the entire cervical portion of the trapezius muscle has been documented consistently, based on this dominant pedicle. Raising the flap is described in Operative Technique 10.3.

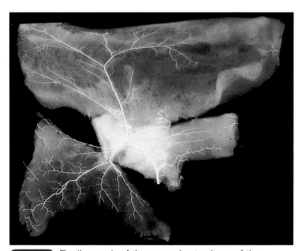

10.14 Radiograph of the vascular territory of the prescapular branch of the superficial cervical artery. The vascular pedicle is in the centre. The trapezius muscle is shown in the lower left, a segment of the omotransversarius muscle in the centre, and the cutaneous territory in the upper portion.

The trapezius muscle is broad and flat and, therefore, lends itself well to the cosmetic reconstruction of many wounds. The bulk of the flap also rapidly diminishes due to denervation atrophy (Figure 10.15). Vascular density of muscle flaps has been shown to be maintained despite progressive muscle atrophy.

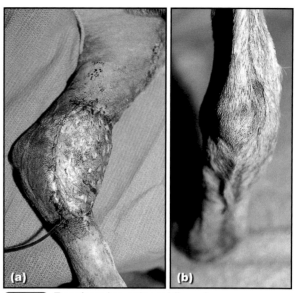

10.15 Transferred muscle rapidly undergoes neurogenic atrophy. **(a)** Bulky appearance of a trapezius muscle transfer with overlying skin graft immediately after transfer. **(b)** Appearance of the same flap, in profile, 6 weeks after transfer.

Latissimus dorsi muscle flap

The latissimus dorsi muscle is a large, relatively flat muscle. It is used commonly for the reconstruction of large soft tissue deficits in human patients and has been used to a limited extent in dogs and cats. It has a Type V vascular supply; the thoracodorsal artery and vein serve as the dominant vascular pedicle and enter the muscle near its insertion. Survival of the entire muscle based solely on this dominant vascular pedicle has been documented. Raising the flap is detailed in Operative Technique 10.4.

Vascularized bone grafts

The indications, contraindications and clinical utility of non-vascularized cortical allografts are well established. They provide immediate structural integrity in instances of segmental bone loss. Ultimate success of non-vascularized allografts, however, is dependent upon revascularization followed by a process of graft resorption and new bone production that requires years. The risk of infection, delayed union, implant loosening or graft collapse is substantial.

Vascularized autogenous cortical bone grafts are immediately revascularized following transfer, and have the advantage of providing viable cellular elements that contribute actively to bone healing. They are more resistant to infection and heal more rapidly than do non-vascularized cortical allografts. After transfer, vascularized grafts rapidly remodel and hypertrophy, according to the stresses placed upon them at the recipient site. They have the disadvantage of necessitating the harvesting of a segment of cortical bone from a donor site, with an attendant risk of morbidity. Experience using microvascular transfer of cortical bone is limited in veterinary medicine, and few experimental studies exist. However, several potentially useful vascularized bone grafts have been described.

Vascularized fibular graft

The canine fibula has been used as an experimental model for the study of the biology of vascularized bone grafts:

- The fibular graft is based on either the caudal tibial or the popliteal vascular pedicle
- The popliteal artery branches into a larger cranial tibial and a smaller caudal tibial artery. The caudal tibial artery continues deep to the flexor hallicus longus muscle within the interosseous space
- The nutrient artery of the fibula arises from the caudal tibial artery, entering the fibula medially in its proximal third
- Dissection of the vascularized fibular graft, as with all vascularized bone grafts, is performed to include a surrounding myoperiosteal cuff of tissue. The flexor hallicus longus muscle belly is preserved with the graft, ensuring the integrity of the caudal tibial artery and vein.

Transfer of the fibula with the caudal tibial artery and vein results in a relatively short vascular pedicle of limited diameter. Dissection to the level of the popliteal artery and vein yields a more substantial vascular pedicle, but necessitates ligation of the cranial tibial artery and vein. Iatrogenic damage to the peroneal nerve must be avoided during proximal dissection.

Microvascular free transfer of the fibula is probably of limited use in the dog. The fibula has a small diameter and would provide little of the structural integrity needed for long bone reconstruction. However, the fibula may prove useful for augmentation of more traditional fracture repairs, or for the management of non-union fractures.

Vascularized rib graft

Microvascular transfer of the canine rib has been reported experimentally. As with the fibula, the rib is likely to be of minimal benefit to the veterinary surgeon performing reconstructive surgery, due to its curved shape and poor structural integrity. The rib is harvested with the intercostal artery and vein. The pedicle may be formed either by the dorsal intercostal artery and vein or by the ventral intercostal artery and vein. Dorsal dissection includes the nutrient artery and vein, while ventral dissection yields a graft solely dependent upon its myoperiosteal vascular supply for survival.

Vascularized ulnar graft

The ulna derives its blood supply from the caudal interosseous artery and vein (Figure 10.16). The common interosseous artery arises from the median artery at the level of the proximal radius. After entering the interosseous space from the medial side, the common interosseous artery bifurcates into caudal and cranial interosseous branches. The cranial interosseous artery emerges from the interosseous space laterally and gives rise to muscular branches to the extensor carpi ulnaris and the lateral and common digital extensor muscles. The caudal interosseous

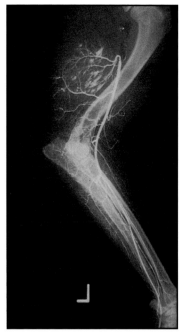

10.16

Perfusion patterns of the forelimb in a specimen after injection of barium into the brachial artery. The ulna derives its vascular supply from the caudal interosseous artery, which arises from the short common interosseous artery and extends distally in the interosseous space between the radius and the ulna.

vessels continue distally in the interosseous space, and give rise to the nutrient arteries of the radius and the ulna at the junctions of their proximal and middle thirds. Multiple periosteal branches arise throughout its course.

Vascularized ulnar transfers based on either a proximal or distal dissection have been described in dogs:

- The ulna is harvested through a caudolateral curvilinear skin incision for both proximal and distal dissections
- Fasciotomy is performed on both the extensor and flexor muscle groups to facilitate their elevation and retraction.

The proximal ulnar graft is based on the common interosseous vascular pedicle. Retraction of the extensor carpi ulnaris and lateral digital extensor muscles proximally reveals their muscular branches. These muscular branches serve as a landmark for the level of the common interosseous pedicle.

Both proximal and distal ulnar grafts are harvested with a myoperiosteal sleeve, including the ulnar head of the deep digital flexor, the pronator quadratus and the abductor pollicis longus muscles. The nutrient artery of the ulna is incorporated in the proximal dissection, while distal dissection results in preservation of the myoperiosteal blood supply only. Both result in predictable survival. Proximal dissection has the disadvantage of requiring osteotomy of the ulna near the elbow joint. The dissection procedure is detailed in Operative Technique 10.5.

Fixation of vascularized grafts at the recipient site deserves special mention. Since vascularized grafts depend substantially or wholly upon the integrity of their myoperiosteal blood supply, it is imperative that fixation techniques be used that minimize embarrassment of this vasculature. Therefore, external skeletal fixation is recommended

Compound flaps

Compound flaps refer to flaps that incorporate more than one type of tissue, e.g. myocutaneous, osteocutaneous, myo-osseous flaps. As with all microvascular flaps, the only prerequisite is that all the tissues are nourished by a single source artery and vein. A detailed knowledge of vascular anatomy allows a great deal of flexibility in flap design.

The trapezius flap may be harvested as a myocutaneous flap by preserving the direct cutaneous branch of the superficial cervical artery and vein. The associated axial pattern skin flap is then included with dissection of the trapezius muscle. Skin is used either to resurface the muscle or, dissected free of the underlying muscle, to resurface portions of the wound bed adjacent to the muscle flap.

The latissimus dorsi flap may be harvested as a myocutaneous flap by inclusion of the direct cutaneous vessels arising from the thoracodorsal artery and vein. The thoracodorsal axial pattern skin flap is then used in a manner similar to that described for the trapezius myocutaneous flap (see Chapter 9). Skin directly overlying the latissimus dorsi muscle can also be included as a myocutaneous flap without preservation of the direct cutaneous artery of the thoracodorsal skin flap. This region of skin is supplied by intercostal cutaneous perforators and does not mandate inclusion of the direct cutaneous artery and vein in the flap design.

The scapular spine has been successfully included with the trapezius flap, resulting in the formation of a myo-osseous or osteomusculocutaneous flap. The scapular spine does not lie within the primary angiosome of the superficial cervical vessels, but survives based on blood flow through 'choke vessels'. These are small-calibre vascular channels that connect adjacent angiosomes. In the event of vascular injury, choke vessels increase in size, allowing a redistribution of blood supply. The trapezius–scapular spine myo-osseous flap may be used for the reconstruction of small bone defects (such as metatarsal or metacarpal injuries) associated with extensive soft tissue trauma.

References and further reading

Basher AWP, Fowler FD, Bowen CV *et al.* (1990) Microneurovascular free digital pad transfer in the dog. *Veterinary Surgery* **19**, 226–231

Brown K, Marie P, Lyszakowski T *et al.* (1983) Epiphysial growth after free fibular transfer with and without microvascular anastomosis. *Journal of Bone and Joint Surgery (Br)* **65B**, 493–501

Degner DA, Walshaw R, Fowler JD, *et al.* (2004) Surgical approaches to recipient vessels of the head and neck for microvascular free tissue transfer in dogs. *Veterinary Surgery* **33**, 200–208

Degner DA, Walshaw R, Fowler JD et al. (2005) Surgical approaches to recipient vessels of the fore- and hindlimbs for microvascular free tissue transfer in dogs. Veterinary Surgery **34**, 297–309

Degner DA, Walshaw R, Lanz O *et al.* (1996) The medial saphenous fasciocutaneous free flap in dogs. *Veterinary Surgery* **25**, 105–113

Fisher J and Wood MB (1987) Experimental comparison of bone revascularization by musculocutaneous and cutaneous free flaps. *Plastic Reconstructive Surgery* **79**, 81–90

Fowler JD, Miller CW, Bowen V *et al.* (1987) Transfer of free vascular cutaneous flaps by microvascular anastomosis: result in six dogs. *Veterinary Surgery* **16**, 446–450

Levitt L, Fowler JD, Longley M *et al.* (1988) A developmental model for free vascularized bone transfers in the dog. *Veterinary Surgery* **17**, 194–202

Miller CW, Chang P and Bowen V (1986) Identification and transfer of free cutaneous flaps by microvascular anastomosis in the dog. *Veterinary Surgery* **15**, 199–204

Miller JM, Lanz OI, Degner DA (2007) Rectus abdominis free muscle flap for reconstruction in nine dogs *Veterinary Surgery* **36**, 259–265

Moens NMM and Fowler JD (1997) The microvascular carpal foot pad flap: vascular anatomy and surgical technique. *Veterinary and Comparative Orthopaedics and Traumatology* **10**, 183–186

Nicoll SA, Fowler JD, Remedios AM *et al.* (1996) Development of a free latissimus dorsi muscle flap in cats. *Veterinary Surgery* **25**, 40–48

Ostrup LT and Fredrickson JM (1974) Distant transfer of a free, living bone graft by microvascular anastomoses. *Plastic and Reconstructive Surgery* **54**, 274–285

Philibert D and Fowler JD (1993) The trapezius osteomusculocutaneous flap in dogs. *Veterinary Surgery* **22**, 444–450

Philibert JD, Fowler JD and Clapson JB (1992) Free microvascular transplantation of the trapezius musculocutaneous flap in dogs. *Veterinary Surgery* **21**, 435–440

Szentimrey D and Fowler D (1994) The anatomic basis of a free vascularized bone graft based on the canine distal ulna. *Veterinary Surgery* **23**, 529–533

OPERATIVE TECHNIQUE 10.1:
End-to-end anastomosis

Positioning
Depends on location.

Assistant
Essential

Equipment extras
Operating microscope and instruments for microvascular surgery (see text).

Surgical technique

1. Place the donor and recipient vessels into approximation, using a double microvascular approximating clamp.
2. Check the lengths of the dissected vessels to ensure they are not twisted or kinked. Excessive tension and vessel redundancy must be avoided.
   - If vessels are too long, transect them at an appropriate length.
   - Inadequate vessel length presents a more difficult problem: the intervening space must be bridged using a vein graft.
3. Once the vessel ends have been trimmed and placed into the approximating clamp, adjust the clamps along the slide bar, such that the vessels are not quite in contact with one another. This allows for easy identification of the vessel lumen during suture placement, but prevents undue tension on the sutures while tying.
4. Place a contrasting background material beneath the vessels to facilitate handling and visual identification.

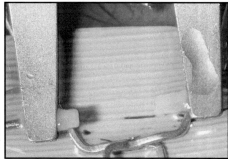

Vessel ends in approximation, held in a double microvascular approximating clamp.

5. Adventitial tissue is extremely thrombogenic and must be dissected from the vessel ends to avoid its incorporation into the anastomosis. This is most easily accomplished by grasping the loose adventitial tissue with jewellers' forceps and placing traction on the vessel. Pull the adventitial tissue beyond the level of the vessel end in a 'shirt-sleeve' fashion. The vessel end is easily identified through the translucent adventitia, and the excess adventitia is amputated at the level of the vessel end. Allow the adventitia to retract back on to the vessel, leaving the terminal few millimetres of the vessel free of adventitia.

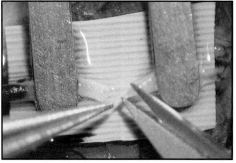

Loose adventital tissue is excised from the vessel ends.

6. After adventitial dissection, flush the vessels with a heparin/saline solution, prepared at a concentration of 10 IU heparin per 1 ml saline, to remove debris and blood elements.

OPERATIVE TECHNIQUE 10.1 continued:
End-to-end anastomosis

7. Suturing. The size of needle and suture material is critical (see Figure 10.4). Several suturing techniques have been described for end-to-end anastomosis, but the 'front wall' technique is most commonly employed:
   i. Divide the vessel lumen into thirds. With the 12 o'clock position defined as the centremost position of the superior vessel wall, place simple interrupted sutures at the 10 and 2 o'clock positions. Use jewellers' forceps to place counterpressure gently against the vessel wall during needle placement. The full thickness of the vessel wall should not be grasped since this will cause intimal injury at the anastomosis.

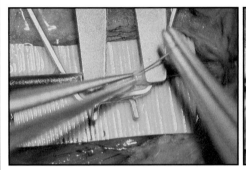 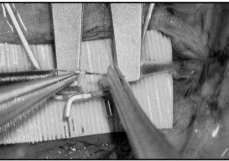

Suture placement at 10 and 2 o'clock.

   ii. Place a third simple interrupted suture at the 12 o'clock position.
   iii. Place further sutures as needed to complete apposition of the 'front wall' .

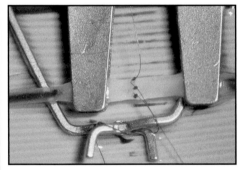

The 'front wall' is completed.

   iv. Turn over the microvascular approximating clamp such that the previous 'back wall' is brought into the superior position. Inspect the previously placed sutures to ensure they are placed properly.

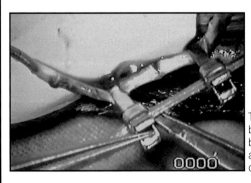

The 'back wall' is brought into view by inverting the approximating clamp.

   v. Place a simple interrupted suture at the central point of the remaining defect.
   vi. Complete the anastomosis by placing additional simple interrupted sutures.

OPERATIVE TECHNIQUE 10.1 continued:
End-to-end anastomosis

8. Release the clamps in this order:
    i.   Donor vein
    ii. Recipient vein
    iii. Donor artery
    iv. Recipient artery.

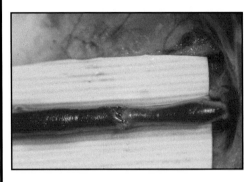

Closure is complete and the approximating clamp has been removed.

9. Confirm blood flow a few minutes after clamp release, and again at 15 minutes after clamp release (see text for details).

Postoperative care
See text.

OPERATIVE TECHNIQUE 10.2:
End-to-side anastomosis

Positioning
Depends on location.

Assistant
Essential.

Equipment extras
Operating microscope and instruments for microvascular surgery (see text).

Surgical technique

1. End-to-side anastomosis is performed when dealing with a marked size discrepancy, the recipient vessel being larger than the donor vessel. Dissect adventitial tissue from the donor vessel as described for end-to-end anastomosis (see Operative Technique 10.1) and place a single microvascular clamp, if needed, across the donor vessel to facilitate handling and prevent passive efflux of blood from the vessel during anastomosis.
2. Dissect the recipient vessel wall free of adventitial covering for a length of several millimetres at the proposed site of anastomosis. Place a double microvascular approximating clamp on to the recipient vessel, such that one clamp is situated proximal and one distal to the site of anastomosis.
3. Make an opening into the recipient vessel to accommodate the donor vessel. The size and precision of this opening is critical to the success of the anastomosis.
   i. Grasp the vessel wall using jewellers' forceps and make a full-thickness cut into the vessel at an angle of approximately 45 degrees (obliquely in the wall of the vessel) using fine dissection scissors. The depth of the cut should be sufficient to result in an opening approximately 50% of the size of that required.
   ii. Make a matching cut from the opposing side, planned such that the terminal ends of each cut meet precisely. The resulting opening will assume a round to oval configuration due to tensile forces from the vessel wall.

With the recipient vessel secured in a double microvascular approximating clamp, adventitial tissue is dissected and an opening made for the donor vessel.

4. Use heparinized saline to lavage blood elements and debris gently from the donor and recipient vessels.

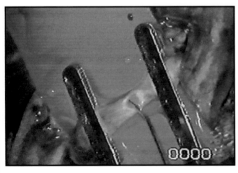

Blood is flushed from the recipient vessel using heparinized saline.

OPERATIVE TECHNIQUE 10.2 continued:
End-to-side anastomosis

5. Bring the donor vessel into approximation with the recipient vessel.
6. Suturing. Place simple interrupted sutures at the 3 and 9 o'clock positions. Place a third suture at the 12 o'clock position and use interposing sutures to complete the anastomosis along one side of the vessel. Retraction of the donor vessel by the assistant facilitates suture placement. Finally, place a suture at the 6 o'clock position to complete the anastomosis.

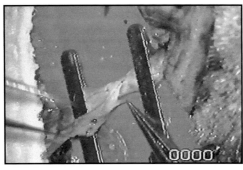

Simple interrupted sutures are placed at the 3 and 9 o'clock positions.

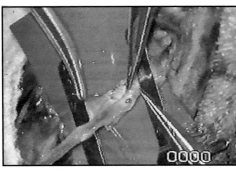
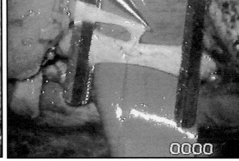

Retraction of the donor vessel in one direction facilitates closure of one side of the anastomosis. Retraction in the opposite direction allows completion of the anastomosis.

7. Release the clamps in this order:
   i. Donor vein
   ii. Recipient vein
   iii. Donor artery
   iv. Recipient artery.
8. Confirm blood flow a few minutes after clamp release, and again at 15 minutes after clamp release (see text for details).

Postoperative care
See text.

OPERATIVE TECHNIQUE 10.3:
Raising a trapezius muscle flap

Positioning
Lateral recumbency.

Assistant
Essential

Equipment extras
Operating microscope and instruments for microvascular surgery (see text).

Surgical technique

1. Dissect the trapezius muscle flap through a curvilinear incision beginning approximately 2 cm cranial to the point of the shoulder, extending dorsally parallel to the scapular spine and curving cranially below the dorsal midline.

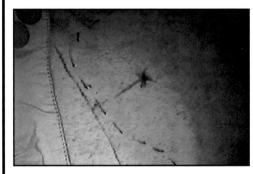

Anatomical landmarks. X = position of direct cutaneous artery. Dashed line = proposed incision. The dog's head is in a direction towards upper right.

2. Elevate a flap of skin, subcutaneous tissue and superficial cutaneous musculature from the underlying trapezius muscle.

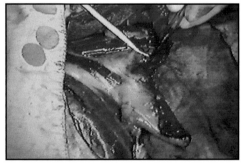

Elevating the trapezius muscle along its dorsal and fascial attachments. Vascular branches are identified on the deep surface of the muscle. Branches extending into deep cervical musculature are ligated.

3. Identify the direct cutaneous branch of the superficial cervical artery (the vascular pedicle of the superficial cervical axial pattern skin flap) and ligate it as it exits the septum formed by the trapezius, the omotransversarius and the cleidocervicalis muscles.
4. Incise the cervical portion of the trapezius muscle from its attachment to the scapular spine. Incise dorsal fascial attachments and ligate or cauterize bleeding vessels as required.
5. Elevate the muscle gently; identifying, ligating and transecting several vascular branches extending to deep musculature. At this point the superficial cervical vascular system is readily visualized. In some dogs the vessels adopt a course immediately beneath the body of the trapezius muscle; in others, the vessels parallel the cranial border of the trapezius muscle. Dissection in the latter group must be performed cautiously to preserve the integrity of the vascular pedicle.

OPERATIVE TECHNIQUE 10.3 continued:
Raising a trapezius muscle flap

6. Continue dissection towards the vascular pedicle, incising between the trapezius and cleidocervicalis muscles. One or two small vascular branches to the omotransversarius muscle are identified, ligated and transected, completing elevation of the trapezius muscle.

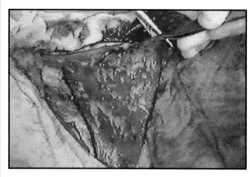

After identification of the vascular pedicle, cranial and ventral dissection of the trapezius muscle is completed.

7. Skeletonize the artery and vein for a length of at least 2–3 cm. The prescapular lymph node is intimately associated with the vascular pedicle and may be incorporated in the dissection, or cautiously dissected free of the vascular pedicle. Inclusion of the lymph node in the dissection will result in a bulky vascular pedicle and may cause difficulty in closing incisions overlying the vascular pedicle at the recipient site.

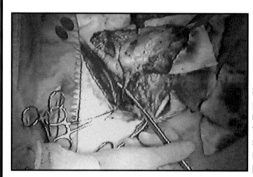

Skeletonized vascular pedicle. Perfusion is maintained with the flap protected in moist sponges until the recipient site is prepared.

See Operative Techniques 10.1 and 10.2 for anastomosis techniques.

OPERATIVE TECHNIQUE 10.4:
Raising a latissimus dorsi muscle flap

Positioning
Lateral recumbency.

Assistant
Essential.

Equipment extras
Operating microscope and instruments for microvascular surgery (see text).

Surgical technique (demonstrated using a cadaver)

1. Approach the muscle through a curvilinear incision beginning at the axilla and extending dorsally and caudally to the level of the muscle's origin (see Chapter 9).

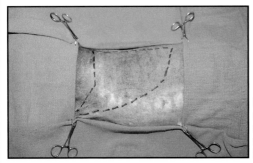

Landmarks for dissection. Ventral dotted line = proposed skin incision. The head is to the left.

2. Elevate the skin, subcutaneous tissue and cutaneous trunci muscle.

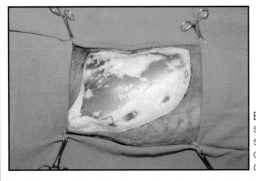

Elevation of the skin reveals the superficial aspect of the latissimus dorsi muscle.

3. Transect the latissimus dorsi muscle along its fascial origin caudally and dorsally.
4. Elevation of the muscle reveals several segmental vascular branches extending from the intercostal vessels. Electrocauterize or ligate and transect these vessels to allow continued dissection of the muscle toward its origin.

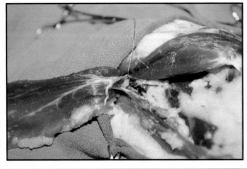

The muscle is dissected from its origin towards its insertion. Several segmental intercostal vessels must be ligated and transected near the muscle's origin. The thoracodorsal vascular pedicle is shown on the deep surface of the muscle near its insertion.

OPERATIVE TECHNIQUE 10.4 continued:
Raising a latissimus dorsi muscle flap

5. The dominant thoracodorsal artery and vein are easily seen as they course along the deep surface of the muscle.
6. After identification and protection of the vascular pedicle, transect the tendinous insertion of the latissimus dorsi muscle.

PRACTICAL TIP
The size of the thoracodorsal pedicle in the cat is <0.8 mm; therefore, dissection of the vascular pedicle to the level of the subscapular artery and vein is recommended in this species.

7. Skeletonize the vascular pedicle along its length in preparation for transfer.

See Operative Techniques 10.1 and 10.2 for anastomosis techniques.

OPERATIVE TECHNIQUE 10.5:
Harvesting a vascularized ulnar graft

Positioning
Lateral recumbency, with donor limb on padded surface.

Assistant
Essential.

Equipment extras
Operating microscope and instruments for microvascular surgery (see text).

Surgical technique (demonstrated using a cadaver)

Proximal ulnar graft

1. Incise the skin over the caudolateral aspect of the forelimb.

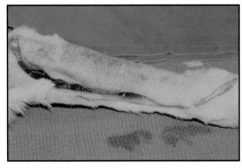

Arcuate skin incision over caudolateral aspect of forelimb.

2. Incise the lateral radial periosteum along the cranial surface of the abductor pollicis longus muscle, and continue subperiosteal dissection of the radius into the interosseous space.

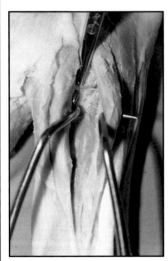

Fasciotomy of extensor and flexor muscle groups facilitates their evaluation. Vascular branches to the extensor muscles are identified laterally and mark the level of the medially located common interosseous vessels.

OPERATIVE TECHNIQUE 10.5 continued:
Harvesting a vascularized ulnar graft

3. Incise and elevate the medial radial periosteum in a similar manner.

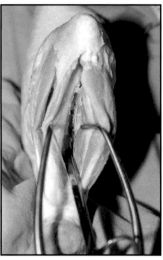

Medial dissection of the ulna is carried into the interosseous space, taking care to preserve a myoperiosteal soft tissue cuff surrounding the bone.

4. Determine the appropriate length of bone graft according to the requirements of the recipient site. The location of the proximal osteotomy is determined immediately proximal to the common interosseous pedicle; the location of the distal osteotomy is calculated based on measurement from that point.
5. Perform distal osteotomy first – locating, ligating and dividing the caudal interosseous vessels within the interosseous space.
6. Perform circumferential subperiosteal elevation of the ulna at the level of the proximal osteotomy prior to its being osteotomized.

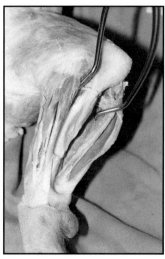

Osteotomy.

7. After completion of both osteotomies, continue subperiosteal elevation of the radius in the interosseous space. Sharp transection of the interosseous ligament is required.

OPERATIVE TECHNIQUE 10.5 continued:
Harvesting a vascularized ulnar graft

8. Identify the common interosseous artery and vein, and dissect them to their points of origin from the median artery and vein, respectively, after elevation of the ulna.

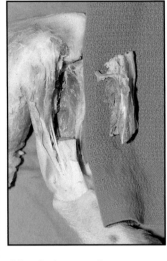

Dissection of the specimen has been completed. The short common interosseous vascular pedicle is shown.

Distal ulnar graft

1. Identify, ligate and transect the caudal interosseous vessels as they exit the interosseous space distally and caudally.
2. Perform circumferential dissection of the ulna and osteotomy immediately distal to this level.
3. Incise and elevate the medial and lateral radial periosteum as described for the proximal ulnar graft.
4. Perform proximal osteotomy of the ulna at a level that will yield 2–3 cm greater length than is required at the recipient site. Dissect the ulna carefully subperiosteally at this level to avoid trauma to the interosseous vessels, and perform proximal osteotomy.
5. Elevate the ulna carefully, ligating and transecting the caudal interosseous artery and vein.
6. Dissect the caudal interosseous artery and vein under the operating microscope for a length of 2–3 cm from the proximal osteotomy, and excise the 'extra' length of ulna to provide the length needed for reconstruction.

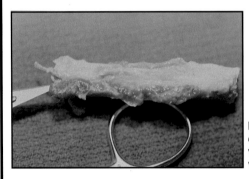

Distal ulnar graft. The caudal interosseous vessels form the vascular pedicle.

See Operative Techniques 10.1 and 10.2 for anastomosis techniques.

11

Special considerations in wound management

Jacqui D. Niles

Introduction

This chapter considers a number of specific types of wound that may require surgical management, such as pharyngeal stick injuries, chronic draining sinuses, bullet, burn and bite wounds. It also discusses the surgical management of some specific skin conditions such as skin fold pyoderma and perianal fistulas.

Chronic draining sinus tracts

- **Sinus tracts are fibrous tissue tracts lined by poor-quality oedematous granulation tissue. Bacterial (and fungal in some countries) infections are common and are usually associated with pain and inflammation together with a purulent, serous or serosanguineous discharge.**
- **A fistula differs from a sinus tract in that it connects the skin surface with the mucosal surface of a viscus and may be lined with epithelium.**

Causes of sinus tracts include bacterial infection, penetrating foreign bodies (e.g. plant awns, wood splinters, insect mouth parts), bone sequestra, surgical implants (e.g. sutures, meshes, orthopaedic implants) and neoplasia. Sinus tracts can occur at many locations on the body, depending on the cause, its point of entry/location and any migratory path. The interdigital spaces, ear canals, oral mucosa, conjunctiva and nares are common points of entry.

All sinus tracts should be thoroughly investigated and explored surgically to determine and eliminate (if possible) the cause. It is important to develop a systematic approach to the investigation of sinus tracts (Figure 11.1).

> **WARNING**
> **The clinical signs associated with sinus tracts (pain, swelling, discharge) may be ameliorated and can subside completely when treated with courses of antibiotics. However, the tract and clinical signs will recur after the medication is stopped.**

1. A thorough history – for example, working gundogs may be more prone to foreign body penetration from working in thick undergrowth.
2. Thorough clinical examination, looking for evidence of concurrent disease – especially if neoplasia is suspected.
3. Palpation and probing of the tract with the patient under general anaesthesia – may be useful in giving some idea as to the extent, but can be inaccurate as some tracts may appear to be blind-ended.
4. Plain/survey radiographs of the area – it may be necessary to radiograph some distance away from the exit site as some tracts can extend considerable distances. Plain radiographs may reveal radiodense foreign bodies, bone sequestra, areas of discospondylitis or surgical swabs (sponges) inadvertently left following some previous surgery. However, in many cases changes other than soft tissue swelling are not identified.
5. Sinography, using instillation of sterile iodine-based water-soluble radiopaque contrast material – can be useful in some cases, where it may allow delineation of a foreign body (filling defect in the tract) and allow the full extent of the tract to be shown. Contrast radiography can be frustrating in some cases as the contrast material does not always remain in the tract and may leak out, especially if injected under pressure. If the tract is wide enough a Foley catheter can be inserted and the bulb gently inflated (to prevent leakage); for narrow tracts a 16 or 18 gauge intravenous catheter can be used. It is helpful even when a Foley catheter is used to apply some digital pressure to the proximal tract to reduce backflow.
6. Magnetic resonance imaging and/or computed tomography – very useful for identifying the extent of sinus tracts and may identify foreign bodies that cannot be seen on radiography.
7. 'Woundoscopy' – the use of a suitable gauge flexible endoscope inserted into the opening of the sinus tract. Foreign bodies can be removed with forceps, or deep tissue biopsy can be performed. This is rarely as useful as thorough surgical exploration.
8. Surgical exploration –
   - Prior to surgery, clip and aseptically prepare a **large** area around the tract, especially if the extent of the tract is unknown. Explore and excise all tracts encountered. Depending on anatomical area it is often helpful to explore tracts from midline surgical incisions, particularly if sinus tracts are bilateral, rather than following the tracts from the discharging skin wound.
   - If foreign material is found, look for more!! There is nothing more frustrating than a patient being presented some weeks or months later due to recurrence of a problem that was thought to have been solved.
   - All previously implanted surgical materials should be removed and tissues should be thoroughly lavaged.
   - If no foreign material is found, dissect out the tract and close the wound. In some cases foreign material has been broken down but the sinus tract caused by it still remains. Submit the tract for bacteriological culture and sensitivity as well as for histopathology.
   - Owners should be warned that recurrence may happen, in which case further surgical exploration is usually recommended.

11.1 Clinical approach to the investigation of a chronic sinus tract.

If the cause is not eliminated, the problem will recur. Chronic sinus tracts can be extremely frustrating to manage for the patient, client and veterinary surgeon, as small fragments of foreign material can be elusive and repeated surgical intervention may be required.

Dermoid (pilonidal) sinus

A dermoid sinus is a neural tube defect that results from incomplete separation of the skin and neural tube during embryonic development. The lesion is congenital and heritable in some breeds, and is most commonly seen in Rhodesian Ridgebacks. It has also been reported in Shih Tzus, Boxers, English Bulldogs, Chow Chows, Siberian Huskies, Yorkshire Terriers and Springer Spaniels. In Ridgebacks the mode of inheritance is though to be simple recessive, and affected dogs should not be bred.

The sinus is a tubular skin indentation that extends as an epithelium-lined blind sac from the dorsal midline to varying depths in the underlying tissues. They have been classified by their depth of penetration (Figure 11.2):

- Class I: Sinus extends to the supraspinous ligament, where it is attached
- Class II: Sinus extends into muscular or subcutaneous tissue and is connected to the supraspinous ligament by a fibrous band
- Class III: Sinus extends into muscular or subcutaneous tissue but is not connected to the supraspinous ligament
- Class IV: Sinus extends to the spinal canal and is attached to the dura mater.

Investigation

Diagnosis is usually made based on the breed and age at presentation: usually young dogs with an opening found amidst a whorl of hair on the dorsal midline. Most sinus tracts are found in the cervical or cranial thoracic region but they have also been reported in the lumbosacral area. When a fold of skin is elevated in the area of the sinus, a tubular structure can be palpated as a thin cord coursing towards the spine. The sinus opening provides a portal of entry for bacteria; secondary infection is common and can lead to cellulitis and abscessation. If the sinus communicates with the dura (Class IV), meningitis or encephalitis may result, with subsequent neurological abnormalities.

The full extent of the tract can be defined by performing a sinogram using a non-ionic iodine-based water-soluble contrast medium, though it may not always follow a tract all the way to the dura if the tract narrows significantly or is blocked with sebaceous material. If there is communication with the spinal cord a cervical myelogram may also be valuable.

> **PRACTICAL TIP**
> CT and MRI are the most useful imaging techniques when neural involvement is suspected.

Treatment

Surgical excision of the tract is the treatment of choice but should only be performed once the depth of the sinus has been determined by advanced imaging, since a laminectomy may be required to access the dura. A dorsal midline approach is employed. In the majority of cases the tracts narrow at, or just dorsal to, the nuchal ligament. Occasionally it is necessary to split the nuchal ligament, ideally longitudinally, but transection may be unavoidable. If this is done, then on closure the ligament should be re-apposed using a modified Kessler locking loop suture pattern using a non-absorbable suture material (e.g. polypropylene). A proportion of tracts will stop immediately dorsal to a vertebral spinous process, the dorsal portion of which should be excised with the tract. If the tract does extend into the dura mater, a dorsal laminectomy is required and the part of the dura connecting with the sinus is excised with it. Samples of tract should be submitted for both bacteriological culture and histopathology.

Postoperatively, seroma formation is common at this site and drainage must be established, preferably with closed suction (see Chapter 5).

The prognosis is good for cases with no evidence of meningiomyelitis; if there are neurological signs the prognosis is more guarded.

Nasal dermoid sinus cyst

This is a congenital lesion found on the nasal midline and is thought to represent a similar embryological failure of neuroectodermal separation to a pilonidal sinus. These cysts have been reported in Golden

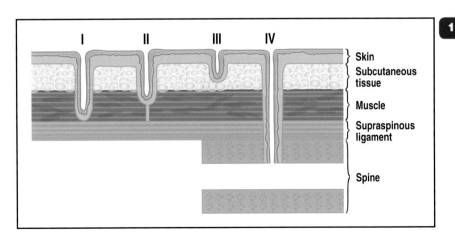

11.2 Classification of dermoid sinuses.

Skin
Subcutaneous tissue
Muscle
Supraspinous ligament
Spine

Retrievers, Spaniels and in an English Bull Terrier. Dogs are usually presented for management of sebaceous discharge immediately caudal to the nasal planum. The lesion should be dissected from the dorsal nasal midline, where it may end in the nasal septum. Communication with the meninges and consequent meningitis is recorded in human cases, and the potential for extension into the cranial vault should always be considered.

Oropharyngeal stick injuries

Penetrating injuries to the canine pharyngeal region are uncommon but are potentially very serious events. In dogs the pharynx is susceptible to wooden stick injury, particularly in those breeds that chase or carry sticks. Injuries are most commonly described in young, medium- to large-breed dogs, especially collies and German Shepherd Dogs. There has been one case reported in a young Bengal cat. Pharyngeal stick injuries can present acutely, within a short time of the injury occurring, but in the majority of cases they present chronically with a discharging sinus tract (see above).

Clinical signs

Acutely presenting patients will either have a known history of stick injury, or be presented within a few days of trauma with dysphagia and pharyngocervical pain due to temporomasseteric trauma or pharyngeal laceration and secondary cellulitis. Some dogs present in acute distress due to penetration of the stick into the oesophagus or thoracic cavity. The potential track taken by a stick entering the oropharynx has been well described; two common routes are shown (Figure 11.3). Sites of oropharyngeal penetration include:

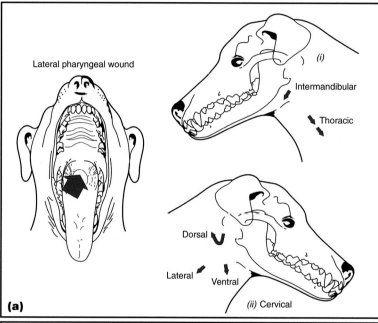

11.3

Potential paths of pharyngeal stick injuries: **(a)** from lateral wound; **(b)** from dorsal wound.

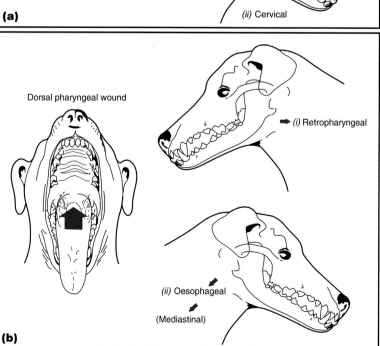

- Sublingual region (most common)
- Lateral pharyngeal wall
- Tonsillar region
- Rostral pharynx
- Dorsal pharynx.

Crepitation due to subcutaneous air accumulation may be noted within a few hours, occurring secondary to pharyngeal or oesophageal lacerations.

Investigation
Radiography is valuable, especially in acute cases. Radiographs of the thorax should be taken in addition to the oral/cervical region. The films should be reviewed carefully for any evidence of air in the fascial planes of the neck, soft tissue swelling, a radiopaque foreign body, pneumomediastinum or mediastinitis. Contrast radiography may be used to reveal tears (Figure 11.4).

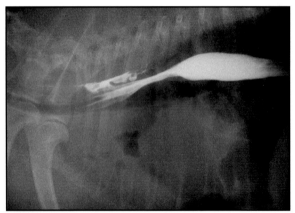

11.4 Positive contrast oesophogram showing leakage of contrast from an oesophageal tear. (© Alison L. Moores)

Treatment
Prompt and aggressive treatment of acute pharyngeal penetration injuries is necessary. A fresh pharyngeal or suspected pharyngeal laceration should be explored immediately, in order to minimize the development of chronic complications; this is especially important if oesophageal penetration has occurred. In the author's experience, oesophageal lacerations should be explored with 24 hours of trauma, otherwise wound dehiscence with subsequent death of the patient is common.

A penetrating foreign body can drive bacteria deep into the soft tissues, which may give rise to an abscess, even if the foreign material is removed. Culture of the deep tissues of the wound should be performed in all cases. Prior to obtaining results of culture and sensitivity testing, broad-spectrum intravenous antibiotics should be instituted, with the addition of metronidazole to combat anaerobic infection.

In some cases foreign material can be retrieved via an oral approach, although surgical exploration of the wound tract should still be performed to remove residual foreign material and bacteria. For all suspected dorsal or lateral pharyngeal penetration injuries, a ventral midline cervical approach should be used. This will allow the full extent of the injury to be established, the area to be fully explored for

fragments of foreign body and the lavage of affected tissues. Care should be taken to avoid damaging vital structures, such as the recurrent laryngeal nerve, during dissection.

Pharyngeal and oesophageal lacerations (Figure 11.5) should be debrided, sutured with 1.5 or 2 metric (4/0 or 3/0 USP) synthetic absorbable material (the oesophagus can be closed with one or two layers of simple interrupted or continuous sutures) and the oesophageal wound supported either by suturing the cranial portion of the sternothyroid muscle to the wound or with lengthened omentum (see later). If oesophageal damage is extensive, a gastrostomy tube should be placed (see below) for 7 days to allow healing to occur. Wound drains should be placed in the area of the dissection.

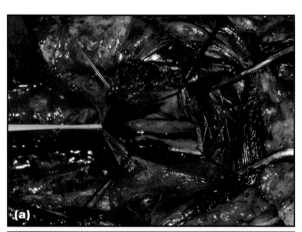

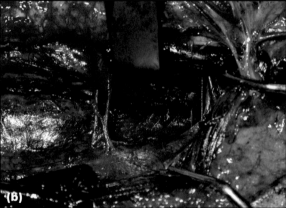

11.5 **(a)** Cervical oesophageal laceration due to a penetrating stick injury in a dog. The oesophageal stethoscope can be seen in the oesophageal lumen. **(b)** The laceration has been repaired with full thickness appositional sutures. (© Alison L. Moores)

Where the stick has penetrated the retrobulbar area, drainage is achieved via the oral cavity, using a haemostat to enlarge the wound or by penetrating the pharyngeal mucosa caudal to the last molar.

Perianal fistulation (anal furunculosis)

Canine perianal fistulation (PAF) or anal furunculosis is a poorly understood disease encountered commonly in German Shepherd Dogs and Border Collies, with sporadic occurrences being seen in other large and medium-sized breeds. It is characterized by chronic infection and ulceration of the perianal tissues (Figure 11.6) and can progress to 360-degree involvement of the perianal skin. There are often deeply infiltrating sinus tracts that in some cases can form true fistulae with the rectum. The underlying cause of this disease is unknown, but factors that have been proposed as perpetuating the problem include anal sacculitis, so the anal sacs should be removed if surgical treatment is pursued. The conformation of the German Shepherd Dog – allowing the broad base of the tail to remain in close contact with the anus, allowing accumulation of faecal material and moisture over the perineal region – is also thought to be a perpetuating factor.

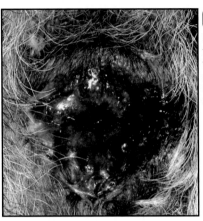

11.6
Perianal fistulas (anal furunculosis) in an 8-year-old German Shepherd Dog.

Clinical signs
The range of clinical signs seen with perianal fistulation varies immensely.

- Mild cases may show few signs apart from licking of the perianal region.
- In some advanced cases damage and scarring of the anal sphincter and rectum cause fibrous stricture formation, which prevents normal dilation of the anus. These dogs can show severe faecal tenesmus, dyschezia, weight loss and pain.
- Conversely, some dogs with severe anal furunculosis lose the ability to close the anal sphincter and become faecally incontinent.

Treatment
The treatment of perianal fistulas has consisted of both medical and surgical intervention, but it remains a frustrating disease to manage due to poor response to treatment, a high rate of recurrence and morbidity associated with surgical excision.

> **WARNING**
> **Whatever treatment modality is chosen for perianal fistulas, including surgery, owners need to be aware that the condition requires life-long vigilance and management, and that complete and permanent resolution is rare.**

Drug therapy
An immune-mediated aetiopathogenesis has been postulated and there is some evidence that there is an association with inflammatory bowel disease, as there is in human Crohn's disease patients who have concurrent perianal fistulas. This has prompted investigation into immunosuppressive therapy, e.g. with ciclosporin. Ciclosporin causes immuno-suppression by inhibition of T lymphocyte activation. In two studies resolution of perianal fistulas occurred in >85% of dogs treated with ciclosporin, lending support to PAF being an immune-mediated disease. Unfortunately, the widespread use of ciclosporin is limited by its high cost.

Two other medical treatment protocols deserve mention. One involves the use of a tapering dose of oral prednisolone (2 mg/kg q24h for 2 weeks; then 1 mg/kg q24h for 4–6 weeks; 1 mg/kg q48h until resolution). This is usually coupled with feeding a novel protein diet such as one based on fish and potato (Harkin *et al.,* 1996). The author has had some success with this protocol but some dogs need to stay on higher doses of prednisolone for longer than the original study describes and this increases the risk of iatrogenic Cushing's disease.

The second protocol uses tacrolimus, a relatively new immunosuppressive drug, which is applied topically to the perianal region. Tacrolimus is 10 to 100 times more potent than ciclosporin, but with fewer side effects. It is in the form of a 0.1% ointment that is applied to the perianal region once or twice daily until resolution occurs (Misseghers *et al.,* 2000). The author has also had success with this treatment.

The recent advances in medical management all hold promise and such medical management has much to commend it, but issues still surround long-term efficacy and morbidity as well as affordability. Despite the promising results achieved with ciclosporin and other immunosuppressive drugs, no single technique has been shown to result consist-ently in a cure.

Surgery
The role of surgery is controversial, given the suggested underlying immune-mediated process, but the author has found that in those dogs that do not respond well to medical therapy, or those that respond initially but whose lesions do not completely resolve, surgery can significantly improve quality of life.

> **PRACTICAL TIP**
> **Perform a rectal examination under anaesthesia prior to surgery to evaluate the anal sphincter for fibrosis and stricture.**

Open excision of the anal sacs should be performed (see Operative Technique 11.1), combined with sharp dissection of the sinus tracts, and all abnormal tissue, followed by primary wound closure. Resins and other materials to pack the anal sac are to be avoided, as they may leak into surrounding tissues producing a chronic focus for infection.

Bite wounds

Bite wounds occur frequently in dogs and cats and can be amongst the most serious injuries seen in small animal practice. The canine teeth of dogs and cats penetrate tissues deeply, whilst the molars and premolars are designed for shearing. The jaws of larger dogs can generate tremendous crushing forces, from 150–450 psi, resulting in severe crushing, avulsion and devitalization of tissues beneath the skin. Bites can also crush the airway or penetrate the abdominal or thoracic cavities, resulting in life-threatening injuries. Small dogs and cats are particularly at risk because most portions of their body can be grasped by a large dog. Many of these victims of a 'big dog–little dog' interaction are lifted and shaken violently, causing both direct and indirect trauma to internal organs (Figure 11.7). Thus, it is extremely important to assess the patient as a whole, because trauma to the upper airway, oesophagus or thorax must be dealt with promptly. The kidneys in small animals are particularly at risk from bites over the back.

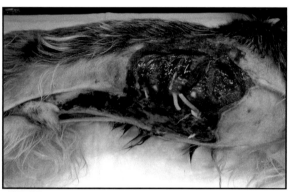

11.7 A 2-year-old Yorkshire Terrier with a chronic body wall wound secondary to bites sustained during an attack by a Rottweiler. Note the fractured ribs.

Stabilization and initial assessment

Prior to wound assessment it is necessary to stabilize the patient. Blood loss, shock, respiratory distress (resulting from laryngeal, tracheal and chest wall injuries, pneumothorax, haemothorax and pneumomediastinum) are conditions that require emergency intervention before the rest of the examination is completed.

Dogs and cats with suspected bite wounds should be clipped over the area of trauma to determine the full extent of contusions and to find small puncture wounds, which can be readily masked by hair (Figure 11.8). Orthogonal view radiographs may help assess

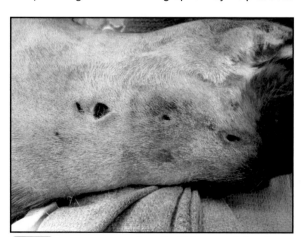

11.8 The area around cervical bite wounds has been clipped to allow thorough assessment.

the extent of the damage. Further assessment and management considerations will be determined by the anatomical location of bite wounds (Figure 11.9).

Bite wound site	Considerations
Head	Cranial nerve and CNS evaluation should be performed
Neck	Consider injury to the larynx (Figure 11.10), pharynx, cervical trachea, major vessels and oesophagus
Thorax	Evaluate for pneumothorax, lung contusions or lacerations, haemothorax or thoracic tracheal trauma. Thoracotomy with positive pressure ventilation may be required
Abdomen	If trauma to the kidneys or ureters is suspected, an intravenous excretory urogram should be obtained. Radiography and diagnostic peritoneal lavage may not always help identify significant intra-abdominal trauma, especially in acute cases. Coeliotomy should be performed to define the extent of visceral organ damage and body wall hernias, and to allow repair
Perineal	Evaluate for concurrent injury to the rectum and lower urinary tract
Limbs	Assess viability of limb: consider presence of bleeding from a cut toenail, peripheral pulse oximetry or Doppler ultrasonography to assess blood flow. Following stabilization, carry out a full orthopaedic and neurological examination

11.9 Considerations arising from anatomical locations of bite wounds.

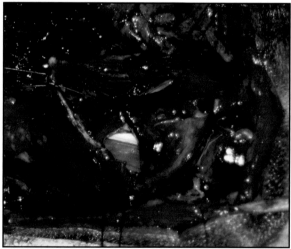

11.10 Bite wounds to the neck of a young Dachshund resulted in severe laryngeal trauma. Following a ventral surgical approach, the endotracheal tube can be seen through a ventral defect in the larynx.

WARNINGS
- **All suspected bite wounds should be carefully examined. Trivial puncture marks seen at the initial presentation are usually just the 'tip of the iceberg' with respect to damage to the underlying structures. In some cases skin puncture wounds do not**

> occur despite extensive damage to deeper structures. Failure to explore bite wounds can lead to marked tissue necrosis, infection and even death.
> • All bite wounds are contaminated and must be managed as such. As teeth penetrate, the wound is inoculated with bacteria. The mouths of both dogs and cats are heavily contaminated with aerobic, anaerobic, Gram-positive and Gram-negative bacteria. In cats and dogs *Pasteurella multocida* and *P. canis* are the most common pathogens cultured from the oral cavity.

Bite wound exploration and management

All bite wounds should be explored further under anaesthesia and debrided.

1. Administer intravenous antibiotics (e.g. cephalosporins) that rapidly achieve effective plasma levels.
2. Temporarily cover open wounds with sterile saline-soaked gauze swabs (sponges).
3. Clip a wide area around the bite wound. Consider the possibility of an exploratory thoracotomy or laparotomy (Figure 11.11) and clip accordingly. Prepare and drape aseptically.

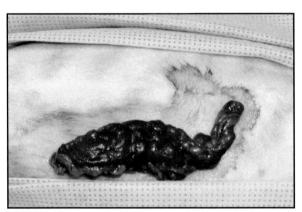

11.11 A 12-week-old kitten attacked by a Jack Russell Terrier has omentum protruding from an abdominal bite wound and has been clipped, prepared and draped for exploratory laparotomy.

4. Puncture wounds should be excised and then a sterile haemostat inserted into the wound and spread, to help identify underlying tissue damage. Skin incisions may need to be extended widely if there is extensive damage.
5. Take deep tissue cultures and submit them for aerobic and anaerobic bacteriological culture and sensitivity testing.
6. Remove hair or foreign material from the wound.
7. Wounds with little or no damage may be lavaged and either left open to heal by second intention or closed with one or two sutures.
8. In cases with more significant tissue damage, excise macerated or necrotic tissue.
9. Debridement and closure should ideally occur in one stage when the thoracic or abdominal

cavities are involved. In less critical areas, such as the limbs, a more conservative approach can be adopted, using principles of open wound management and staged debridement, followed by delayed primary closure, secondary closure or healing by second intention (see Chapter 4).
10. Wound drainage is required, especially after aggressive debridement of contaminated bite wounds. Closed suction drains or Penrose drains should be used (see Chapter 5).

> **WARNING**
> **Assessment of skin viability may be difficult to determine on initial presentation as tissue necrosis may take 5–7 days to become evident.**

Burns management

Burn injuries in small animals can result from heat, sun, flames, scalding liquids, friction, chemicals, electricity and the effects of radiation. The causes and classification of burn wounds are discussed in depth in Chapter 2.

- **It is essential to deal immediately with any life-threatening problem the patient may have, including airway damage from smoke inhalation or direct thermal injury.**
- The airway should be checked and maintained and any evidence of burn shock should be treated by fluid administration.
- It is important to provide pain relief; opioids should be the first choice. The use of corticosteroids and non-steroidal anti-inflammatories is controversial.
- In cases of ingestion, emesis is contraindicated since oesophageal contact will be worsened and gastric perforation is a significant risk. Neutralizing the corrosive solutions may lead to an exothermic reaction strong enough to cause significant thermal damage. Inactivated charcoal is of no benefit, so the best option for treatment involves dilution and supportive treatment.

Airway injury

Any animal suffering severe oropharyngeal oedema will require emergency intubation or, more likely, emergency tracheostomy tube placement.

In some cases tracheal mucosal sloughing is so severe that the debris may physically obstruct the lower airways. This may also be associated with the development of pulmonary oedema (Figure 11.12), usually within 72 hours of the inhalational injury; its occurrence is associated with a high mortality rate. Currently the best option for management of smoke inhalation is bronchodilators in conjunction with humidified oxygen delivered by positive pressure ventilation.

Carbon monoxide poisoning requires therapy with 100% oxygen supplied by mask or via a tracheostomy tube to reduce the level of carboxyhaemoglobin.

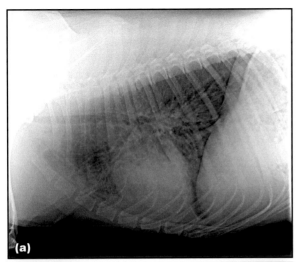

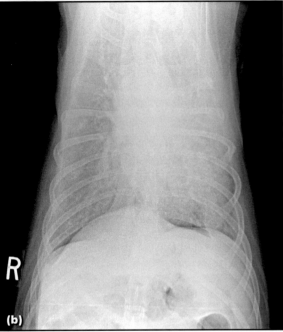

11.12 Lateral and VD radiographs of a young male Labrador rescued from a house fire. Smoke inhalation had caused severe pulmonary oedema.

Fluid therapy

Following severe burns varying degrees of capillary damage will lead to increased capillary permeability at the burn site and throughout the body, resulting in loss of plasma, electrolytes and plasma proteins into the extravascular space. This extracellular fluid (oedema) forms in direct proportion to the severity of the burn. The leakage is maximal during the first 8 hours after burning and gradually decreases over 48–72 hours until the animal creates enough fluid to compensate. For burns affecting up to 20–30% of total body surface area (TBSA) the leakage tends to be local to the wound site, whereas if >30% of TBSA is affected the increase in capillary permeability tends to be generalized. Even with a 20% TBSA burn, 28% of the plasma volume of a dog can be lost within 6 hours. When >40% of TBSA is affected, an animal may lose up to 50% of its plasma volume within 2–3 hours. As it is not possible to stem the leakage of fluid it is essential to maintain the patient's circulating

volume; otherwise hypovolaemic shock, with the potential for renal failure, will occur.

- Lactated Ringer's (Hartmann's) solution should be used during the first 24 hours
- An initial shock dose of 90 ml/kg may be indicated during the initial presentation
- To maintain normal renal function, fluid administration rates are adjusted to maintain a urine output of 1 ml/kg/h. The rate of fluid administration can be calculated based on a number of different formulae.

Anaemia

Anaemia is a common consequence of burns and occurs due to a number of mechanisms:

- Thermal destruction of red blood cells, followed by physiological lysis some hours later. Some red cells will, in addition, be so morphologically damaged that they will be filtered out by the spleen
- Erythrocyte membrane damage due to various catecholamines, prostaglandins and altered plasma lipids reduces the lifespan of the cells
- Reduced erythropoietin levels, which depresses erythropoiesis and results in a normocytic normochromic anaemia.

Whole blood or packed red cells should be given to maintain a haematocrit above 25% and supplemental oxygen therapy is recommended in seriously burned patients.

Management of skin burns

Animals with burns are often not presented to the veterinary surgeon immediately after injury because the owner may not know a burn occurred or may fail to recognize the extent of the injury. The severity and extent of the burn must be identified in order to develop a proper medical and surgical plan. However, this can be difficult in the initial phase of injury and when in doubt a 'wait and reassess' approach is usually indicated.

The goals of burn patient management are to:

- Prevent further thermal injury – remove the heat source as quickly as possible and rapidly cool tissue with cold water or ice
- Minimize contamination and infection – large wounds should be covered during transportation; 'clingfilm' is a suitable covering that will help protect the wound
- Provide adequate analgesia – applying a dressing to the affected area will produce some local analgesic effect
- Remove dead tissue
- Reconstruct the wound.

> **PRACTICAL TIP**
> **Debridement using wet-to-dry dressings and aggressive surgical debridement are essential to remove necrotic tissue, to control sepsis and to promote formation of a viable vascular bed suitable for surgical closure.**

Though topical dressings are beneficial in burn wound management, it is current practice to undertake surgical debridement of large or deep wounds at an early stage, and to graft or reconstruct the wound as soon as possible. Large areas of full-thickness skin necrosis (Figure 11.13a) impede granulation bed formation and dramatically increase the risk of infection. With conservative treatment, several days to several weeks may pass before spontaneous separation of the necrotic tissue occurs. Surgical excision has the potential to eliminate all necrotic tissue in a single stage; once debrided, the wounds should be managed by the use of dressings. Dressings should maintain a moist wound environment and be non-adherent (see Chapter 4), allowing a healthy granulation bed to form over 5–7 days, suitable for closure (Figure 11.13b) or application of an axial pattern flap (see Chapter 7) or skin graft (see Chapter 8). Systemic antibiotics should not be used unless infection is present and should be selected based on results of microbial culture and sensitivity tests.

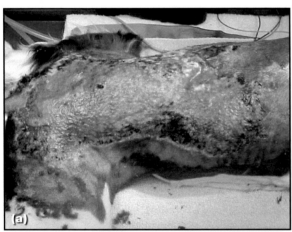

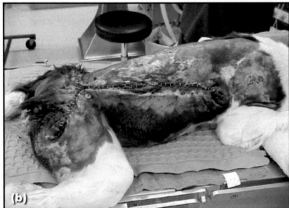

11.13 Extensive burn wounds on a Springer Spaniel. **(a)** The burn covers much of the dog's back. **(b)** Following aggressive debridement and wound closure. (Courtesy of Dr Brad Coolman)

Superficial and partial-thickness burns are not routinely excised; topical management is used to control infection, debridement and epithelialization. A variety of topical agents are available, which can be applied to the burn directly or beneath a bandage. The most useful is a 1% silver sulfadiazine cream that has a broad spectrum of activity against Gram-positive and Gram-negative bacteria and also against *Candida*.

Complications

The two most common complications are excessive scarring (Figure 11.14) and wound contracture. If major cutaneous losses occur areas subject to constant motion are the most susceptible to the development of wound contracture. Owners should be warned of these potential complications, some of which may require additional surgery such as Z-plasty, pedicle grafts and scar excision followed by free skin grafting (see Chapters 6, 8 and 12).

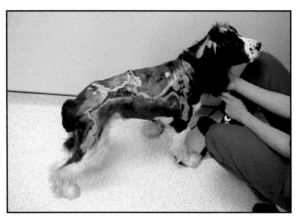

11.14 The dog in Figure 11.13 photographed 12 weeks after initial presentation. Note the extensive hairless scar tissue. There are still some areas of the wound where granulation tissue has not yet epithelialized. (Courtesy of Dr Brad Coolman)

Nutritional support

If a burns patient is unable to eat, particularly if it is suffering from oropharyngeal oedema, non-oral enteral feeding techniques (oesophageal or gastrostomy tube) should be considered. Total parenteral nutrition should be considered only if there is intestinal dysfunction, due to the risk of introducing infection in an already immunocompromised patient. The diet should provide at least 4 g of protein per 100 kcal in dogs and at least 6 g per 100 kcal in cats. The injured patient should be fed at least 1.5 times its resting energy requirement (RER). The RER can be calculated using appropriate formulae:

- Patient 2– 45 kg: RER (kcal) = 30 x bodyweight (kg) + 70
- Patient <2 kg or >45 kg: RER = 70 x bodyweight (kg) $^{0.75}$

Projectile injuries

The causes and classification of firearm injuries are discussed in Chapter 2.

All ballistic wounds are grossly contaminated, with potential for large amounts of devitalized tissue, therefore all wounds should be explored and debrided (Figure 11.15). The entry and exit wounds should be located, explored, debrided and lavaged. In general, entrance wounds are smaller than exit wounds due to deformation of the bullet through the tissues; small entrance wounds can be easily missed beneath the fur of dogs and cats. Once the wounds have been

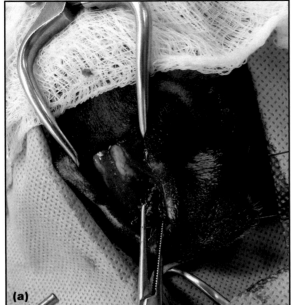

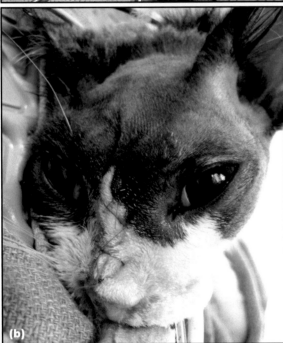

11.15 (a) Bullet fragments being removed from the frontal sinus of a cat. (b) Closure of the wound following removal of the bullet fragments.

located the fur should be clipped away. Bullets that are relatively superficial should be removed, although those that are inaccessible are probably best left unless they involve a vital structure. The affected area(s) should be radiographed and a baseline complete blood count and biochemistry profile should be performed in the seriously injured patient.

The majority of low- and high-velocity gunshot wounds (see Chapter 2) will also require open wound management before attempting closure, due to the high level of contamination. This is especially true of high-velocity injuries.

Thoracic ballistic injuries, as in humans, can, following debridement of the superficial wounds, be left unexplored unless there is evidence of

haemothorax or pneumothorax. In these cases a thoracostomy tube may need to be placed; exploratory thoracotomy may be required if there is continuous accumulation of air or blood within the thorax.

Limb injures that involve shattered bone are best addressed by open wound management and application of an external fixator, although the choice of stabilization may vary depending upon the individual fracture. In cases with extreme trauma to a limb, amputation may be considered. Penetration of joints requires an arthrotomy to remove metallic debris and fragments of bone and cartilage.

Gunshot wounds to the neck are frequently associated with lacerations of the trachea or oesophagus, which will require prompt repair following debridement. Around 90% of abdominal gunshot wounds will have associated visceral injury and will require extensive surgical exploration. Confirmation of the need to perform laparotomy can be obtained by abdominal imaging, abdominocentesis and diagnostic peritoneal lavage.

If there is any evidence of haemorrhage, peritonitis, food or air within the abdominal cavity, surgical exploration should be performed as soon as the patient is stable. If findings are equivocal, radiography and diagnostic peritoneal lavage can be repeated several hours later.

WARNING
The risks of peritonitis secondary to visceral trauma are extremely high and a laparotomy is always indicated for penetrating abdominal wounds.

Exploratory laparotomy should be thorough and well planned, with the patient clipped and prepared for extension of the incision into the thorax if necessary. Any major haemorrhage should be dealt with and then a systematic exploration carried out for evidence of lacerations, starting with the diaphragm and liver and then examining the gastrointestinal tract in its whole length, running from stomach aborally to the descending colon. It is also important to assess the pancreas, spleen, kidneys, ureters and bladder. Small single lacerations of the viscera should be debrided and closed. Large defects may require partial excision of tissue, such as partial hepatic lobectomy, splenectomy, nephrectomy or enterectomy. If there are multiple lacerations of the intestinal tract it may not be possible to resect all affected areas and multiple serosal patching should be performed. If there has been extensive contamination of the peritoneal cavity, open abdominal drainage should be considered (see *BSAVA Manual of Canine and Feline Abdominal Surgery*).

Redundant skin folds and skin fold pyoderma (intertrigo)

Redundant skin folds are a characteristic of some breeds and can occur in many sites. The most commonly encountered include the labial, facial, vulvar, tail, head and leg folds. Friction arises from the skin-to-skin contact at these sites and an altered skin microenvironment. Ventilation of, and evaporation from, the skin surface are reduced; secretions (sebaceous, saliva, faeces, urine, vaginal) accumulate and result in bacterial and fungal overgrowth. This leads to inflammation, pain and a foul-smelling exudate forming in the depths of the fold. The most frequently involved organisms include species of *Staphylococcus*, *Streptococcus*, *Pseudomonas*, *Proteus*, *Candida* and *Escherichia coli*. In mild cases patients may respond to medical therapy, including cleansing of the affected area with topical antiseptic solutions, antibiotic therapy and weight loss in those patients in which the skin folds are a result of obesity.

> **PRACTICAL TIP**
> **Skin fold resection is the most effective treatment for skin fold dermatitis.**

Lip fold pyoderma

Dog breeds with large heavy lips, such as Saint Bernards, Newfoundlands, Spaniels, Retrievers and Irish Setters, most commonly develop lip fold pyoderma. As food and saliva accumulate in the redundant lip folds, dogs rub and paw at their faces, leading to inflammation of the skin and associated pruritus and halitosis.

A cheiloplasty should be performed on affected animals by making an elliptical incision around the infected skin, excising it and apposing the healthy skin edges with non-absorbable suture material (Figure 11.16). In dogs that drool excessively, an antidrool cheiloplasty has been described to reduce the loss of food and saliva from the lateral vestibules of the oral cavity (see *BSAVA Manual of Canine and Feline Head and Neck Surgery*).

Nasal fold pyoderma

The prominent nasal folds that occur across the bridge of the nose in brachycephalic dogs and Persian cats can lead to chronic pyoderma and a foul odour. In some cases, hairs on the skin fold can rub on the cornea and cause keratitis, ulceration and pain.

1. Make an elliptical incision around the base of the skin fold. The caudal extent of the incision should be 1 cm away from the medial canthus of the eyes.
2. Undermine and remove the skin fold, taking care not to damage the facial vessels during dissection. Care must also be taken not to excise too much skin, since this can cause ectropion.
3. Prior to closure, lavage the area copiously with sterile saline.
4. Appose the subcutaneous tissue and suture using 1.5 metric (4/0 USP) absorbable suture material with buried knots.
5. Close the skin with simple interrupted sutures of non-absorbable suture material. Cut the ends short and place them so as to avoid corneal irritation.

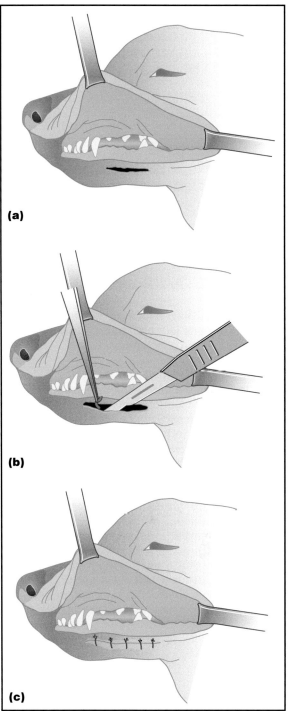

(a)

(b)

(c)

11.16 Cheiloplasty. **(a)** The upper lip is retracted to expose the lower lip. Placing a gag between the canine teeth can be useful to aid exposure. **(b)** A scalpel is used to make an elliptical incision and the infected material is excised. **(c)** Healthy skin edges are apposed and sutured using a simple interrupted pattern.

Vulvar fold pyoderma

Vulval folds occur in obese females and in animals with juvenile recessed vulvas. Vaginal secretions and urine become trapped by the skin fold, resulting in moist dermatitis and in some cases chronic or recurrent urinary tract infections (Figure 11.17).

The skin fold should be surgically excised via an episioplasty. In one study of 31 bitches presenting with either perivulvar dermatitis or chronic/recurrent

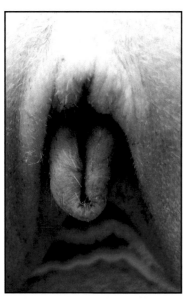

11.17
Prominent dorsal
skin fold over the
vulva in a bitch with
a history of recurrent
urinary tract
infections.

urinary tract infections, there was complete resolution
of all clinical signs for both groups following episioplasty (see Operative Technique 11.2).

Screw tail pyoderma

Screw tail pyoderma, also termed ingrown tail or tail
fold pyoderma, occurs predominantly in the English
Bulldog due to the spiral and ventral deviation of the
caudal coccygeal vertebrae. This causes the stubby
tail to bury itself in the skin folds of the dorsal perineal
skin. Other brachycephalic breeds are less frequently
affected and the condition has also been reported in
Manx cats. The depth of the skin folds varies,
depending on the animal's size and weight and on
the degree of vertebral deviation.

Moist dermatitis develops in the folds and
becomes exacerbated by faecal contamination,
licking and scooting. Signs include perineal pruritus,
pain, odour, ulceration and sinus tracts. Cleansing
the area and antibiotic therapy may palliate the
disease but the condition is likely to recur. Resolution
of the problem can be achieved by resection of the
skin folds and tail in most cases (see Operative
Technique 11.3).

Footpad surgery

The footpads are specialized structures designed to
absorb shock and withstand the rigours of weight
bearing and the shear stresses created by ambula-
tion. The stratum corneum is highly specialized and is
usually pigmented, thick and keratinized. It overlies
a fibrovascular pad cushion that anchors the dermis
to the underlying bone. Footpad injuries include laceration, degloving, burns and tumours.

> **WARNING**
> **Footpad injuries may not heal well as a result
> of the weightbearing forces placed upon the
> region and loss of pad tissue. Weightbearing
> areas without pads are likely to ulcerate.**

Simple lacerations

Lacerations of the footpads, if not managed
appropriately, can turn into chronic non-healing
wounds due to the forces applied across the pads
when walking. The depth of the laceration should be
assessed (full *versus* partial thickness) and the wound
lavaged, sutured and bandaged to provide support.
The deepest layers of the pad should be sutured with
buried simple interrupted sutures of a monofilament
absorbable material such as polydioxanone. The
epithelial surface is then closed taking large bites,
several millimetres from the cut edges. The foot
should be kept bandaged until the pad has healed
completely and the sutures have been removed. If
pad lacerations are left unsutured granulation tissue
tends to fill in the wound and protrude from the wound
edges, resulting in some loss of pad function.

More severe wounds

In some cases more advanced surgical techniques
are required to reconstruct severe footpad wounds.

Fusion podoplasty (see Operative Technique
11.4) is a technique involving removal of the interdigital and interpad tissue and fusion of the phalanges,
by suturing the remaining strips of skin on the dorsum of the paw and suturing the pads together on the
ventral aspect. It is a salvage procedure and is used
to treat chronic interdigital pyoderma or severed
flexor tendons.

Phalangeal fillet (digital pad transfer) (see
Operative Technique 11.5) involves removal of the
proximal, middle and distal phalanges from a digit, so
that the free pad and associated skin can be used to
replace or fill a defect in the metacarpal or metatarsal
pad. Usually the metacarpal/metatarsal pad is
reconstructed using the skin and pad from either the
second or fifth digit. The technique can also be used
as a salvage procedure when patients have sustained
considerable digital trauma to the bony structures of a
digit, with skin deficits of adjacent digits.

Footpad grafts (see Operative Technique 11.6)
are useful for resurfacing an extensive area of paw
pad loss. They are small, full-thickness segments of
pad tissue that are placed in a granulation tissue bed
around the edges of a wound when the weightbearing
pad tissue is missing.

A dispensible footpad with an area of surrounding
skin can be dissected, based on its neurovascular
pedicle, and transferred to a central weightbearing
location, where it is revascularized by microvascular
anastomosis to a recipient artery and vein. Further
details on microvascular footpad transfer are given in
Chapter 10.

Mammary gland surgery

Mammary neoplasia is the commonest reason for
performing mammary gland surgery, although
infrequently severe trauma, bite wounds or chronic/
recurrent mastitis may warrant removal of one or
more mammary glands. The dog has five pairs of
mammary glands, all of which can develop one or
more benign or malignant tumours; 41–53% of

mammary tumours in dogs prove to be malignant. The cat has four pairs of mammary glands; whilst the overall incidence of mammary tumours in cats is lower than in dogs, >80% are malignant.

Surgery is the treatment of choice for all dogs with mammary tumours, with the exception of those with inflammatory carcinoma or distant metastasis. The type of surgery (Figure 11.18) depends upon the extent of the disease, but there is little evidence that one type of surgical procedure results in a better prognosis than any other; thus, the primary goal of surgery in canine mammary tumour removal is to remove all the tumour by the simplest procedure.

Technique	Indications
Lumpectomy/ Nodulectomy (local excision)	Small (<0.5 cm) nodules that are firm, superficial and non-adherent
Mammectomy (removal of one gland)	For lesions located centrally in a gland, >1cm, ± fixation to the skin or fascia
Regional mastectomy (removal of tumour plus glands associated with vascular and lymphatic drainage)	Tumours involving glands 1, 2 or 3 are removed en bloc. Tumours involving glands 4 and 5 are removed en bloc plus inguinal lymph node
Uni- or bilateral mastectomy	Glands 1–5 are removed as a unit if multiple tumours or several large tumours preclude rapid and wide removal by a lesser procedure
Lymph node removal	Axillary lymph nodes: do not remove prophylactically; only remove if fixed, adherent and large. Inguinal lymph node: remove whenever gland 5 is removed, since they are intimately associated

11.18 Surgical techniques for resection of canine mammary tumours.

Surgery is also indicated in cats, where wider surgical margins are associated with improved survival; hence, unilateral (see Operative Technique 11.7) or bilateral mastectomy is recommended. For a complete discussion on canine and feline mammary neoplasia the reader is referred to the *BSAVA Manual of Canine and Feline Oncology*.

Wound bed vascular augmentation using omentum

The first account of omental anatomy was by Hippocrates, followed by Aristotle (384–322BC) describing it as 'a fatty material present in all warm-blooded animals'. In 1906 the British surgeon Rutherford Morrison recognized that the greater omentum had an extraordinary capacity for the formation of new blood vessels and first used the term 'policeman of the abdomen'.

The canine and feline omentum is extremely well developed and is folded on itself to form a flattened sac, with superficial and deep leaves that intervene between the intestinal mass and the abdominal floor.

The omental bursa exists as a potential space between the two leaves of the omentum. In dogs and cats the major arterial supply to the greater omentum is via the epiploic branches of the right and left gastroepiploic arteries. In addition to the anastomosis between epiploic vessels, there is a rich collateral circulation provided by small vessels and capillaries. The venous drainage mimics that of the arterial vessels.

The omentum has been used extensively in the management of a variety of intra-abdominal problems. It also provides a flap of tissue that can be readily transposed outside of the abdomen, and wider applications for the omentum have now been found in virtually every subspecialty of human surgery. In veterinary surgery, omentum can be used to: aid reconstruction of wounds; provide drainage of lymphoedema; seal abdominal (and thoracic) viscera; and aid in the management of prostatic abscesses and retention cysts. Reports also exist describing its use to treat the subcutaneous accumulation of chyle following thoracic duct ligation in a dog and for the drainage of chylothorax.

Omental transposition in the pelvis

Pelvic fistula repair
Since the first description of repair of a vesicovaginal fistula in 1935 by the Mayo Clinic, omental transposition has gained in popularity for repair of pelvic fistulae involving the bladder, urethra, vagina and rectum. In oncological surgery these fistulae commonly follow radical radiotherapy, with or without previous surgery; they are often large or multiple, and the surrounding tissues are usually scarred and rigid. Using a combined abdominoperineal approach, a tunnel is created to interpose the apex of the omentum between the involved structures.

Extra-abdominal omental transposition
For extra-abdominal use an omental pedicle can be created, which allows it to reach potentially even to the extremities of the patient. The pedicle is created by detaching the dorsal omental leaf from the pancreas and the spleen, thus doubling the length of available omentum, allowing it to be used from the axilla to the proximal pelvic limbs. Occasionally it may be useful to create a pedicle that reaches the distal thoracic or pelvic limbs or the head of an animal. In such cases omentum is incised in an inverted 'L' shape, starting immediately caudal to the gastrosplenic ligament. In most cases it is sufficient to extend only the dorsal portion.

> **WARNING**
> In some cases the omentum may be congenitally absent or rudimentary, or it may have been previously surgically removed or used already.

The omentum can be used in managing chronic non-healing wounds in two ways: one relies on primary wound closure over the site; and the other uses the omentum as a vascular bed for a free skin graft.

Chronic wounds in cats are common in clinical practice, occuring over pressure points or in high motion areas such as the axilla and thigh (Figure 11.19a). The most common cause is from the thoracic limb becoming entrapped through the collar resulting in ischaemic necrosis of the skin, subcutaneous tissue and muscle in the axillary area.

- The wound is debrided or excised.
- A vascularized omental pedicle is created via a midline or paracostal laparotomy incision.
- The omentum is tunnelled subcutaneously from the abdomen to the wound (Figure 11.19b). Care is taken when handling the omentum to avoid tearing it, and its vascular pedicle must not be

rotated since this could compromise its blood supply and lymphatics.
- The laparotomy incision is closed and the exit hole should be left large enough so as to cause no vascular damage while ensuring visceral herniation does not occur. Alternatively the omentum is exited via a lateral abdominal incision and the midline incision is closed completely.
- The omentum is sutured into the wound site. Skin is then mobilized, e.g. a rotational flap, and closed over the omentum (Figure 11.19c,d).

The use of combined omental pedicle grafts and thoracodorsal axial pattern flaps for the reconstruction of chronic axillary wounds has also been described.

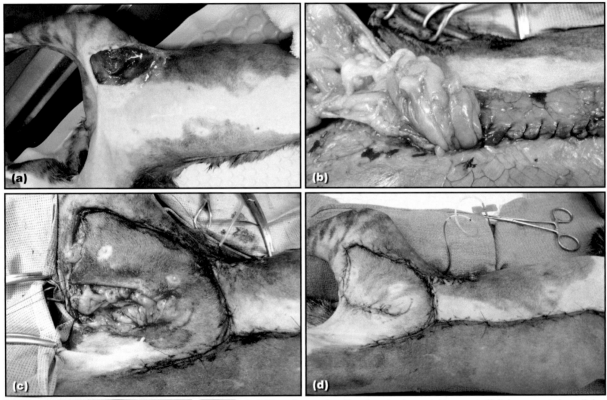

11.19 **(a)** Chronic non-healing inguinal wound in a cat. **(b)** An omental pedicle has been exteriorized from the abdomen and used to augment the wound bed. **(c)** A caudal superficial epigastric axial pattern flap (see Chapter 7) has been rotated to cover the omentalized wound. **(d)** Flap sutured in place. **(e)** Healed wound 2 weeks after surgery and just prior to suture removal.

References and further reading

Basher AW, Fowler JD, Bowen CV *et al.* (1990) Microneurovascular free digital pad transfer in the dog. *Veterinary Surgery* **29**, 226–231

Bray JP, White RA and Williams JM (1997) Reconstruction and omentalization: a new technique for the management of prostatic retention cysts in dogs. *Veterinary Surgery* **26**, 202–209

Bright SR, Mellanby RJ and Williams JM (2002) Oropharyngeal stick injury in a Bengal cat. *Journal of Feline Medicine and Surgery* **4**, 153–155

Brockman DJ, Pardo AD, Conzemius MG *et al.* (1996) Omentum-enhanced reconstruction of chronic non-healing wounds in cats: techniques and clinical use. *Veterinary Surgery* **25**, 99–104

Griffiths LG, Tiruneh R, Sullivan M, Reid SWJ (2000) Oropharyngeal penetrating injuries in 50 Dogs: a retrospective study. *Veterinary Surgery* **29**, 383–388

Harkin KR, Walshaw R and Mullaney TP (1996) Association of perianal fistulation and colitis in the German Shepherd dog: response to high dose prednisone and dietary therapy. *Journal of the American Animal Hospital Association* **32**, 515–520

Kehoe A and Elmore M (1999) Woundoscopy: a new technique for examining deep non-healing wounds. *Ostomy Wound Management* **45**, 23–40

Lascelles BD, Davison L, Dunning M *et al.* (1998) Use of omental pedicle grafts in the management of non-healing axillary wounds in 10 cats. *Journal of Small Animal Practice* **39**, 475–480

Lascelles BD and White RA (2001) Combined omental pedicle grafts and thoracodorsal axial pattern flaps for the reconstruction of chronic, nonhealing axillary wounds in cats. *Veterinary Surgery* **30**, 380–5

Lightner BA, McLoughlin MA, Chew DJ *et al.* (2001) Episioplasty for the treatment of perivulvar dermatitis or recurrent urinary tract infections in dogs with excessive perivulvar skin folds: 31 cases (1983–2000). *Journal of the American Veterinary Medical Association* **219**, 1577–1581

Mann GE and Stratton J (1966) Dermoid sinus in the Rhodesian Ridgeback. *Journal of Small Animal Practice* **1**, 631

Mathews KA, Ayres SA, Tano CA *et al.* (1997) Ciclosporin for the treatment of perianal fistulas in dogs. *Canadian Veterinary Journal* **38**, 39–41

Mathews KA and Sukhiani HR (1997) Randomized controlled trial of ciclosporin for treatment of perianal fistulas in dogs. *Journal of the American Veterinary Medical Association* **211**, 1249–1253

Misseghers BS, Binnington AG and Mathews KA (2000) Clinical observations of the treatment of canine perianal fistulas with topical tacrolimus in 10 dogs. *Canadian Veterinary Journal* **41**, 623–627

Pavletic MM (1999) Management of specific wounds. In: *Atlas of Small Animal Reconstructive Surgery, 2nd edn*, ed. MM Pavletic, pp.65–106. WB Saunders, Philadelphia

Ross WE and Pardo AD (1993) Evaluation of an omental pedicle extension technique in the dog. *Veterinary Surgery* **22**, 37–43

White RAS and Williams JM (1995) Intracapsular prostatic omentalization: a new technique for management of prostatic abscesses in dogs. *Veterinary Surgery* **24**, 390–395

Williams JM and Niles JD (1999) Use of the omentum as a physiological drain for the treatment of chylothorax in a dog. *Veterinary Surgery* **28**, 61–65

CASE EXAMPLE 1:
Management of a shotgun injury to the face

History
A 2-year-old male intact Coon Hound had escaped from the back garden and was found by the neighbour chasing chickens. The dog had been shot in the face with a shotgun. He was stabilized by the referring veterinarian with intravenous fluids, opioid analgesia and broad-spectrum antibiotics. A defect in his right upper lip was sutured on initial presentation. Ten days after he was shot, a large area of necrosis had developed that involved most of his right upper lip.

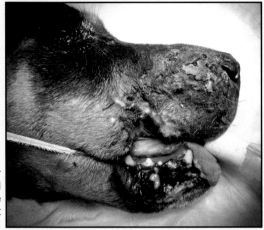

On presentation the area of the right upper lip delineated by the sutures was cold and had a leathery feel. There was a large amount of scabbing with purulent exudates beneath it.

Assessment
On general clinical examination the dog was bright and alert. Blood was taken for haematology and biochemistry and results were within normal limits. A CT scan of the head revealed numerous shotgun pellets. Necrosis of the tissues had occurred secondary to vascular injury caused by the shotgun blast and had resulted in a large flap of dead tissue.

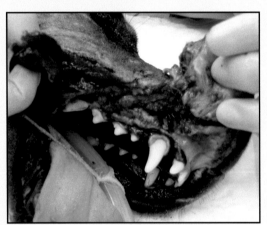

Note the devitalized flap of lip that is purple. A large fistula can be seen above the canine tooth, extending up into the nasal cavity.

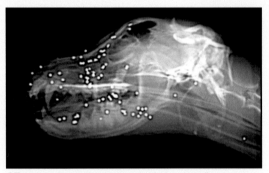

CT scan, showing numerous shotgun pellets.

Treatment
Under anesthesia, the area was clipped and cleaned. The necrotic flap of skin was excised and the edges of the wound were debrided. A sample was taken from the wound and submitted for bacteriological culture and sensitivity. The wound was packed with sterile gauze swabs soaked in sterile saline.

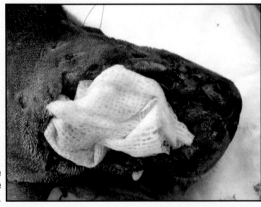

Note the multiple puncture wounds caused by the shotgun pellets.

Case Example 1 continues ▶

CASE EXAMPLE 1 continued:
Management of a shotgun injury to the face

A wet-to-dry dressing was placed and changed once daily. At each bandage change the wound was lavaged copiously.

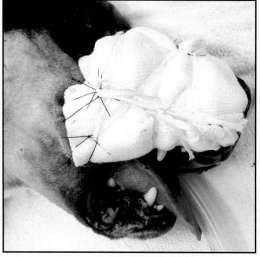

A tie-over bandage technique was used to hold the wet-to-dry dressing in place.

By day 6 the wound had started to epithelialize and granulation tissue was forming; this progressed over the next week.

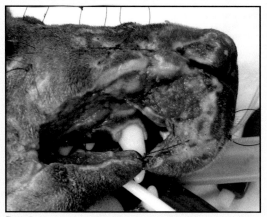

Day 6.

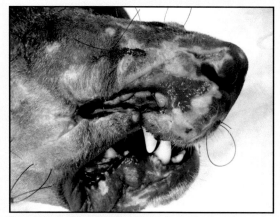

Day 11.

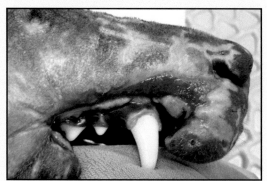

Day 14.

By day 14, the wound was significantly more healthy but a defect still existed in the lip. On day 16 a sliding lip flap procedure was performed.

Case Example 1 continues ▶

CASE EXAMPLE 1 continued:
Management of a shotgun injury to the face

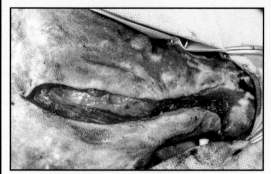

Lip flap raised.

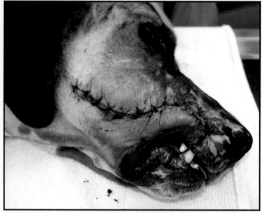

Immediately postoperatively.

One small area at the tip of the flap dehisced and a local repair was performed.

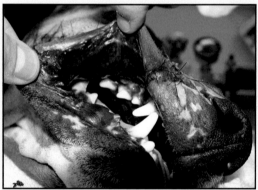

The dehisced flap has been repaired.

Outcome
The wound healed and the defect in the lip was repaired.

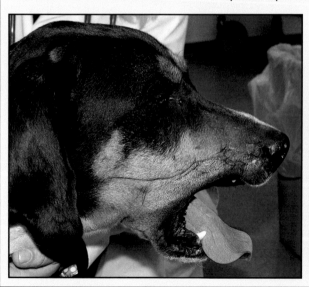

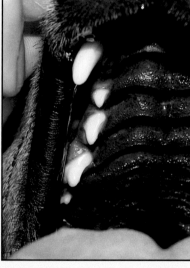

The dog 4 weeks after surgery.

OPERATIVE TECHNIQUE 11.1:
Anal sacculectomy

Preparation
The area is clipped and prepared as aseptically as possible. Enemas are avoided to prevent perianal leakage of liquid faeces; gauze swabs soaked in 1% povidone–iodine may be inserted per rectum and the perineal area is draped out.

Positioning
Surgery is carried out with the patient placed in sternal recumbency with the tail tied upward and forward and the hindlimbs hanging over the end of the table.

> **PRACTICAL TIPS**
> * **The tail can be held upward and forward by placing strips of adhesive tape, e.g. micropore, from one side of the table to the other, passing over the tail.**
> * **To facilitate surgery, the table can be tipped at an angle to raise the animal's tail end, taking care not to exceed 25–30 degrees (a tilt greater than this may compromise respiration, due to cranial shift of the abdominal organs).**

Assistant
Not essential.

Equipment extras
Sterile surgical probe; electrocautery. Gelpi self-retaining retractor may also be helpful.

Surgical technique

1. Insert a small haemostat, scalpel guide or probe through the anal sac opening and incise on to it with a No.15 scalpel blade. This is a simple technique with little risk of damaging the deep portion of the anal sphincter muscle or the caudal rectal branch of the pudendal nerve.

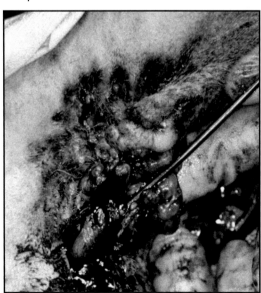
Probe in anal sac.

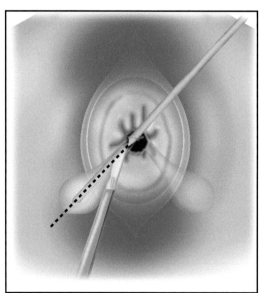
Incising on to the probe.

2. Using fine thumb forceps, grasp the anal sac lining and dissect it free from the surrounding tissues. In severe disease it is common to find only remnants of the anal sacs, which must be removed.

OPERATIVE TECHNIQUE 11.1 continued:
Anal sacculectomy

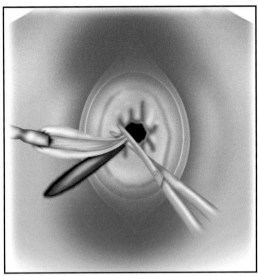

Anal sac removal.

3. Carry out sharp excision of any sinus tracts, paying careful attention to haemostasis. It may be necessary in severe cases to excise part or all of the external anal sphincter muscle. Owners should be warned of this possibility with its attendant risk of postoperative faecal incontinence.
4. Suture the deep tissues with 2 metric (3/0 USP) absorbable monofilament and close the skin with 2 metric (3/0 USP) monofilament nylon in a simple interrupted pattern.

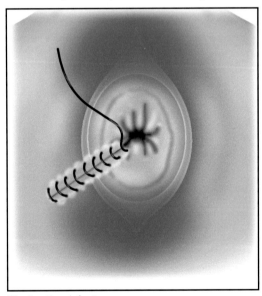

Closing the defect.

Postoperative care

- Postoperative analgesia should be provided using an opioid together with a non-steroidal anti-inflammatory drug. The intraoperative use of epidural analgesia can be invaluable in the immediate postoperative period.
- An Elizabethan collar should be placed postoperatively.
- Wound dehiscence may occur but can be allowed to heal by second intention if it is not excessive.

OPERATIVE TECHNIQUE 11.2:
Episioplasty

Positioning
Perineal stand with pelvic limbs positioned over the end of a well padded table. Place a purse-string suture around the anus prior to surgery to avoid faecal contamination of the surgical field.

Assistant
Not required.

Equipment extras
Electrocautery; skin marker; self-retaining retractor (Gelpi).

Surgical technique

1. Estimate the amount of skin removal required to expose the vulva.
2. Make an initial skin incision adjacent to the vulva. The incision begins ventral and lateral to the vulva and continues dorsally, curving around to the contralateral side of the vulva.

> **PRACTICAL TIP**
> **This incision can be made in the fold created by the junction of the skin covering the vulva and the perineal skin.**

3. Make a second concentric incision, lateral and dorsal to the first incision.

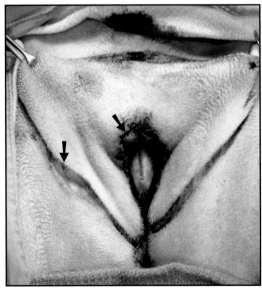

Two concentric crescent-shaped incisions (arrowed).

4. Additional skin can be removed if required, but the dorsal extent of the skin defect created should remain 2–3 cm ventral to the anus.

> **PRACTICAL TIP**
> **If insufficient skin is removed initially to improve the conformation of the vulva satisfactorily, additional skin is removed to achieve the desired effect. If excessive skin is removed initially it may be difficult to close the resultant defect or excessive elevation of the vulva may occur.**

OPERATIVE TECHNIQUE 11.2 continued:
Episioplasty

5. Excise excess subcutaneous tissue.

> **WARNING**
> **Be careful not to penetrate the dorsal wall of the vagina as you excise subcutaneous fat.**

6. Approximate skin edges to evaluate excisional effect.

> **WARNING**
> **The surgeon should be confident that the resulting wound can be closed without tension.**

7. Close the incision in two separate layers. The subcutaneous tissue is closed with absorbable monofilament suture material. The skin is closed with a non-absorbable monofilament suture material. Pre-place initial skin sutures at the 12, 3 and 9 o'clock positions. Appose remaining skin and suture with a simple interrupted pattern.

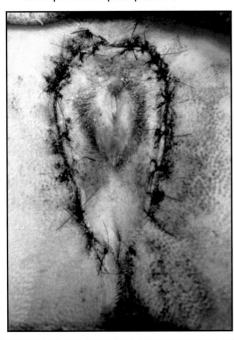

Closure of the primary wound without tension.

Postoperative care

- Elizabethan collars are recommended for bitches until suture removal to avoid self-mutilation.
- Antibiotics are continued postoperatively if necessary to resolve pyoderma.

OPERATIVE TECHNIQUE 11.3:
Caudectomy

Preoperative planning
Preparation of the surgical site can be difficult due to the deep skin folds and tail deviation. The anal sacs should be expressed and a purse-string suture placed in the anus to prevent faecal contamination during surgery. The area should be clipped and aseptically prepared for surgery. Perioperative antibiotics should be given and continued postoperatively.

Positioning
Sternal recumbency. Tilting the table 10–15 degrees may facilitate the surgical approach.

Assistant
Ideal but not essential.

Equipment extras
Electrocautery.

Surgical technique

1. Make a teardrop-shaped incision around the entire tailbase.

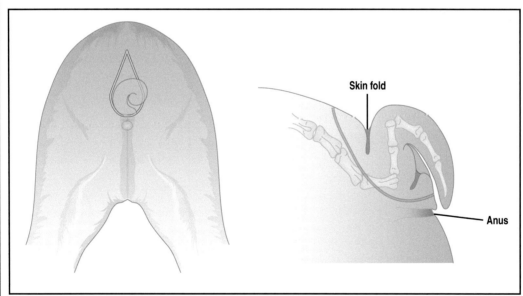

Teardrop-shaped incision around the tailbase.

2. Dissect the tissues down to and around the deviated vertebrae. Care should be taken during ventral dissection to avoid iatrogenic damage to the rectum and muscles of the pelvic diaphragm.
3. It is useful to manipulate the tail with a towel clamp. Resect the tail and skin folds *en bloc*, cranial to the deviated vertebrae. If the intervertebral space cannot be identified, the bone may be transected using bone-cutting rongeurs.
4. Lavage the area copiously prior to closing and insert closed suction drainage if deemed necessary.
5. Close the subcutaneous tissue with 1.5 or 2 metric (4/0 or 3/0 USP) absorbable suture material.
6. Close the skin with 1.5 or 2 metric (4/0 or 3/0 USP) nylon.

Postoperative care
The area should be kept clean and free of faecal contamination by applying warm, moist compresses for 10–15 minutes two or three times a day for the first few days.

OPERATIVE TECHNIQUE 11.4:
Fusion podoplasty

Preoperative planning
The paw should be clipped and aseptically prepared.

Positioning
Dorsal or lateral recumbency.

Assistant
Ideal but not essential.

Equipment extras
Electrocautery.
A half-inch Penrose drain or a sterile roll of bandage can be used to fashion a tourniquet.

Surgical technique

1. Once the foot has been clipped and aseptically prepared, place a tourniquet around the distal limb.
2. Excise the interdigital web skin, along with the skin between the digital and metacarpal/metatarsal pads, taking care not to damage the digital vessels and nerves. A sterile marker pen can be used to outline the interdigital skin to be removed. Preserve 2–3 mm of skin adjacent to the nails. When dissection becomes difficult close to the web fold, discontinue the dissection and move to an adjacent interdigital space.

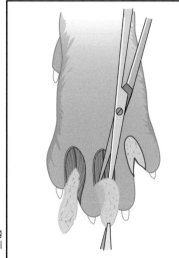

Excising interdigital web skin.

3. Once all the interdigital spaces have been dissected, move on to dissect the caudal aspect of the digital pads and the base of the metacarpal/metatarsal pads.

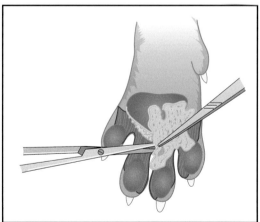

Dissecting the footpad.

OPERATIVE TECHNIQUE 11.4 continued:
Fusion podoplasty

4. Remove the tourniquet and control any haemorrhage using pressure, ligation and electrocautery.
5. Lavage the wound thoroughly prior to closing and place an active suction drain.
6. Suture the digital pads together with simple interrupted sutures, using 2 or 3 metric (3/0 or 2/0 USP) monofilament nylon. Do the same for the skin strips on the dorsum of each digit. The areas at the very ends of each digit are not sutured to allow for drainage.

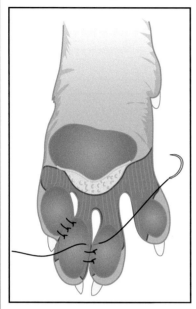 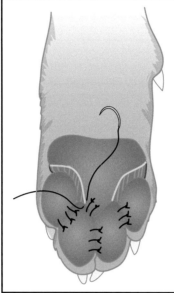 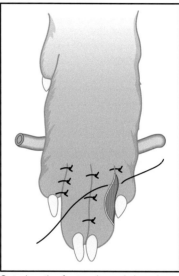

Suturing the footpads and dorsal skin strips.

PRACTICAL TIP
If the dog needs surgery on all four feet, perform surgery on the worst two feet first and allow complete healing to occur before operating on the other two feet 3–4 weeks later.

Postoperative care
The wound should be covered with a splint and bandage which should be changed daily. Sutures are removed 14–20 days after surgery and the foot should be kept bandaged until healing is complete.

Antibiotics should be given, based on culture and sensitivity test results, for an appropriate period. At any bandage change, if the paw has the characteristic odour of *Pseudomonas* infection the paw can be soaked in 0.5% chlorhexidine solution before rebandaging.

Complications
The most common complication of this surgery is dehiscence of the suture line between the digital pads and the metacarpal/metatarsal pad; use of a spoon splint in the bandage helps to prevent this.

The owners should be warned that if non-healing wounds or draining tracts recur, additional surgery may be required.

OPERATIVE TECHNIQUE 11.5:
Phalangeal fillet (Digital pad transfer)

Preoperative planning
The paw should be clipped and aseptically prepared.

Positioning
Dorsal or lateral recumbency.

Assistant
Ideal but not essential.

Equipment extras
Electrocautery.

Surgical technique

1. Make a ventral midline incision over the second or fifth phalanx and dissect out the bones, staying as close to the bones as possible. The skin and pad are preserved on their neurovascular pedicle.

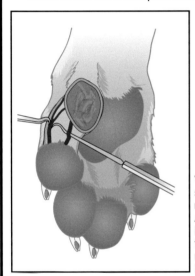

Ventral aspect of the paw, showing a large defect in the metacarpal or metatarsal pad. A ventral midline incision has been made to allow access to the phalangeal bones. The neurovascular pedicle should be identified and preserved.

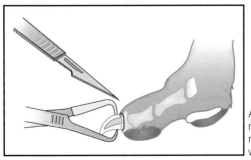

A circumferential incision is made around the base of the nail to allow it to be removed with the bones of the phalanx.

2. Gently debride the edges and surface of the metacarpal/metatarsal pad defect.
3. Transpose the digital flap into position to fill the defect.
4. Close the skin with simple interrupted sutures using 2 or 3 metric (3/0 or 2/0 USP) monofilament nylon. The area where the nail was removed is left open for drainage.

OPERATIVE TECHNIQUE 11.5 continued:
Phalangeal fillet (Digital pad transfer)

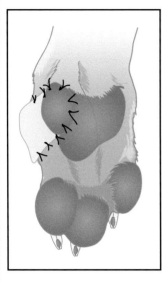

Digital pad sutured in place.

Note: An alternative technique for phalangeal fillet uses a staged approach, via a dorsal skin incision. Following removal of the digits, the dorsal skin incision is closed and the foot is bandaged for 14 days, with periodic bandage changes. After 14 days the dorsal skin sutures are removed and a ventral, rectangular skin incision is made to allow the pad to be transposed into place. This technique is easier but takes longer since it is a two-step procedure.

Postoperative care
The flap should be protected by a well padded bandage and, ideally, by placing the dog in a non-weightbearing sling. If the dog will not tolerate a non-weightbearing sling, a splint and bandage will suffice. The bandage should be changed daily until drainage subsides and then the wound rebandaged every 3–4 days. Sutures are removed between 14 and 20 days after the operation.

OPERATIVE TECHNIQUE 11.6:
Footpad grafts

Preoperative planning
The paw wound needs to undergo a period of open wound management to the point where a healthy bed of granulation tissue has developed. The paw should be clipped and aseptically prepared.

Positioning
Dorsal or lateral recumbency.

Assistant
Ideal but not essential.

Equipment extras
Electrocautery.

Surgical technique

1. Footpad grafts are harvested from healthy footpads on the same animal, using a 4–6 mm skin biopsy punch or by excising rectangular sections of pad tissue from donor sites using a No.11 or No.15 scalpel blade. If a blade is used, strips should be harvested that are 10–15 mm long and 5–10 mm wide, depending on the size of the dog.

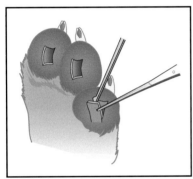
Harvesting rectangular footpad grafts.

2. Close the donor sites using cruciate or mattress sutures, or leave them to heal by second intention. Protect with padded bandages for 10 days.
3. Prepare the grafts by excising the subcutaneous tissue to the level of the deep surface of the dermis using a No.11 scalpel blade. Pass fine monofilament nylon suture material through each footpad graft. ***Pad grafts must be kept moist at all times with sterile saline***.

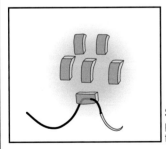
Suture material passed through the graft.

4. Excise an area of tissue on the recipient metatarsal/metacarpal pad wound to match the size of the graft. Place the graft into this area and stabilize it with one or two mattress sutures of monofilament nylon. Grafts should be placed around the perimeter of the defect so that re-epithelialization progresses towards the centre of the wound.

OPERATIVE TECHNIQUE 11.6 continued:
Footpad grafts

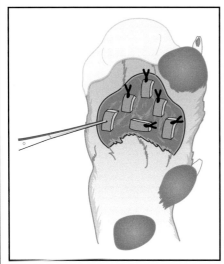

Grafts secured in
the granulation bed.

Postoperative care
The grafts should be bandaged using a non-adherent bandage and the animal placed in a non-weightbearing sling. The stratum corneum usually sloughs in 5–7 days, leaving a pinkish graft from which epithelialization and generation of new stratum corneum proceed over a period of approximately 3 weeks.

OPERATIVE TECHNIQUE 11.7:
Mastectomy

Preoperative planning and preparation
Plan excision around the number of glands involved. The ventral abdomen should be clipped and prepared aseptically.

Positioning
Dorsal recumbency.

Assistant
Not required.

Equipment extras
Electrocautery is useful.

Surgical technique

1. Combine a ventral midline incision with elliptical incisions around the lateral aspects of the glands to be removed, to create wide margins. Continue the incision through the subcutaneous tissues to the fascia of the external abdominal wall.

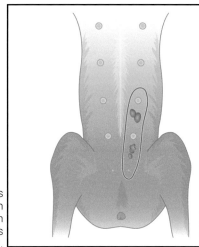

Midline incision is continued in an elliptical fashion around the glands to be excised.

2. For *en bloc* excision, elevate one edge of the incision, dissecting subcutaneous tissue from the pectoral and/or rectus fascia. Traction on the elevated skin segment facilitates dissection, which proceeds in a cranial to caudal direction in most cases. The abdominal and inguinal glands are loosely attached by fat and connective tissue to the underlying rectus fascia and are easily separated, although the inguinal fat and inguinal lymph node should be removed *en bloc* with the fifth mammary gland. The thoracic glands are more tightly adherent to the pectoral muscles with very little intervening fat or connective tissue. Major vessels encountered include the cranial and the caudal superficial epigastric vessels. These should be identified, ligated and transected.

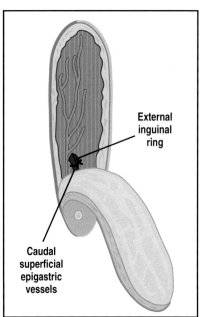

External inguinal ring

The cranial border of the wound is elevated and dissection continued along the abdominal fascia. The caudal superficial epigastric artery and vein are ligated as close to the inguinal ring as possible.

Caudal superficial epigastric vessels

OPERATIVE TECHNIQUE 11.7 continued:
Mastectomy

PRACTICAL TIP
Fascia should be excised if the tumour has invaded the subcutaneous tissue. If the tumour has invaded the abdominal musculature, a portion of the abdominal wall will also need to be excised.

3. Close the defect (after a simple, regional or complete unilateral mastectomy), taking into account the considerable dead space created. The subcutaneous tissue can be sutured to the abdominal wall using 'walking sutures' to help relieve tension and close the dead space.

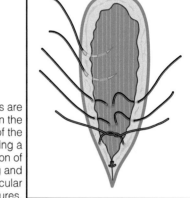

Wound edges are apposed in the middle of the wound using a combination of walking and subcuticular sutures.

If much dead space still remains, as is often the case in the inguinal region, a Penrose or closed suction drain can be placed. The skin should then be apposed with subcutaneous sutures, followed by skin closure using sutures or staples.

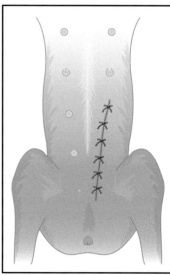

Wound edges sutured with an appositional pattern.

Postoperative care
A padded circumferential bandage can be placed to help compress dead space and support the wound for the first 2–4 days postoperatively.

12

Complications of wound healing

Ed Friend

Why and how do complications occur?

Wound healing complications are often difficult to deal with, as there are so many factors involved in the wound healing process and an almost infinite variety of wound type. Furthermore, the complication may be as a result of surgical intervention, and there may be extra pressure from an owner for the problem to be resolved, as it may be perceived as being the fault of the veterinary surgeon.

There is no generic formula or 'recipe' that can be applied to any one type of wound. This chapter finishes with a description of the causes and treatment of some wound complications, with specific guidance. It is important to remember that these general principles, discussed in the first section, can be applied to any type of wound.

Complications of wound healing may arise through:

- Factors related to the wound itself
- Factors related to the patient
- Factors arising from surgery/surgeon.

Wound factors

Type of injury

Traumatic wounds: For a wound to heal, the tissues on the edge or within the wound must be healthy and have a good blood supply. The subcutaneous fat has been shown to have a role in normal wound healing (Bohling *et al.*, 2006). Any type of traumatic wound will disrupt these tissues to a greater or lesser extent, and crush or tear injuries may be particularly damaging. Thermal injuries will also damage tissues, and are especially problematic as there is often a delay of 5–10 days before the full extent of injury is apparent.

There is a natural desire to close a wound as quickly as possible after an injury, in order to return the animal back to normal life at the earliest opportunity. Many wounds are sutured fairly soon after an injury, when the tissue may be swollen and inflamed, and there may be vasospasm in vessels at the edges of the wound. These conditions are unfavourable to wound healing, and therefore it is preferable to allow the tissues time to recover from trauma before attempting wound repair (typically 24–72 hours) (see

Chapters 3 and 4). Clinicians should remember that life-threatening concurrent injury or disease always takes priority over wound management.

Surgical wounds: These are generally more likely to heal without complications, as the aim of the surgeon is always to cause as little tissue damage as possible.

Contamination

Surgical procedures have for many years been classified as clean, clean–contaminated, contaminated or infected (see Chapter 3). Studies have shown that, as expected, wound infection rate increases from clean surgery to contaminated or infected surgery.

Traumatic wounds can also be classified as clean–contaminated, contaminated or infected. Chronicity is clearly a factor: the longer a traumatic wound is left untreated, the greater is the chance for bacterial multiplication with the increased risk of infection. This principle has led many to describe a 'golden time' of 6 hours after wounding, during which primary closure can be undertaken.

> **WARNING**
> The 'golden time' does not take into account the degree of gross and bacterial contamination and tissue trauma which, in some cases, may preclude wound closure. It is much better to assess each wound on its own merits and only suture the wound when it is thoroughly debrided. This may be straight after injury or several days later after a period of wound management (see Chapters 3 and 4).

Appropriate treatment and regular bandage changes and wound lavage can halt the increase in bacterial numbers and allow primary closure to be performed when all conditions are favourable (Figure 12.1).

> **WARNING**
> Antimicrobial drugs are indicated in the treatment of traumatic wounds but they are not a substitute for appropriate wound management.

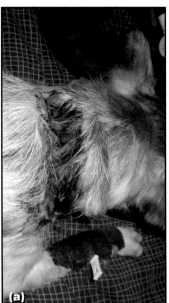

12.1 This 6-year-old neutered female Chihuahua had been attacked by another dog. **(a)** The wound was heavily contaminated and so initially conservative wound management was indicated. **(b)** After 6 days of open wound management, delayed primary closure using active suction drains was performed. The wound healed completely (the other dressings were for further wounds still being managed conservatively).

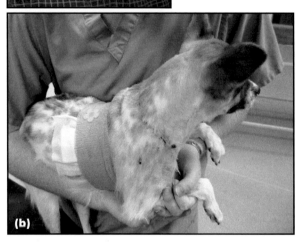

If a wound appears to be infected, colonization by an organism resistant to antimicrobial drugs should also be considered. Resistant organisms may be present in a wound even if an animal has not received veterinary treatment, e.g. cases where the owner has been a carrier of a resistant organism that has already infected the wound. Organisms such as methicillin-resistant *Staphylococcus aureus*, *Nocardia* spp., *Mycobacteria* spp. and, rarely, fungal organisms may compromise wound healing. If these are suspected, a tissue sample should be taken from deep in the wound and submitted for aerobic and anaerobic bacteriological culture and sensitivity testing and for fungal culture. Swabbing the superficial layers of a wound is not beneficial, as commensal organisms that are not significant are most likely to be sampled.

Underlying nidus for infection
A wound infection is much less likely to resolve if there is a focus of infection present, such as road dirt after a road traffic accident or bone sequestrum after a fracture. A nidus for infection offers an area where bacteria can adhere, with a poor blood supply and low oxygen tension. Phagocytes are less likely to clear infection from such an area, and systemic antibiotics will not penetrate effectively.

Anatomical area
Wound complications are more commonly seen in some areas of the body, including high-motion areas (joints, proximal limb skin folds) and pressure points (especially elbows and hocks; Figure 12.2).

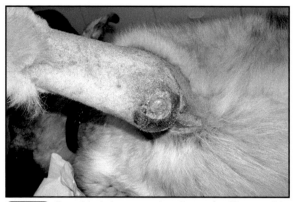

12.2 Decubital ulcer over the elbow of a 10-year-old male entire German Shepherd cross. This region is very difficult to treat as it is a pressure point when the animal lies down, as well as being a high-motion area.

Inguinal and especially axillary wounds in cats can be very difficult to manage, and many different treatments have been suggested (Lascelles and White, 2001). Furthermore, there is evidence for fundamental differences in cutaneous wound healing in the cat compared to the dog, which may predispose cats to slower wound healing (Bohling *et al.*, 2004). Footpad injuries may also be slow to heal in both dogs and cats.

Some anatomical areas have particularly tight skin; these include:

- The distal limb (Figure 12.3)
- The face/nose area in some patients
- The proximal limb in some breeds (e.g. Staffordshire Bull Terrier).

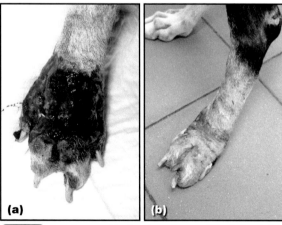

12.3 **(a)** A wound to the dorsal paw of the left pelvic limb in a 2-year-old Italian Greyhound. This area is difficult to treat as there is no redundant skin on the distal limb, and this is a high-motion area as there are underlying joints. A free skin graft was performed after the wound had been prepared for surgery. **(b)** Fourteen days after free skin graft surgery. The application of the skin graft has enabled healing to occur, despite skin tension in the area and motion from the underlying digits.

This results in extra tension being placed on a surgically closed wound, or reduces the wound's ability to contract if healing is by second intention.

> **PRACTICAL TIP**
> **Although some injuries are too extensive for treatment to be successful, and limb amputation or euthanasia is recommended, these cases may benefit from assessment at a referral centre as many severe wounds can be managed successfully.**

Abnormal tissue in the wound

Wound healing may be affected if there are neoplastic cells present, e.g. following incomplete tumour resection or failure to diagnose neoplasia in a chronic wound; healing may also be affected by adjunctive treatment for neoplasia, such as radiotherapy.

Patient factors

Concurrent disease due to trauma

Any trauma that has led to wounding may have affected an animal's systemic health, and must be assessed. In cases of life-threatening concurrent disease, this should be treated appropriately before considering wound management. Factors to consider include:

- The animal may be dehydrated or in shock, which may in itself be life-threatening
- Other specific life-threatening injuries may also be present, such as respiratory compromise or gastrointestinal, biliary or urinary tract rupture
- The trauma may have led to days or weeks of reduced appetite, and poor nutritional status will influence wound healing
- Traumatic injury may have led to consumption of platelets and clotting factors, and haemostasis may be affected.

Pre-existing concurrent disease

The systemic health of any patient suffering from wound healing complications should be assessed. Underlying diseases should be diagnosed from thorough clinical history taking, physical examination and use of appropriate diagnostic tests. A wide variety of underlying diseases or conditions may affect wound healing (Figure 12.4).

Diabetes mellitus
Hyperadrenocorticism
Hypothyroidism
Infectious agents, e.g. FIV/FeLV, feline coronavirus (FIP)
Anaemia
Uraemia
Hypoproteinaemia
Neoplastic disease
Coagulopathies
Poor nutritional status

12.4 Pre-existing concurrent diseases that may affect wound healing.

Pre-existing medication

An owner should always be questioned to see whether their animal is on any medication, even when the animal is presented as an emergency after a trauma. Medications such as corticosteroids or chemotherapeutic agents may have an adverse effect on wound healing.

Surgeon factors

The surgeon can have an effect on the likelihood of wound complications. One of the most important aspects of this is initial decision-making (see Chapter 3). Decisions to be considered are:

- Is surgical management appropriate or should a conservative treatment plan be adopted?
- If surgical closure is used, at what stage is this done?
- Do advanced techniques for wound closure need to be employed?
- Should referral to a specialist be advised?

The surgeon must also pay particular attention to good surgical technique when closing wounds.

> **WARNING**
> **Inappropriate or poor surgical technique can increase the incidence and severity of wound complications.**

Factors to consider to minimize the risk of complications include:

- Care should be taken not to use potentially cytotoxic wound lavage solutions. In most cases, use of sterile saline or lactated Ringer's solution is best for preparing a wound for surgery (see Chapters 3 and 4)
- Surgical debridement may be required, particularly if the wound has not undergone debridement with dressings
- Tissues should be handled gently to avoid injury and vasospasm of vessels that will supply the healing edges (see Chapter 3)
- Meticulous haemostasis should reduce the incidence of postoperative haematoma formation, but excessive use of electrocoagulation must be avoided to minimize tissue damage and the build-up of carbon in the wound, which can be a nidus for infection
- Appropriate and minimal use of implants is indicated. More advanced surgical techniques should be used with care as they may themselves cause further injury (Figure 12.5)
- Dead space should be closed by the accurate apposition of tissues and the use of surgical drains if appropriate, to prevent seroma formation
- Skin edges should be apposed without excessive tension
- The judicious use of antimicrobial agents and/or anti-inflammatory agents will aid wound healing where bacterial load or swelling may be a problem

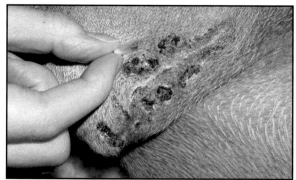

12.5 A small benign neoplasm had been removed from the skin overlying this elbow. The surgeon had used pieces of plastic tubing as a way of relieving tension in the skin but the tubing had itself caused pressure necrosis of the underlying skin. This would have complicated further surgery had the original wound not healed.

- Surgical time should be as short as possible, without compromising surgical technique, as prolonged anaesthetic as well as surgical time is associated with increased rates of wound infection (Beal *et al.*, 2000). Prolonged investigations (such as radiographic procedures) should ideally be performed under a separate period of anaesthesia from that used to close the wound.

Managing complications of conservative (non-surgical) wound management

Delayed or incomplete wound healing

Delayed and incomplete wound healing are really degrees of the same process. Each is difficult to define as every wound will heal at a different rate, but while a wound is being appropriately treated, if there is absolutely no progression of wound healing over a 7-day period, delayed wound healing should be diagnosed.

Most wounds left to heal by second intention when treated with appropriate dressings will heal over a period of 2–6 weeks, depending upon the size of the defect and the location. If all progress has stopped over a period longer than this, incomplete wound healing can be diagnosed. Second intention healing is more rapid in locations where there is plenty of loose skin. Some surgeons advocate leaving wounds covered with granulation tissue without dressings on, although wound hydration cannot be maintained and owners may be less likely to keep the animal under veterinary supervision.

There are many possible causes of incomplete healing. The wound should be assessed for all the reasons outlined above under 'Wound factors'. Similarly, the patient must be assessed for conditions detailed under 'Patient factors'. Particular attention should be paid to skin tension in the area (is there enough loose skin for the wound to be able to contract?), general health and nutritional state of the patient, and whether appropriate wound management is being used.

Treatment

- The patient should be **re-assessed** through clinical examination and blood sampling for haematology/biochemistry and viral status (cats).
- **Nutritional status** should be considered:
  - In theory, energy expenditure increases in trauma victims and surgical patients, but there may also be a decrease in the basal energy requirement (BER) so that the new energy requirements are often similar to pre-trauma levels. The exception is burns victims, where energy requirements are increased
  - The aim is to ensure the animal is receiving sufficient food to maintain bodyweight in hospital without aiming for weight gain until an animal is in the recovery phase, usually after hospital discharge
  - In the author's experience, most animals referred with chronic or severe wounds have lost weight, and tube-feeding at least double the calculated BER is needed to maintain bodyweight in hospital
  - Monitoring the weight of a patient is useful, especially as many wounded animals are hospitalized for prolonged periods, and veterinary surgeons and nursing staff may not notice deteriorating body condition. An increase in feeding should be implemented if weight loss over several days is noted, but is limited to a 10–20% increase in calorie content only in those animals that have been shown to tolerate supplemental feeding
  - Repeating measurements of blood proteins can be helpful, although as the half-life of albumin is approximately 7 days there will be a delay after the onset of malnutrition before levels fall
  - Cyproheptadine is an antihistamine that can act as an appetite stimulant in dogs and cats, and is useful in animals that are inappetent due to the stress of hospitalization. However, it is not a substitute for good nursing care
  - Animals that are undergoing daily sedation or anaesthesia may not have sufficient time in the day to eat enough food for their nutritional requirements. Pre-anaesthetic starvation for 6 hours is recommended and unnecessary delays in procedures should be avoided. If an animal will not or cannot take sufficient food by mouth, enteral feeding should be considered. A naso-oesophageal tube is convenient, but is usually of such a narrow gauge that it is not realistic to get sufficient food into the animal. An oesophagostomy or gastrostomy tube is preferred as these are larger gauge, making feeding easier. Placement of oesophagostomy tubes in particular can be performed quickly and is especially useful in cats that will require daily anaesthesia. It may be preferable to place the tube under anaesthesia on the second day of treatment, as duration of anaesthesia is usually less than on the first day.

- If there is obvious wound **infection** present, samples should be taken for aerobic and anaerobic bacteriological and fungal cultures, and diagnostic imaging considered to look for underlying causes of persistent infection (e.g. foreign body or sequestrum).
- **Biopsy** should be considered to rule out an underlying neoplastic cause for non-healing.
- **Changing local management of the wound** should be considered, e.g. reverting to daily or twice-daily flushing and wet-to-dry debriding dressings for a few days.
- The **patient's environment** may need altering to aid wound healing, e.g. cage rest for an overactive animal.
- If there is adequate skin around the area and there is not significant secondary infection, changing the management plan to a **(delayed) primary closure** should be considered.
- If there is inadequate tissue around the wound for second intention healing, an **advanced surgical closure technique** may have to be used (e.g. advancement or rotation skin flaps (see Case Example 1); use of thoracodorsal flap combined with omentalization for non-healing axillary wounds in cats).

Wound contraction

Complications arising from the wound contraction associated with conservative wound management are sometimes seen.

- If contraction occurs over a joint surface, it may limit range-of-motion of the joint and cause a mechanical lameness.
- Contraction may lead to deviation, stenosis or even complete closure of anatomical 'openings' such as the preputial orifice, vulva, ear or eye (Figure 12.6).
- The epithelium resulting from second intention healing is often thin and weak, and so can be easily traumatized. This potential for damage is compounded by the lack of hair growth in this type of tissue, which makes the area further exposed and vulnerable.

Treatment

Prevention is better than cure: wounds should not be left to heal by second intention if over a joint surface, or if the contraction may compromise openings of the urogenital tract, ear or eye. A defect of >50% of the circumference of a limb is unlikely to heal by second intention due to excessive tension, and may cause distal oedema owing to a tourniquet effect resulting from contracture.

The only option for treating a wound where contraction is causing a problem is surgical resection of the contracted epithelium, replacing it with a layer of normal skin that will not contract. The most convenient way to do this is usually with advanced surgical techniques such as local subdermal plexus flaps, axial pattern flaps or free skin grafts (see Chapters 6, 7 and 8). It should be remembered that fibrous tissue forms underneath the epithelium and is

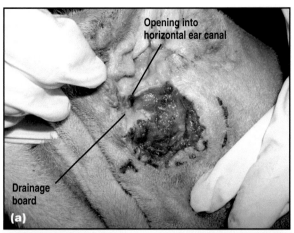

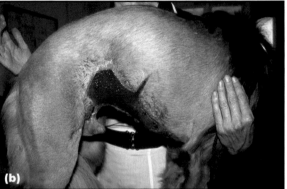

12.6 Contraction. **(a)** A 10-month-old male Shar Pei, 10 days after lateral wall resection. Two sides of the closure around the drainage board have dehisced due to excessive tension on the skin. If more of the area around the drainage board had dehisced, leaving the wound for second intention healing may have risked stenosis or closure of the external ear canal. **(b)** A middle-aged Collie cross with loss of ventral and lateral abdominal skin following bite wounds. The wound was left for second intention healing and eventually healed completely. The resulting epithelium was thin and sparsely haired, however, and so prone to damage. Contraction also led to lateral deviation of the prepuce.

difficult to remove completely, thus joint movement may still be limited. In these cases a guarded prognosis should be given if such revision surgery has to be undertaken. Furthermore, if the wound contraction has occurred over a joint and is causing limited range of motion, irreversible 'stiffening' of the joint may already have occurred.

Managing complications of surgical wound management

Haemorrhage and haematoma

Relatively minor bleeding in the perioperative and immediate postoperative period may lead to complications of wound healing. These complications are most likely to occur in the first few hours after surgery, although animals with coagulation disorders may start bleeding several days after surgery. Careful haemostasis should be maintained throughout any surgical procedure, and the wound should be checked again prior to closure for smaller bleeding vessels.

The surgeon must use appropriate haemostatic techniques during surgery to reduce the risk of bleeding and haematoma formation:

- Direct pressure
- Electrocautery
- Clamping with mosquito forceps
- Ligation
- Topical application of adrenaline
- Use of collagen sponge.

Haematoma will have a negative effect on wound healing for the following reasons:

- Mechanical disruption to edges of healing tissues
- Physical obstruction to invading macrophages and other cells that can engulf bacteria, as well as to invading blood vessels. This poor blood supply leads to a lower oxygen tension, which favours the growth of some bacteria
- Haemoglobin also has a direct inhibitory effect on phagocytic cells, predisposing a wound to infection
- Haematoma provides a nutrient source for bacteria.

Postoperative haemorrhage/haematoma is usually not a serious complication, although more serious haemorrhage may be life-threatening. In these cases, concern for the wound is overtaken by the need to stabilize the patient. This degree of haemorrhage is likely to be associated with a disorder of haemostasis, and so the animal should be screened thoroughly. Ideally, thorough clinical history taking and physical examination before surgery should increase the surgeon's index of suspicion for a clotting problem, so this can be investigated and appropriate steps taken. Investigations for possible clotting disorders are summarized in Figure 12.7. More detail is given in the *BSAVA Manual of Canine and Feline Emergency and Critical Care*.

Thrombocyte count
Blood smear and manual count/cytology
Prothrombin time (OSPT)
Activated partial thromboplastin time (APTT)
Activated clotting time
von Willebrand factor assay
Buccal mucosal bleeding time

12.7 Diagnostic tests for investigation of clotting disorders.

A dilutional coagulopathy has been described in animals that have received large volumes of intravenous colloids. This is occasionally of significance in animals wounded as a result of trauma, as they may have received life-saving intravenous fluid therapy on initial presentation. Trauma may also have contributed to consumption of platelets and clotting factors, further reducing haemostatic function.

Treatment

- Prevention is favoured – a thorough assessment of the patient prior to surgery (see above) and appropriate haemostatic technique intraoperatively.
- If there is minor bleeding or haematoma formation postoperatively, a conservative approach is preferred, as any intervention may increase the chance of introducing infection into the wound:
  - Initially direct pressure or a light bandage can be applied to the site (if anatomically possible), as some pressure will be enough to stop haemorrhage from most small blood vessels. Large amounts of padding should be used to prevent bandage-related injury, and the bandage should be changed or removed after no more than 12 hours
  - Patient movement should be limited by cage confinement or appropriate bandaging
  - Investigation for an underlying disorder of haemostasis (see above) should be considered, with serial monitoring of packed cell volume. Physical examinations should be repeated frequently if the bleeding is severe, to ensure the animal is not becoming hypovolaemic
  - If bleeding is ongoing, especially if clotting times are prolonged, fresh-frozen plasma should be administered to supply additional clotting factors. Whole blood should be used if the packed cell volume is low
  - Once haemostasis is achieved, bandages can be removed and the wound monitored for infection. A course of prophylactic antibiotics should be commenced, especially if some degree of wound dehiscence has occurred.
- Surgery is not often indicated for postoperative haemorrhage and should be used only when absolutely necessary. Some indications for surgery would be:
  - Arterial bleeding that is severe or is not responding promptly to conservative management with a bandage
  - Significant partial or complete wound dehiscence because of pressure from the haematoma. Under general anaesthesia and aseptic conditions, the source of bleeding should be identified and ligated, and the wound flushed with sterile isotonic solution such as lactated Ringer's, followed by careful wound reconstruction
  - Severe secondary infection of the haematoma, although this may take several days to become clinically apparent. Under general anaesthesia and aseptic conditions, the wound should be opened, infected and necrotic tissue debrided and the wound flushed. The tissues should be checked carefully for bleeding vessels. Placement of a drain should be considered if there is any possibility of further fluid production, before the tissues are carefully apposed again. Open wound management followed by delayed primary closure should be considered if there is remaining infection.

Dehiscence and infection

Wound dehiscence can occur within a few hours after surgery (often due to patient self-trauma) or up to several weeks later.

> **PRACTICAL TIP**
> **Clinical signs of dehiscence are the wound apposition becoming disrupted with swollen and/or necrotic wound edges. There is usually a serosanguineous discharge that may become more purulent as secondary infection develops (see Figure 12.6a).**

Some degree of infection is usually present when a wound breaks down, and it is up to the clinician to decide whether this infection is the primary cause of dehiscence (Figure 12.8) or secondary to the dehiscence. Infection undoubtedly plays a role in wound breakdown, as bacteria release proteolytic enzymes and other substances that inhibit normal wound healing. It should never be *assumed*, however, that an infection is the primary cause of dehiscence, or of any other wound complication such as delayed healing.

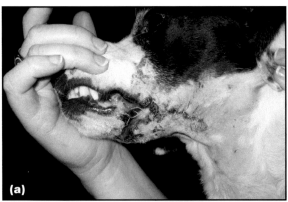

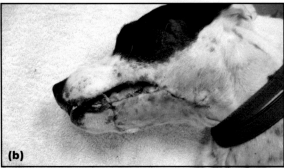

12.8 A 2-year-old male Terrier cross that had a jaw wound sutured following a fight with another dog. **(a)** The wound dehisced 5 days postoperatively due to infection and excessive tension at the site. **(b)** After open wound management, the wound was closed with an advancement skin flap, eliminating tension as a possible cause for further dehiscence.

Obvious causes of dehiscence, such as patient self-trauma, use of drugs that inhibit wound healing (e.g. chemotherapeutic agents or corticosteroids) or other therapies (e.g. radiotherapy), should be ruled out. In addition, excessive skin tension or movement of the area should be considered (see above). Dehiscence can also be secondary to the formation of oedema, seroma or haematoma (see other sections of this chapter). Only after recognition and treatment of an underlying cause will the wound be able to heal effectively.

> **PRACTICAL TIP**
> **Partially immobilizing a wound with a bandage may help prevent dehiscence.**

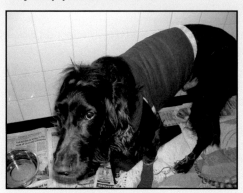

Infection as a primary cause

If infection is thought to be the primary cause, the clinician should review his/her surgical technique. Operating facilities and failure in sterile practice should also be examined as a possible cause of postoperative infection, especially if it occurs in multiple patients.

The systemic health of the patient should be reviewed if a primary wound infection has developed, as systemic disease may affect local and systemic immune response. The history from the owner should be taken again, general physical examination repeated, and further investigations (such as haematology and biochemistry tests) performed if there is a suspicion of a more generalized problem.

Pathogenic organisms such as meticillin-resistant *Staphylococcus aureus* (MRSA), *Pseudomonas aeruginosa* or *Proteus* spp. may be involved, so a tissue sample from deep within the wound should be taken for aerobic and anaerobic bacteriological culture and sensitivity testing.

The finding that MRSA is present in a wound does not mean that the clinician should assume the infection is a primary cause. MRSA may have been carried by the animal, its owner or hospital staff as a commensal organism, and invaded the wound as an opportunist bacterium. The wound should be assessed, like any wound, for other potential underlying causes of wound dehiscence.

> **WARNING**
> **Particular care should be taken when handling animals with infected wounds to prevent transmission of infection to other animals.**

Delayed wound infection

It is possible to have wound infection without dehiscence, although this is uncommon. Signs of infection may become apparent weeks or months after the surgery, after the overlying tissues have already healed. Swelling and pain over the site are initially seen, although eventually a draining sinus may develop.

Diagnosis of delayed wound infection is by:

- History of previous surgery in the anatomical area
- Clinical examination findings of swelling, heat or pain on palpation
- Fine-needle aspiration and cytology (presence of pus on aspiration)
- Diagnostic imaging (radiography, ultrasonography, CT/MRI)
- Surgical exploration and tissue biopsy (histopathology, aerobic/anaerobic bacteriological culture) will give the definitive diagnosis.

Infection of a wound weeks to months after the injury is most commonly caused by infection of surgical implants, such as orthopaedic implants, non-absorbable mesh implants or braided non-absorbable suture material. These materials can harbour bacteria in an environment where blood supply is poor and phagocytic cells cannot easily function.

Another possible cause may be failure of adequate debridement at the first surgery, for example:

- Failure to remove a bone sequestrum, or to fully remove debris (such as road debris, or hair) following a traumatic incident
- Inadequate debridement of the middle ear during a total ear canal ablation and lateral bulla osteotomy, leading to formation of a para-aural abscess (Figure 12.9).

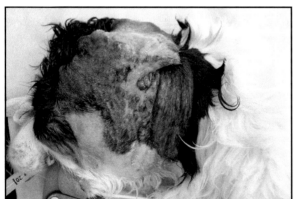

12.9 A non-healing wound developed caudal to the pinna base 4 months after total ear canal ablation and lateral bulla osteotomy had been performed in a 10-year-old neutered female Cavalier King Charles Spaniel. It was surgically explored, and infected aural epithelium was found in the middle ear. The wound healed uneventfully following thorough debridement.

Treatment

The decision to opt for conservative or surgical management is one that needs to be assessed on a case-by-case basis. Owners may be reluctant to consent to further surgery, as they often prefer to avoid further anaesthesia for their pet and/or the costs involved with surgery. For conservative management the animal may require sedation to allow dressing changes, especially if it is a reluctant patient, and this

may not be feasible if daily or twice-daily changes are required. Conversely, surgical management may be associated with the risk of further complications, so the clinician should consider whether referral to a surgical specialist is advisable.

PRACTICAL TIP
It should be remembered that prolonged conservative management might be more expensive than a successful definitive surgery.

Conservative management: (see Chapter 4 for management of open wounds)

- The underlying primary cause of dehiscence should be investigated and addressed.
- The animal should be systemically well, but if there is any evidence on history or physical examination of generalized disease, blood should be taken for haematology and biochemical testing.
- A sample should be taken (ideally by deep tissue biopsy) for aerobic and anaerobic bacteriological culture and sensitivity testing.
- Broad-spectrum antibiotics that are also effective against anaerobes (e.g. potentiated amoxicillin) should be given; if necessary, they should be changed, according to sensitivity testing results. Antibiosis should continue for 14–28 days, or at least 5 days after resolution of clinical signs.
- Hair should be thoroughly clipped from around the wound, after moist sterile swabs or sterile aqueous gel are placed in or over the wound to prevent the clipped hair entering the wound. Hair acts as a barrier to the ingress of macrophages, fibroblasts and finally epithelial cells, as well as acting as a nidus for bacterial growth
- Physical debridement may be useful, i.e. flushing twice daily with copious amounts of sterile isotonic solution (e.g. lactated Ringer's solution) followed by wet-to-dry dressings changed once or twice daily (see Chapter 4). This should be continued until there is a good covering of granulation tissue, which is highly resistant to infection
- The use of an adjunctive flushing solution such as Tris-EDTA has been recommended, as it disrupts bacterial cell walls (particularly those of *Pseudomonas aeruginosa)* and makes them more sensitive to antibacterial agents
- Delayed closure of the wound can be performed once granulation tissue has started to develop, as this process suggests that contamination in the wound is minimal. It may be more appropriate in many cases to continue conservative management until the wound is fully closed by second intention healing (see Case Example 2)
- Strict hygiene practices, including hand washing before and after handling the wound and the patient and use of sterile gloves to handle the wound, will minimize the risk of infection from other organisms and transfer of infection to wounds in other patients.

MRSA and other multiple-antibiotic-resistant infections: Conservative management is usually the preferred route in cases of multiple-antibiotic-resistant organisms. If MRSA or another multiple-antibiotic-resistant infection is suspected or confirmed, the animal should be placed in isolation facilities, and staff entering the area should use barrier nursing techniques as follows:

- Disposable gloves, overshoes, facemasks and plastic aprons should be worn
- Jewellery, mobile phones and other personal effects should not make contact with the animal. Other hospitalized patients that are not affected should be treated first to reduce the incidence of cross-contamination
- Separate materials and equipment (mops, buckets, thermometers, stethoscopes, etc.) should be used exclusively for that animal, and should be cleaned and disinfected after use, and sterilized if possible
- Food bowls should be sterilized in an autoclave after use, and bedding should be soaked in disinfectant for 30 minutes before separate washing on a 65°C cycle using a biological detergent. Soiled bedding, urine, faeces and bandage materials should be removed and disposed of as quickly as possible
- Polymeric biguanide solution (e.g. Trigene; Medichem International) at 1:50 dilution is effective against MRSA, and should be used to clean all surfaces in the isolation facility twice daily and up to 48 hours after the animal has been discharged from the hospital
- Hands should be cleansed before and after handling the patient, with either 70% ethanol or chlorhexidine disinfectant. This is also good practice when handling any hospitalized veterinary patient
- Sterile gloves should be used when treating the wound itself (in common with all wounds) and dressings should be changed at least twice daily
- Any tube or catheter is a possible source of ongoing infection and so their use should be minimized in any patient with a wound. Intravenous catheters and all indwelling tubes (e.g. PEG, cystostomy) should be cleaned twice daily with chlorhexidine solution after hand cleansing and glove changing
- Urethral catheters or cystostomy tubes, if used, should be drained continuously as a closed system, to reduce the incidence of ascending infection but also to prevent transmission of infection via the urine.

Although MRSA is resistant to many antibiotics, there is often an antibiotic found on bacteriological sensitivity testing to which the organism is sensitive. This should be administered, if safe to do so, as soon as results are available. The animal should be weighed to ensure an adequate dose is administered.

Physical debridement of the wound is more important in these cases than in others, as the organism may become more drug-resistant during treatment.

An intensive treatment of daily, or ideally twice-daily, flushing with balanced isotonic solution should be commenced, along with debriding dressings.

Basic open wound management principles, by diluting and flushing away the bacteria, and removing necrotic tissue that the bacteria are being harboured in, should be the mainstay of treatment for these resistant infections.

The owners should be informed if a multiple-antibiotic-resistant infection is isolated from their animal's wound. In most cases these do not pose a risk to owners, and animals can be discharged home when the wound has been successfully treated, even if the wound remains colonized by the bacteria in question. However, certain individuals, including those with compromised immune systems, should not come into contact with infected wounds. Owners are advised to seek advice from their GP or medical specialist. In cases where there is a higher risk of developing a multiple-antibiotic-resistant wound infection, e.g. degloving injuries that will be associated with long hospital stays and open wound management, it may be beneficial for the clinician to discuss the risk of infection with owners prior to commencing treatment.

Veterinary clinicians should be aware that multiple-antibiotic-resistant bacteria can colonize skin and granulation tissue in a way which is not the same as infection. Such colonization of granulation tissue, which is highly resistant to bacterial invasion, does not need to be treated with antibiotics unless overt signs of infection develop. Similarly, repeated bacteriological culture of swabs taken from the surface of granulation tissue is unnecessary unless clinical infection is suspected.

Surgical management:

- Underlying causes for wound dehiscence should be investigated and addressed. The area should be clipped and the wound flushed, and broad-spectrum antibiotic therapy commenced as described above for conservative management
- In all cases, the wound should be thoroughly debrided before closure is performed. This can be done surgically immediately before closure, or by conservative management as described above. The latter is often the preferred method, as the clinician can be more assured the wound is no longer significantly contaminated when healthy granulation tissue is present
- Any focus for infection such as haematoma or surgical implants should be removed
- Tissue samples should be taken from deep in the wound and submitted for aerobic and anaerobic bacteriological culture and sensitivity. Antibiotics should be changed if necessary depending on sensitivity results
- The veterinary surgeon should consider a different surgical plan to counteract any underlying cause for the dehiscence:
  - If excessive tension is one of the factors implicated, a different *closure technique* may have to be used. This may involve simple techniques, such as walking sutures or

tension-relieving suture patterns, or the use of advanced surgical closure techniques such as an axial pattern flap (Figure 12.10). In distal limb wounds, it may be necessary to allow a healthy granulation tissue bed to form before performing a free skin graft
- The use of a surgical drain or *drains* may be indicated if the dehiscence was associated with seroma formation. The drain may be passive or active, and will drain fluid from below the wound while healing takes place. It helps the tissue planes to remain apposed, allowing the ingress of phagocytic cells for removal of bacteria and necrotic tissue. Veterinary surgeons may use drains as an adjunct to management of contamination or infection. However, if the surgeon is not experienced in this aspect of wound management it may be preferable to manage wound infections via open wound management only, to avoid complications
- *Postoperative management* may need to be altered if the clinician is suspicious that excessive movement may have contributed to the dehiscence. This may mean bandaging the area to prevent movement and/or self-trauma, or confining the animal within the house or a cage
- A *complete change* of management plan may be required, such as allowing second intention healing to occur
- Referral to a specialist should be considered.

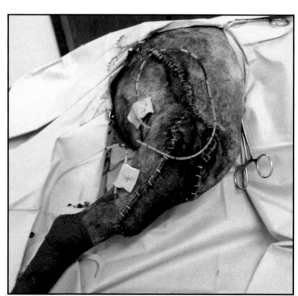

12.10 Closure of skin defects in areas of tight skin can be challenging, especially in the distal limb. In this case, a lateral genicular axial pattern flap has been used to close a skin defect between the stifle and hock. Two active suction drains have been placed.

Seroma formation

A seroma is an accumulation of sterile fluid (a filtrate of blood) underneath a wound. The fluid is often straw-coloured but may be blood-tinged; it can be differentiated from a haematoma or an abscess by gross appearance and cytological examination.

Clinical signs are of a swelling that usually develops 2–5 days after surgery, is soft, and is non-painful on palpation. A seroma can sometimes feel firmer if it becomes more chronic, or if the fluid is trapped in an anatomical space such as under a muscle belly.

> **WARNING**
> **If there is heat and pain on palpation, the clinician should be suspicious of possible infection.**

It is not always possible to tell why a seroma develops postoperatively. It is important for the surgeon to consider causes of seromas, both to help with their treatment and to help prevention. Some potential causes or factors involved are:

- The creation of excessive 'dead space' during surgery, or failure to adequately eliminate it. This may be as a result of excessive undermining of tissues (especially skin) during surgery, or because an area of tissue, such as a tumour, has been resected
- Poor surgical technique, where tissue trauma is excessive
- Excessive movement of the animal or the anatomical area postoperatively
- Idiosyncratic reaction to suture material, or of tissues sliding over underlying suture knots. It may also be seen after use of some other implants such as surgical mesh
- It is possibly more commonly seen after some types of tumour resection, e.g. mast cell tumours. This may be related to the release of inflammatory/vasoactive substances from the tumour during resection. In some instances it can occur due to the effect of tumour remaining in the wound bed after incomplete tumour resection.

A seroma does not always have a catastrophic effect on a wound, but the reasons it is desirable to avoid one are:

- Phagocytic cells find it harder to function in the presence of a seroma. This is due to a lack of chemoattractants, and a lack of tissue surface to move across. Some of the constituents of a seroma may provide a nutrient source for bacteria. The net result is an increased chance of infection, rather like with haematoma (see above)
- The formation of a seroma under a wound may have a mechanical effect on the wound. If the pressure of the fluid exceeds the bursting pressure of the tissues and/or suture material, the tissue apposition may be disrupted and the wound may dehisce.

Diagnostics
The swelling should be differentiated from other wound complications (haematoma, oedema, infection, herniation (Figure 12.11)) by history, clinical examination, diagnostic imaging (if herniation suspected), and cytology of a fine-needle aspirate (Figure 12.12).

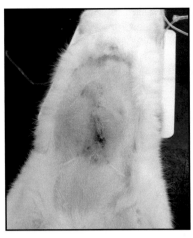

12.11

Wound swelling 6 days after exploratory laparotomy in a 10-year-old neutered male DSH cat. This was initially diagnosed as a likely seroma, but on ultrasound examination an incisional hernia through the body wall was demonstrated.

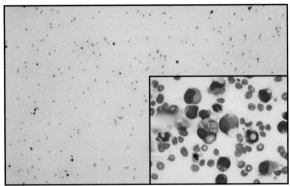

12.12 Cytological preparation of neat seroma fluid (modified Wright's stain; original magnification X100); inset: concentrated preparation (x1000) showing erythrophagocytic macrophages. (Courtesy of Oliver Coldrick, TDDS Laboratories)

Treatment

Conservative management is preferred if possible. Surgery is indicated if:

- There is wound disruption or dehiscence
- There is a chance the seroma is developing a secondary infection
- The animal is not suitable for conservative management as it is difficult to handle
- The seroma is proving refractory to conservative treatment.

Conservative management:

- If the clinician is sure of the diagnosis, the wound is not disrupted and the animal is otherwise well, then no treatment at all is required and the seroma will resolve by the resorption of fluid. Monitoring of the wound by the owner and clinician is indicated until the problem has fully resolved, which may take several weeks
- A pressure bandage over the area may help prevent the progression of a seroma. This needs to be changed every 48–72 hours, but needs to be maintained for at least 7 days to allow fibrosis to eliminate the dead space. It is not always anatomically possible to bandage a wound, or patient compliance may prevent it, and care should be taken to prevent a bandage-related injury

- Cage or small-room confinement may be necessary to prevent an active animal from moving excessively
- The seroma can be drained with a sterile needle, either as a single procedure or intermittently until fully resolved. This must be performed with a sterile needle and syringe following clipping of the hair from the area and surgical aseptic preparation. The disadvantages are: the dead space is still present and so the seroma will often reform, although bandaging may in some cases prevent this; and the formation of 'pockets' means that drainage cannot always be performed. The reported advantage of needle drainage is that it is diagnostic as well as potentially therapeutic; though as a therapeutic procedure it has little to commend it.

> **WARNING**
> **Needle drainage SHOULD ONLY be performed if the seroma is making the animal uncomfortable because of its size, as there is a large associated risk of introducing infection.**

Surgical treatment:

1. Open the wound and remove all necrotic tissue, surgical implants and sutures. Samples should be taken where appropriate for bacteriology and histopathology, to confirm the diagnosis of seroma and rule out infection.
2. Thoroughly lavage the site with sterile isotonic solution (e.g. lactated Ringer's).
3. If the skin or tissues have been stretched excessively by the seroma, excise any excess tissue with a scalpel blade.
4. Carefully appose the dead space using synthetic absorbable suture material. Avoid excessive use of sutures
5. If the dead space cannot be eliminated adequately, a surgical drain should be placed (Figure 12.13). This may be either a passive or an active suction drain (see Chapter 5).

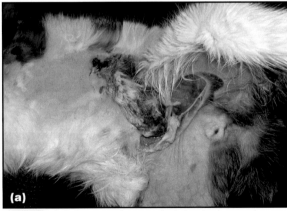

(a)

12.13 **(a)** A traumatic ventral abdominal wound was sutured in a 5-year-old neutered male DSH cat. Seroma formation over 3–4 days postoperatively caused disruption of the suture line and dehiscence, followed by necrosis of adjacent skin. At this stage it was impossible to tell that the initial problem was a seroma. (continues) ▶

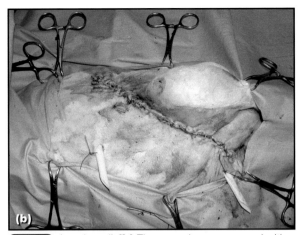

12.13 (continued) **(b)** The wound was managed with debridement and flushing with sterile isotonic solution, followed by placement of Penrose drains and careful apposition of tissues. The wound went on to heal uneventfully.

6. Skin closure is routine.
7. It is not usually necessary to bandage the area postoperatively, but altering the animal's exercise regime (shorter walks or even cage confinement) for 3–4 weeks may be helpful.

Oedema

Oedema is the accumulation of tissue fluid in the interstitial spaces between cells, and so is a more diffuse collection of fluid than a seroma. Oedema can form for many reasons, but in the context of wounds it is usually a result of damage to lymphatic or blood vessels due to trauma or surgery. Alternatively, it may form in an extremity (distal limb, tail or pinna) secondary to proximal vascular occlusion (which may be partial or complete), such as the application of over-tight sutures in the skin. The formation of oedema may cause wound dehiscence due to a mechanical effect on the wound.

Diagnosis

- Oedematous tissue appears as a diffuse swelling that will 'pit' on digital pressure.
- In most cases it will not be hot or painful to the touch, either of which may be more suggestive of infection or cellulitis.
- If severe or left unchecked, oedema may compromise the blood supply to the overlying skin or more distal tissues, and so the skin may begin to appear bruised and even cold to the touch.
- The local lymph nodes and blood vessels proximal to the oedematous area should be assessed, and a general physical examination performed to look for systemic disease. Angiography or lymphangiography can be used

to investigate this further, but is rarely necessary in the clinical situation.
- If generalized oedema is present, the animal should have causes such as hypoproteinaemia or cardiac disease investigated.

Prevention

Surgery should be delayed on any traumatized tissue until the vascular and lymphatic supply has been re-established, which is when swelling, oedema and bruising start to subside, generally after 2–7 days. Additionally, surgical techniques that constrict the tissues should be avoided, especially in the limb. This often presents a challenge in cases of trauma or following oncological surgery where there is a large skin deficit. There is a temptation to stretch the skin back together using tension-relieving suture patterns, but in many cases it may be better to use other advanced techniques (skin flaps or skin grafts) to close the defect instead.

Treatment

- In mild to moderate cases, conservative management can be used to promote a return of blood flow to the area, e.g. massage, hot and cold packing, physiotherapy.
- Oedema will sometimes resolve given time, although the area should continue to be examined daily to assess for worsening and subsequent necrosis of overlying skin.
- Bandaging the area has been recommended by some clinicians to aid dispersal of the oedema, but this technique should be used with caution as it may further compromise vascular supply.
- Removal of skin sutures or further surgery to release sutures in deeper tissues can be performed in moderate to severe cases. This will usually lead to dehiscence of the sutured area, although this is preferable to the skin sloughing distally. If dehiscence occurs a different surgical technique to close the site should be planned for when the oedema has resolved.

References and further reading

Beal MW, Brown DC and Shofer FS (2000) The effects of perioperative hypothermia and the duration of anesthesia on postoperative wound infection rate in clean wounds: a retrospective study. *Veterinary Surgery* **29**, 123–127
Bohling MW, Henderson RA, Swaim SF *et al.* (2004) Cutaneous wound healing in the cat: a macroscopic description and comparison with cutaneous wound healing in the dog. *Veterinary Surgery* **33**, 579–587
Bohling MW, Henderson RA, Swaim SF *et al.* (2006) Comparison of the role of the subcutaneous tissues in the cutaneous wound healing in the dog and cat. *Veterinary Surgery* **35**, 3–14
Lascelles BDX and White RAS (2001) Combined omental pedicle flaps and thoracodorsal axial pattern flaps for the reconstruction of chronic non-healing axillary wounds in cats. *Veterinary Surgery* **30**, 380–385

CASE EXAMPLE 1:
Management of a non-healing wound

History
A 3-year-old neutered female Miniature Dachshund went missing and returned with skin wounds consistent with a road traffic accident. Initial clinical examination by the veterinary surgeon showed no orthopaedic or neurological injuries, but there were multiple small areas of skin loss over the limbs and head. She was stabilized with intravenous fluid therapy and opioid and non-steroidal anti-inflammatory drug analgesia. Broad-spectrum antibiosis was commenced. The small wounds were managed conservatively with daily dressing changes, but after 3 days a large area of necrosis developed in the skin of the ventral thorax/abdomen, consistent with thermal injury. This was examined under anaesthesia and, after clipping and flushing, an area of necrotic skin approximately 10 cm in diameter was surgically removed. The small wounds healed over the next 7–10 days and the ventral wound had ongoing debriding dressings over the following 7 weeks. Initially the wound contracted well, but there was no appreciable change in the wound in the final 2 weeks.

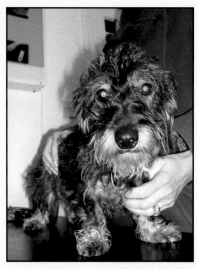

The patient on presentation.

Assessment
On general clinical examination the dog was otherwise well, and was in good body condition indicating the nutritional plane had been adequate. Blood was taken for haematology and biochemical testing; the results were within normal limits, indicating there was not likely to be a systemic cause for delayed/non-healing of this wound. There were two adjacent areas of granulation tissue on the right and ventral thoracic/abdominal wall that were each approximately 3 cm in diameter. The wounds were clean and, as they were covered with granulation tissue, infection was not considered to be a reason for non-healing. On examination, the surrounding skin was very taut and so further contraction of the wound had probably been prevented by excessive tension.

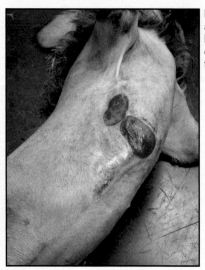

Non-healing ventral abdominal wounds. Note the shiny, thin epithelium caudal to the wounds.

Case Example 1 continues ▶

CASE EXAMPLE 1 continued:
Management of a non-healing wound

Treatment

Ongoing conservative management was unlikely to be effective due to the tension in surrounding skin, and so surgical reconstruction was planned. This tension also meant that simple primary closure would be ineffective and would lead to further wound dehiscence, and so rotation flaps were used. Under general anaesthesia, the granulation tissue and surrounding thin epithelium was resected. Two local subdermal flaps were then raised and rotated to close the defect. An active suction drain was placed to prevent fluid accumulation under the wound. The drain was removed 3 days postoperatively, and the staples were removed 9 days after surgery. The area healed uneventfully.

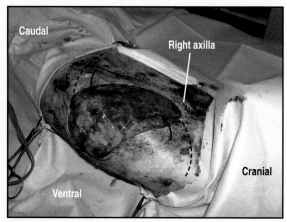

The defect after resection of the granulation bed and unhealthy epithelium.
- - - - - - - Incisions for two rotation flaps.

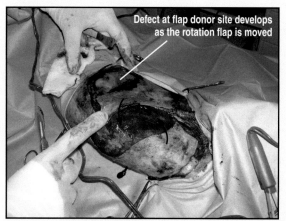

Rotation flaps were carefully raised deep to the subdermal plexus, taking care not to traumatize the tissues. The flap base must be as wide as the widest part of the flap, or blood supply distal to this part may be compromised.

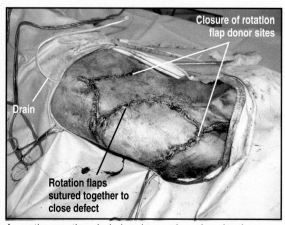

An active suction drain has been placed under the flaps; it does not exit through the base of a flap (which would compromise blood flow). Simple interrupted subcuticular sutures of synthetic absorbable suture material have been placed, followed by surgical skin staples.

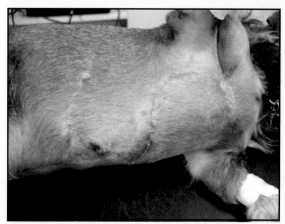

The wounds have healed well by the time of staple removal 9 days postoperatively.

CASE EXAMPLE 2:
Management of a wound dehiscence

History
A 7-year-old male entire Collie cross was presented with an acute laceration in the left precrural fold/inguinal area, suspected to be caused by jumping over barbed wire. It was cleaned and sutured on the same day as the injury, and amoxicillin/clavulanic acid was prescribed along with a non-steroidal anti-inflammatory drug. Over the next few days, the wound became purulent and eventually dehisced.

The wound was cleaned and resutured 8 days after the original injury and surgery, but this time a narrow rotation flap was created from the lateral thigh, which was incorporated into the wound. A Penrose drain was also placed, and antibiotic was changed to cefalexin. The drain was removed 2 days postoperatively, but by day 3 the wound had once again dehisced.

Assessment
There was no history suggestive of systemic illness, and on examination the dog was very bright. He had a very good body condition score, and had been eating well over the period of time that the wounds had been treated. There was a large amount of purulent material within and surrounding the wound. This wound had probably dehisced because of a combination of excessive movement and tension in the skin in this region, with the infection most likely a secondary factor. Barrier nursing was used initially in case of a resistant organism such as MRSA being present in the wound.

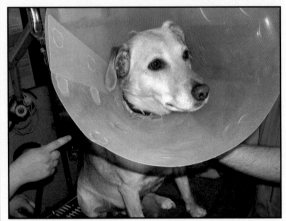

The patient on presentation.

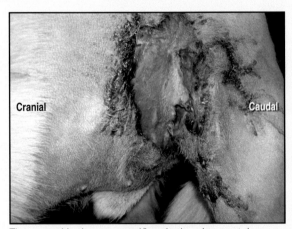

The wound in the precrural/inguinal region contains a large amount of purulent material and the previous suture line has dehisced.

Treatment
With the dog under heavy sedation, the wound was covered with sterile aqueous jelly and the hair from the wound edges and surrounding area clipped. The wound was then explored and a small tissue sample from within the wound removed and sent for aerobic and anaerobic bacteriological culture and sensitivity testing. Large pieces of necrotic tissue were debrided with a scalpel, and all suture material was removed. The wound was lavaged with a large volume of lactated Ringer's solution, and a wet-to-dry dressing applied.

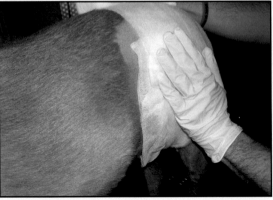

Application of a wet-to-dry dressing. Bandaging a male dog in this area can be difficult, as the penis must be exposed for urination. An indwelling catheter should be avoided because of the risk of ascending infection.

Case Example 2 continues ▶

CASE EXAMPLE 2 continued:
Management of a wound dehiscence

The bacteriology results showed a light growth of non-haemolytic *Escherichia coli*, which was resistant to cefalexin but sensitive to amoxicillin/clavulanic acid, and so this was prescribed. Barrier nursing was then discontinued, although guidelines for managing a patient with a wound were still observed.

The bandage was changed and the wound copiously lavaged twice daily for 2 days, after which the wound was considerably cleaner. Some healthy granulation tissue had started to form, although there was still some necrotic debris within the wound that would inhibit wound healing.

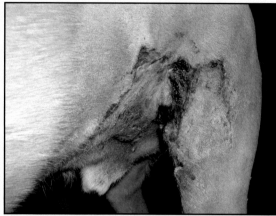

After 2 days of twice-daily debriding dressings granulation tissue is already starting to form in the wound.

Lavage and wet-to-dry dressings were continued once daily. After a further 7 days, the main wound was completely covered with granulation tissue and had contracted considerably.

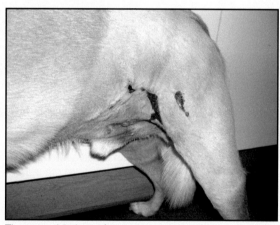

The wound 9 days after conservative management had begun.

Antibiotics were stopped, as granulation tissue is very resistant to infection. Debriding dressings were also discontinued and the wound was simply covered with a light dressing that the owners could change themselves at home. On re-examination 2 weeks later the wound had fully healed.

The original plan for this case was to use debriding dressings until the wound conditions were optimal to perform a primary closure. Motion in this area meant closure with a caudal superficial epigastric flap would have been ideal. Importantly, infection and necrotic tissue had to be removed from the wound first, and time was needed for the blood supply to be re-established in the wound edges following the original trauma and two subsequent surgeries.

The plan changed to ongoing conservative management when the wound progressed so well before surgery was possible. This management would have been very similar if MRSA had been cultured from the wound, except that barrier nursing methods would have been continued until the wound had fully healed.

CASE EXAMPLE 3:
Management of a persistent seroma

History
A 2-year-old neutered female Golden Retriever was presented with swelling and bite wounds on the dorsal thorax after an attack from a smaller dog. The bite wounds were explored, flushed and sutured on the same day and a Penrose drain placed, but the swelling returned after the drain was removed 3 days after surgery. The veterinary surgeon was suspicious of infection, and so fluid was aspirated from the swelling. Cytology confirmed this was seroma fluid.

The seroma was surgically explored and another Penrose drain placed. Tissue was also taken for histopathology, which demonstrated inflammation and no other underlying disease. The drain succeeded in reducing the swelling, but when it was removed 7 days after surgery the swelling returned.

Assessment
The bitch was very bright, and was in good body condition but with a large dorsal swelling. She was uncomfortable moving and on palpation of the swelling. Plain radiographs were taken of the area to ensure there was no obvious underlying cause such as a radiopaque foreign body; these showed no abnormalities. Combined with previous cytology and histopathology results, the diagnosis of a persistent seroma was made.

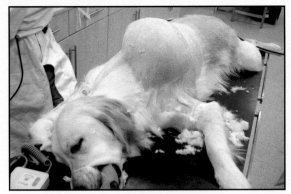

Seroma on the dorsal thorax 10 days after Penrose drain removal.

Treatment
Conservative management was ruled out on welfare grounds as the patient was finding it difficult to move and bend her neck to eat. The area was clipped and prepared for aseptic surgery. An incision was made and the swelling thoroughly explored. Suture material from previous surgeries was removed, and tissue samples were taken for histopathology and aerobic/anaerobic bacteriological culture. This was followed by copious lavage with sterile lactated Ringer's solution.

There was no growth on bacteriological culture. Histopathology once again demonstrated inflammatory changes. Two active suction drains were placed and the skin closed with minimal suture material in the subcuticular layer followed by skin staples.

The drains were activated 6 hours after surgery; negative pressure was maintained by continuous monitoring of the suction bulbs. Initially 600 ml of serosanguineous fluid was removed in total each day; this reduced steadily over a period of 3 weeks. One drain stopped withdrawing fluid after 10 days and so was removed at that stage. The other drain was removed when the volume withdrawn had fallen to about 35 ml/day. There was no recurrence of the seroma thereafter.

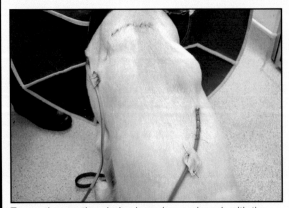

Two active suction drains have been placed, with the bulbs secured to the animal's collar. Hair growth has occurred since surgery.

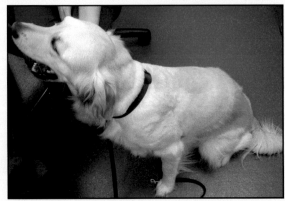

Appearance of the wound 2 weeks after active suction drains were removed. There has been no recurrence of the seroma.

Subject index

Subject index

List of Operative Techniques